ELECTROCARDIOLOGY '91

Warsaw, Poland
24 – 26 August 1991

Proceedings of the
XVIIIth International Congress on Electrocardiology

ELECTROCARDIOLOGY '91

Warsaw, Poland
24 – 26 August 1991

Editors

Józef Jagielski
Mirosław Górnicki

Department of Pathophysiology, Wrocław Medical Academy

World Scientific
Singapore • New Jersey • London • Hong Kong

Published by

World Scientific Publishing Co Pte Ltd
5 Toh Tuck Link, Singapore 596224
USA office: 27 Warren Street, Suite 401-402, Hackensack, NJ 07601
UK office: 57 Shelton Street, Covent Garden, London WC2H 9HE

Library of Congress Cataloging-in-Publication Data is available.

XVIIIth INTERNATIONAL CONGRESS ON ELECTROCARDIOLOGY, 1991

ISBN-13 9789810209476
ISBN-10 9810209479

The XVIIIth International Congress on Electrocardiology was organised under the auspices of the International Council on Electrocardiology:

President:

B. Taccardi, USA

President-elect:

R. Amirov, USSR

Honorary Member:

H. V. Pipberger, USA

Members:

H. Abel	Germany
P. d'Alché	France
Z. Antaloczy	Hungary
A. Bayes de Luna	Spain
K. Harumi	Japan
J. Jagielski	Poland
F. Kornreich	Belgium
J. Liebman	USA
P. Macfarlane	United Kingdom
F. de Padua	Portugal
Z. Pavlov	Bulgaria
P. Rautaharju	Canada
G. Rios	USA
J. Ruttkay-Nedecky	CSRF
E. Schubert	Germany
R. Selvester	USA
L. Titomir	USSR
R. Th. van Dam	The Netherlands
H. Ueda	Japan
R. Wenger	Austria

PREFACE

The present volume is the culmination of the Proceedings of the XVIIIth International Congress on Electrocardiology, organised by the Department of Pathophysiology, Wroclaw Medical Academy, and held in Warsaw on 24–26 August 1991.

These meetings were first initiated by Professor Hugon and Professor Zofia Kowarzyk with a Symposium on Spatial Vectorcardiography, held in Wroclaw in 1959. Since then there have been annual meetings, known as Colloquia Vectorcardiographica, organised in Poland by Professor Hugon and Professor Zofia Kowarzyk, in Czechoslovakia by Professor W. Laufbarger and Professor I. Ruttkay-Nedecky, in Germany by Professor E. Schubert and in USSR by Professor R. Z. Amirov. The 10th International Symposium was held at Jabłonna near Warsaw in 1979. Over the years, the scope of the issues covered broadened and the meetings soon transformed themselves into international congresses on electrocardiology.

The papers presented during the XVIIIth Congress on Electrocardiology and published in this book refer to both the problems of cardiac electric field modelling and activation, done by a computer-aided analysis of ECG, and clinical diagnostics of cardiac mapping, ECG, VCG, as well as the issues associated with coronary heart disease, micropotentials and arrhythmias. During the Congress in Warsaw, we had the opportunity of meeting jointly with the International Society of Computerised Electrocardiology.

We wish to thank the authors for the outstanding standard of the papers submitted and the effort put in the way the papers are worked out.

Professor Józef Jagielski, M.D.
President of the Congress

CONTENTS

Introductory Lecture

Body Surface Potential Mapping in Children

Jerome Liebman, M.D.
Professor Pediatrics (Pediatric Cardiology)
Adjunct Professor Biomedical Engineering
Rainbow Babies and Children's Hospital and
Case Western Reserve University
Cleveland, Ohio 44106

As part of the 14th International Congress of Electrocardiology in Berlin, in 1987, we made a special presentation with the same title as this, Body Surface Potential Mapping (BSPM) in Children[1]. In the four years since then considerable clinical progress has been made using our rapidly applied and processed color calibrated and displayed 180 electrode system, encased in various sized vests[2-10]. A presentation describing the Case Western Reserve University system was made at the 12th International Congress of Electrocardiology in MINSK, USSR[5]. A particular interest has been in the field of cardiac hypertrophy where in children, the potentially confusing effects of coronary disease are usually not a factor. Ventricular conduction defects, particularly on standard ECG may be confused with hypertrophy, so that we have been studying this area in depth as well.

In analyzing our BSPM we utilize what we know about normal activation sequences in animals and humans but recognize that it is possible, perhaps likely, that activation sequences may change in the presence of hypertrophy. We need to know what is being depolarized and when, in both the normal and abnormal. We need to know from direct measurements in humans, what is truly on the epicardium in the patients whose BSPM's are being analyzed. We also must develop accurate solutions to the "forward problem" from known pathology using realistic torso models[11]; and we need to develop accurate inverse problem solutions in order to predict epicardial and even myocardial potentials from the BSPM's on the torso[12]. Until the latter are available, however, we have no choice but to make educational judgements about what the potentials on the torso are predicting. Hopefully these judgements are reasonably accurate.

We have studied a number of normal children[3,4,13] as well as young adults[14] and have included various quantifications of both time and magnitudes. It is rare not to recognize evidence for epicardial right ventricular breakthrough (RVBT) in normal children, indicating that activation has progressed normally through the right bundle, and then from endocardium to epicardium[15]. Being able to recognize this aspect of physiology has been very useful in developing our understanding and diagnostic abilities in interpreting BSPM's[16]. ((In normal adults as well, evidence for RVBT can be seen in more than 90% of cases, (despite the more shallow right anterior superior notch) facilitated by the improved visual resolution provided by the color system[10]). Terminally, in children, four different areas, either alone or together, can be recognized; these are anterior superior, right anterior superior, right posterior and, far less commonly, straight posterior.

A particular clinical use of BSPM has been the differentiation of partial right bundle branch block (RBBB) from right ventricular hypertrophy (RVH) with terminal right conduction delay[17-22].

In patients with right volume overload[19] (atrial septal defect), as well as in pressure overload, (pulmonic stenosis), RVBT occurred, often late, from either the right anterior superior, as in normals, or from the superior. In the patients with right volume overload, once the right ventricle was recognized to the right and anterior, it took as long to complete activation of the right ventricular as it does in partial RBBB (approximately 50 ms). In advanced RBBB[20,21] it takes an average of 100 ms but there is a great spectrum, of both partial and advanced RBBB. In advanced RBBB, evidence for epicardial left ventricular breakthrough is always present, manifest by rapidly moving negative potentials from above and below which appear to separate left ventricular from right ventricular potentials. Once the right ventricle begins activation it moves slowly to the right lateral, then to the right anterior superior. With partial RBBB, in our experience, there has been evidence for epicardial left ventricular breakthrough about three quarters of the time and no evidence for epicardial RVBT. It is possible of course that when there is only a small amount of RBBB, that there would be enough activation via the normal Purkinje system to be able to demonstrate RVBT.

It should be recognized that terminal right conduction delay can be seen in patients with pressure overload. Of interest in pure pulmonic stenosis, where right ventricular pressure can be decreased very quickly utilizing balloon dilatation, we have demonstrated a sudden decrease of the right anterior potentials on the BSPM, when the standard ECG has been unchanged[18].

In patients with severe right ventricular pressure overload we have previously observed that the initial QRS is often directed to the left[23-25]. On the BSPM the initial positive potentials (in normals over the sternum) are often to the left anterior with the negative potentials over the spine or right posterior. This could be reflecting both right septal hypertrophy and very prominent activation of the very thick anterior wall to the left of much of initial septal activation. Initial QRS is seen to the left in other situations as well[26] including severe aortic stenosis[27] where the initial positive potentials are also left anterior. The negative potentials are as in severe pulmonic stenosis but extend to the right anterior very quickly. This is believed to be due to marked hypertrophy of the free posterior wall of the left ventricle which is also normally activated at the same time as the left septum. In advanced LBBB, the initial negative potentials are usually over the sternum with the positive potentials to the left anterior.

Severe aortic stenosis and partial LBBB are often difficult to differentiate electrocardiographically, and it now appears as though the separation will be possible utilizing BSPM. However, many more BSPM's plus correlative studies are needed to separate the types of initial positive and negative potentials in the three lesions, and to understand their pathogenesis.

In LVH investigations continue as to whether pure volume overload can be separated from pure pressure overload (other than in the initial QRS when severe). After normal epicardial RVBT, in both volume and pressure overload, greatly increased peak to peak magnitudes develop with the maximum anterior left, then posterior left. In the last part of QRS there is usually a straight posterior, or right posterior superior maximum, but anterior superior positive potentials can be recognized as well. A possibly more common finding in pressure than volume overload is that the last maximum recognized, at the end of QRS, is frequently right posterior superior (presumably from posterobasal LVH).

Of particular interest in our investigations of LVH was that in a series of patients studied many years after successful surgery for coarctation of the aorta, RVH was found. Of 24 patients who had BSPM (of which 7 had additional aortic stenosis), 8.7 years after the surgery, 19 had RVH, with 9 having additional LVH. On the VCG only 11, and on the standard ECG only 6 of the 19 had the RVH. In 11 of the 24 a cardiac catheterization was done, with just one having an elevation of pulmonary artery pressure (40 mm Hg systolic). The mechanism for the RVH is postulated to involve right ventricular hyperplasia in utero and/or early neonatal life which does not disappear.

Congenital conduction abnormalities [22,28,29] are very common in patients with congenital heart disease and are less well delineated than when acquired as part of surgery. Of great interest and wrongly named for many years is the "abnormally superior vector"[30] formerly called "left axis deviation". It is almost invariably present from birth in patients born with endocardial cushion defects, even when present as part of more complex lesions such as tricuspid (TA) or double outlet right ventricle. Left anterior hemiblock, an acquired condition in adults as well as children, has the same frontal plane ECG in that the initial QRS is inferior after which most of the vector is superior. The initial QRS is inferior because normal initial superior activation is stimulated by the left anterior branch of the left bundle. If the left anterior branch is cut then initial QRS will be inferior. Consistent with this is Durrer's study[31], demonstrating that the earliest activation is the posterobasal left ventricle. In the early BSPM the potentials are negative superior and positive inferior after which there is rapid change to the positive potentials superior and negative potentials inferior.

A striking variety of BSPM's is seen in the three types of hypoplastic right ventricle (HRV). In TA there is a VSD in the endocardial cushion defect position,so that the characteristic BSPM of the abnormally superior vector are present. There is then evidence for epicardial RVBT indicating normal endocardial to epicardial activation, which is usually early since the right ventricle is small. There is also another unusual abnormality in that early negative potentials suggest the possibility of left lateral wall infarction. Negative and positive potentials typical of LVH then remain stable for a long time with extremely high magnitudes (?11000 μv) with the positive posterior. (This latter is the case in all three types of HRV). Of interest is that when

TA is associated with transposition of the great arteries the VSD is not in the endocardial cushion position so that the BSPM shows nothing to suggest the abnormally superior vector. But the other aspects of TA are similar. In the HRV with pulmonary atresia there is no VSD and again nothing to suggest an endocardial cushion type of BSPM. The RV pressure may be very high and the RV wall may be very hypertrophied even though small. Therefore, characteristic positive potentials presumably orginating in the RV are recognized anterior after straightforward late epicardial RVBT from the superior, as seen in RVH. (Finally, in a recent patient with both tricuspid atresia and pulmonary atresia and no VSD, a miniscule right ventricle was recognized after RVBT.

In all of the above cases described we must be very cautious in developing our hypotheses. Confirmation, or changes in concept, must come from direct epicardial mapping in humans, and, especially if the above is not available, successful solutions to the forward and inverse problems.

Bibliography

1. J. Liebman - Body Surface Potential Mapping in Children. *Special Presentation at Proceedings of the 14th Internet. Cong. on Electrocardiology.* Publ. Electrocardiology '87, Academie - Verlag Berlin, 1988, p. 45.

2. R. Plonsey, W. Ko, J. Liebman, et al. *Proc. Internat. Symposium on Body Surface Potential Mapping (Tokyo) (1982) in Advances in Body Surface Potential Mapping* ed. K. Yamada, K. Harumi, T. Musha, Univ. Nagoya Press (1983), p. 77.

3. J. Liebman, C.W. Thomas, Y. Rudy, R. Plonsey et. al. *Proc. 9th Internat. Cong. Electrocardiology* (Tokyo) June 7-11, 1982 publ. Jap. Heart J. **23**(Suppl), 1982, p. 480.

4. J. Liebman, C.W. Thomas, Y. Rudy, R. Plonsey. J. Electrocardiology (1981) **14**: 249.

5. M. Kavuru, H. Vesselle, C.W. Thomas, Y. Rudy, J. Liebman (presented by J. Liebman) *Proceedings XIIth Internat. Cong. Electrocardiology (MINSK)* June 16-19, 1985, p. 29.

6. M. Kavuru, H. Vesselle, C.W. Thomas, Chapter 15 in *Pediatric and Fundamental Electrocardiology*. ed. J. Liebman, R. Plonsey, Y. Rudy, publ. Martinus Nijhoff (1987) p. 315.

7. C.W. Thomas, D. Lee, Chapter 16 in *Pediatric and Fundamental Electrocardiology* ed. J. Liebman, R. Plonsey, Y. Rudy publ. Martinus Nijhoff (1987), p. 329.

8. D. Lee, C.W. Thomas, Y. Rudy, J. Liebman *Proceedings 13th Int. Congress Electrocardiology* (Washington) Sept. 10-12, 1986 p. 17.

9. J. Liebman, C.W. Thomas, Y. Rudy, P.J. Diaz, R. Plonsey. *Proc. 5th Ann. Conf. Frontiers of Engineering and Computing in Health Care in IEEE/Engineering in Medicine and Biology Soc.* Sept. 10-12, 1983.

10. W.P. Huebner, C.W. Thomas, Y. Rudy, J. Liebman. *Proc. 13th Internat. Cong. Electrocardiology* (Washington) Sept. 10-12, 1986, p. 9.

11. R.M. Gulrajani, G.E. Mailloux. Circ. Res. (1983) **52**: 45.

12. Y. Rudy, B.J. Messinger-Rapport in *CRC Critical Reviews in Biomedical Engineering* (1988) **16**: 215.

13. J. Liebman, C.W. Thomas, R. Salamone, Y. Rudy, R. Plonsey. Chapter 19, in *Pediatric and Fundamental Electrocardiography*, ed. J. Liebman, R. Plonsey, Y. Rudy, publ. Martinus Nijhoff (1987), p. 381.

14. L. Widman, J. Liebman, C.W. Thomas, R. Fraenkel, Y. Rudy. *Presented 13th Internat. Cong. Electrocardiology* (Washington) Sept. 10-12, 1986-p. 35, and publ. J. Electrocardiol. (1988) **21**: 121.

15. R.J. Myerberg, K. Nilsson, H. Gelband. Circ. Res. (1972) **30**: 217.

16. J. Liebman. J. Electrocardiol. (1991) **23**:(Suppl), p. 63.

17. J. Liebman Third Internat. *Symposium in Body Surface Mapping*. Nijmegen, The Netherlands, June 11-14, 1985.

18. J. Liebman, C.W. Thomas, R. Franekel, Y. Rudy, A. Ben-Shachar - *Presented 13th Internat. Cong. Electrocardiology* (Washington) Sept. 10-12, 1986, p2.

19. J. Liebman, Y. Rudy, C.W. Thomas, R. Plonsey. Chapter 20 in *Pediatric and Fundamental Electrocardiography* ed. J. Liebman, R. Plonsey, Y. Rudy. publ. Martinus Nijhoff (1987) p. 389.

20. J. Liebman, Y. Rudy, P.J. Diaz, C.W. Thomas, R. Plonsey. Proc. Internat. *Symposium on Body Surface Potential Mapping (Tokyo) (1982) in Advances in Body Surface Potential Mapping* ed. K. Yamada, K. Harumi, T. Musha, Univ. Nagoya Press (1983) p. 217.

21. J. Liebman, Y. Rudy, P.J. Diaz, C.W. Thomas, R. Plonsey. J. Electrocardiol (1984) **17**: 329.

22. J. Liebman, C.W. Thomas, Y. Rudy. Chapter 12 in *Body Surface Potential Mapping in Conduction Abnormalities* ed. D. Mirvis, publ. Martinus Nijhoff, 1988, p. 153.

23. M. Mehranpour, A. Whitney, J. Liebman, G. Borkat. J. Electrocardiol. (1979) **12**: 69.

24. J. Liebman, R. Plonsey, Jap. Heart J. 123(Suppl) 1982. *Presented 9th Internat. Cong. Electrocardiology* (Tokyo) June 7-11, 1982.

25. J. Liebman, Chapter 11 in *Pediatric Electrocardiography*, ed. J. Liebman, R. Plonsey, P.C. Gillette, publ. Williams and Wilkins, 1982 p. 144.

26. J. Liebman, B.L. Miller, I.H. Gessner in Vectorcardiography 1970, *Proc. 11th Internat. Symposium Vectorcardiography*. Ed. R.I. Hamby, E. Glassman, publ. J.B. Lippincott (1971) p. 645.

27. J. Ankeney, T. Tzeng, J. Liebman. J. Thoracic and Cardiovasc. Surg. (1983) **85**: 41.

28. J. Liebman, Chapter 2 in *Pediatric Electrocardiography*, ed. J. Liebman, R. Plonsey, P.C. Gillette, publ. Williams and Wilkins, 1982, p. 15.

29. J. Liebman, Chapter 12 in *Pediatric Electrocardiography*, ed. J. Liebman, R. Plonsey, P.C. Gillette, publ. Williams and Wilkins, 1982, p. 172.

30. J. Liebman, A.S. Nadas. Am. J. Cardiol (1971) **27**, 1977.

31. D. Durrer, J.P. Roos, R.T. Van Dan: Am. Heart J. (1966) **71**: 642.

PART I
Heart Activation Modelling

A STANDARD MODEL OF THE THORACIC GEOMETRY

D. ROMBERG

Institute of Physiology, Humboldt-University
Berlin - Germany
Hessische Straße 3-4, 1040 Berlin

ABSTRACT

For the numerical representation of the thoracic geometry a standard model is presented. A stylized geometry of the cross section area of the thorax was used to construct the model by a regularization procedure. To test the validity of the model, geometrical data for the boundaries of the different compartments were taken from computertomography cross-sectional scans. For reducing the individual variability of the model, the parameters were related to the torso contours at the level of the Processus xiphoideus. This procedure results in a standard torso model for the parameterization of the thoracic geometry.

1. Introduction

The geometry of the volume conductor affects to a large extent the distribution of surface potentials. Consequently, a reasonable accurate representation of the thoracic geometry is necessary to solve the forward as well as the inverse problem of electrocardiology.

Practical considerations require that the model is simple enough to be described analytically and being realized by using a minimum number of geometrical coordinates.

2. Selection of the Model

The human thorax may be regarded, as being composed of piecewise homogeneous compartments (lungs, skeletal muscle, bones, fat tissue - Fig.1).

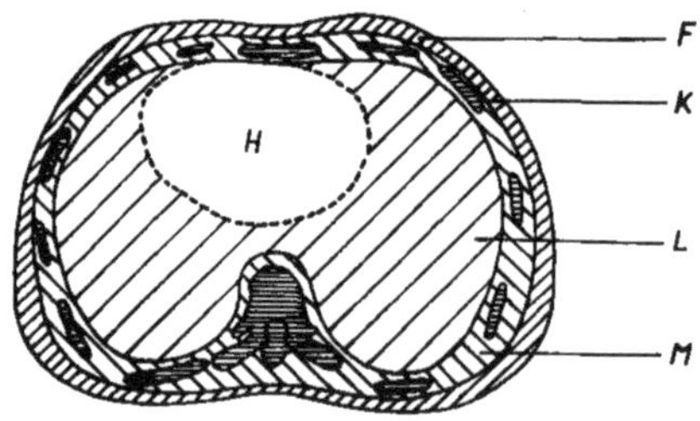

Fig. 1 :
Cross-sectional scan through the thorax

H - heart
L - lung
K - bones
M - muscle layer

For simplification the cross-sectional area of the thorax was approximated by parameterized ellipses (Fig.2), which are conected longitudinally by linear splines. The bones and the subcutaneous fat layer can be neglected because the very high conductivity of these tissues.

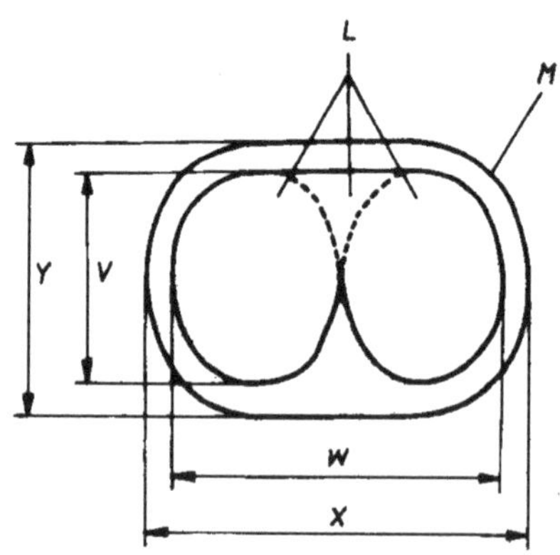

Fig. 2 :
Cross-sectional area of the thorax model

L - lung
M - muscle layer
X,Y,V,W - model parameter

3. Validity of the Model

To test the validity of the model, geometrical data for the boundaries of the different thorax compartments were taken from computertomography cross-sectional scans through the thorax from 28 women and 25 men (Fig.3).

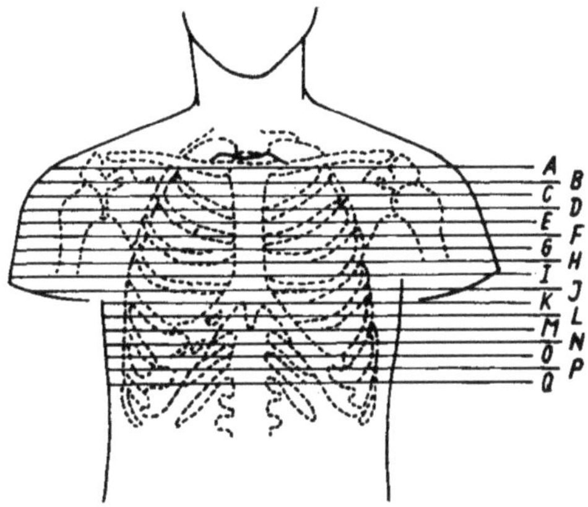

Fig.3 :
Levels of the computer-tomography scans

For reducing the individual variability of the model (Fig.4) the parameters were related to the contours at the level of the Processus xiphoideus. The normalized parameters show only a small variability (Fig.5). Also the differences between the normalized parameters of women and men can be neglected.

Fig.7 shows a standard model of the thorax constructed by the normalized parameters.

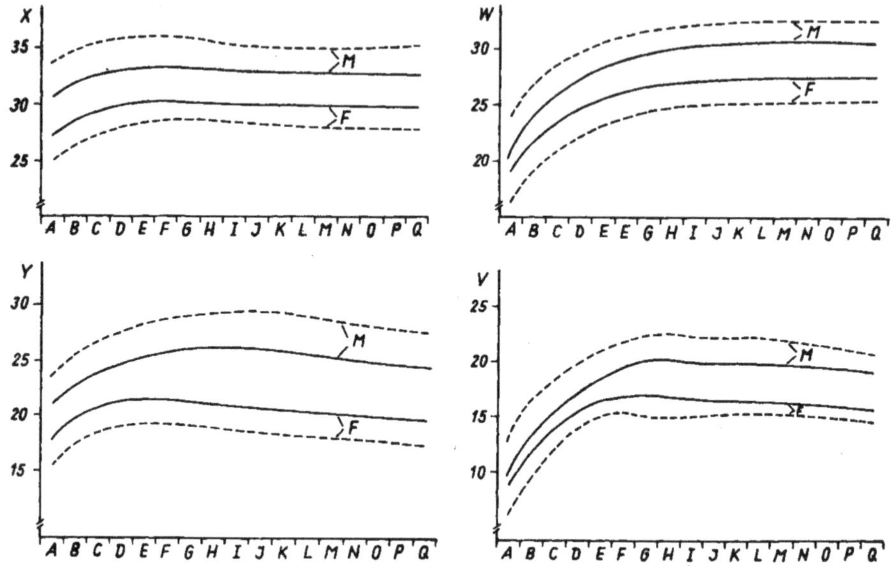

Fig.4 :
Mean (——) and standard deviation (---) of the model parameter (Fig.2) [M - male ; F - female]

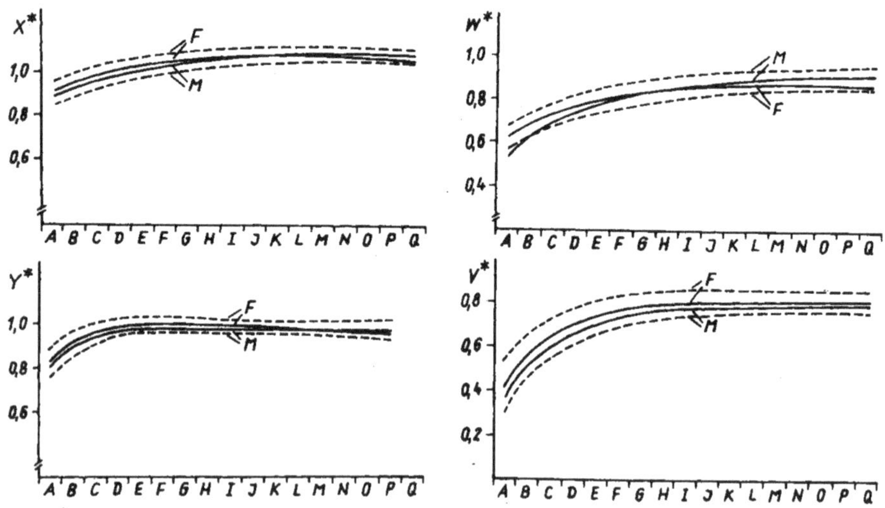

Fig.5 :
Mean (——) and standard deviation (---) of the normalized parameters [M - male ; F - female]

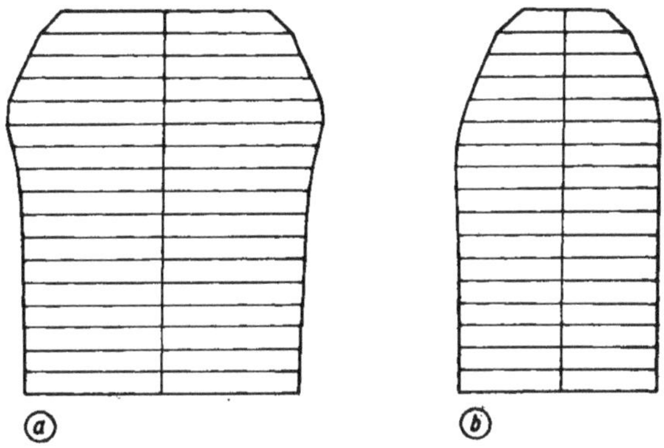

Fig.6 :
Frontal (a) and sagittal (b) view of the thorax model

4. Conclusion

The stylized torso introduced in this work can be discribed by a piecewise smooth, continuous function for the calculation of electrical transfer coefficients. To construct an individualized thorax model, the standard model can be adapted to the individualized torso geometry by linear extension so that its anterior and lateral outlines correspond with those of the subject. This procedure spares the expended designation of the individulized thorax geometry by a full set of geometric measurements.

EFFECT OF THE MYOCARDIAL ANISOTROPY ON THE CARDIAC ELECTRIC AND MAGNETIC FIELDS

L.I.Titomir

Institute for Problems of Information Transmission, Acad. Sci. USSR
Ermolovoy 19, 101447 Moscow, USSR

Influence of the cardiac tissue anisotropy on the extracellular electric and magnetic fields was studied quantitatively using the mathematical bidomain model. In particular, double-layer generator structure simulating an intramural depolarization front was considered. The closed uniform depolarization front in the anisotropic myocardium creates in the external region electric and magnetic fields. In the case of the open double-layer the maximal relative contributions of the higher order terms of the fields caused by the anisotropy are approximately 20 per cent with respect to the dipole term

To evaluate the extracellular bioelectric and biomagnetic fields of myocardium with a propagating depolarization front we have used electrodynamics of stationary currents and classical bidomain model[1]. The extracellular electric potential φ is found using Nicholson's coordinate transformation[2]

$$x' = x\sqrt{\sigma_y\sigma_z}/\sigma, \quad y' = y\sqrt{\sigma_z\sigma_x}/\sigma, \quad z' = z\sqrt{\sigma_x\sigma_y}/\sigma,$$

where

$$\sigma_x = \sigma_{ix} + \sigma_{ex}, \quad \sigma_y = \sigma_{iy} + \sigma_{ey}, \quad \sigma_z = \sigma_{iz} + \sigma_{ez},$$

σ_{ix}, σ_{iy}, σ_{iz} and σ_{ex}, σ_{ey}, σ_{ez} are the effective (spatially averaged) principal conductvities of the intracellular and extracellular spaces, respectively, σ is an arbitrary conductivity, *xyz* and $x'y'z'$ are the initial and transformed frames of reference, respectively.

The conductive medium is supposed to be axially symmetric with respect to z axis and having experimentally determined parameters[3] $\sigma_{ix} = \sigma_{iy} = 0.06$ S/m, $\sigma_{iz} = 0.34$ S/m, $\sigma_{ex} = \sigma_{ey} = 0.08$ S/m, $\sigma_{ez} = 0.12$ S/m. Then extracellular magnetic induction B is calculated as the sum of contributions from the generator itself (impressed currents) and the electric potential field (Coulomb's currents).

The surface generator of depolarization front considered has a small thickness Δn and surface vector density of dipole moment D_s that may not directionally coincide with the normal n to the surface,

$$\bar{D}_s = -\left(\int_{\Delta n}\sigma_{ix}\frac{\partial U}{\partial x}\,\mathrm{d}n\right)\vec{x}^0 - \left(\int_{\Delta n}\sigma_{iy}\frac{\partial U}{\partial y}\,\mathrm{d}n\right)\vec{y}^0 - \left(\int_{\Delta n}\sigma_{iz}\frac{\partial U}{\partial z}\,\mathrm{d}n\right)\vec{z}^0 =$$

$$= U_{\alpha x}\,\sigma_{ix}\,\vec{x}^0 + U_{\alpha y}\,\sigma_{iy}\,\vec{y}^0 + U_{\alpha z}\,\sigma_{iz}\,\vec{z}^0,$$

where U is the transmembrane potential and $\bar{U}_\alpha$ is the vector directed along n and having magnitude U_α equal to the action potential. The shape of the front is approximated as a prolate spheroid with minor semiaxis ϱ_0 and described by the equation

$$x^2 + y^2 + \lambda^2 z^2 = \varrho_0^2 \ ,$$

where $\lambda = \sqrt{\sigma_x \sigma_z}$ is the anisotropy parameter. The aforementioned coordinate transformation changes the spheroid for a sphere, thus facilitating expansion of the electric potential in the series of spherical functions. This analysis, similar to multipole techniques, has been applied to the closed spheroidal front as well as to the open semispheroidal front. The magnetic induction has been calculated straightforwardly from the current density by means of Ampere's net current law. The final expression for low-order terms ($n = 0, 1, 2$) subscribed correspondingly, of the electric potential and nonzero magnetic induction component in xOz coordinate plane for the closed front are

$$\varphi_0 = \varphi_1 = 0\ , \quad \varphi_2 = \frac{U_\alpha K_\varphi}{8}\left(\frac{r_0}{r}\right)^3 \frac{(1 + 2\lambda^2)\cos 2\theta - 1 + 2\lambda^2}{1-(1-\lambda^2)\cos^2\theta}\ ,$$

$$B_{y0} = B_{y1} = 0\ , \quad B_{y2} = \frac{3U_\alpha\,\mu_0\,K_B\,\lambda}{8}\left(\frac{r_0}{r}\right)^3 \frac{\sin 2\theta}{1-(1-\lambda^2)\cos^2\theta},$$

where

$$K_\varphi = -\frac{\sigma_{ix}}{\sigma_x}\,\frac{\lambda\sqrt{1-\lambda^2} + (1-2\lambda^2)\arcsin\sqrt{1-\lambda^2}}{\sqrt{(1-\lambda^2)^3}} -$$

$$-\frac{\sigma_{iz}}{\sigma_z}\,\frac{2\lambda\,(\lambda\sqrt{1-\lambda^2} - \arcsin\sqrt{1-\lambda^2}\,)}{\sqrt{(1-\lambda^2)^3}}\,,$$

$$K_B = \sqrt{\sigma_x\,\sigma_z}\;K_\varphi\,,$$

μ_0 is the magnetic permittivity of vacuum, θ is the angle between the radius-vector of the observation point and z-axis, while the radius-vectors of the generator point and observation point with respective magnitudes r_0 and r have the same orientations. Similarly for the open front

$$\varphi_0 = 0\,,\quad \varphi_1 = \frac{U_a}{2}\left(\frac{r_0}{r}\right)^2 \frac{\sigma_{iz}\,\lambda^2\cos\theta}{\sigma_z\,(1+\lambda)\sqrt{1-(1-\lambda^2)\cos^2\theta}}\,,$$

$$B_{y0} = 0\,,\quad B_{y1} = \frac{U_a\,\mu_0}{2}\left(\frac{r_0}{r}\right)^2 \frac{\sigma_{iz}\,\lambda^2\sin\theta}{(1+\lambda)\sqrt{1-(1-\lambda^2)\cos^2\theta}}\,,$$

the second order terms being exactly half as large in comparison with such terms for the closed front. The ratios of the maximal absolute values of the second order and first order terms of the fields are

$$\frac{\varphi_{2m}}{\varphi_{1m}} = 0.23\,\frac{r_0}{r}\,,\qquad \frac{B_{y2m}}{B_{y1m}} = 0.18\,\frac{r_0}{r}\,.$$

The distributions of the second order fields just near the outside surface of the closed depolarization front for $U_a =$ $= -100$ mV is illustrated by isoline maps in the meridional plane of the generator configuration in the Figure, showing correspondence to another model study[4].

Thus the closed depolarization front in the myocardium creates external electric and magnetic fields that may be essential in experiments with the heart preparations.

1. D.B.Geselowitz and W.T.Miller, Ann. Biomed. Eng. 11 (1983) 191.
2. P.W.Nicholson, IEEE Trans. Biomed. Eng. BME-14 (1967) 55.
3. D.E.Roberts and A.M.Scher, Circ. Res. 50 (1982) 342.
4. N.G.Sepulveda and J.P.Wikswo, Biophys. J. 51 (1987) 557.

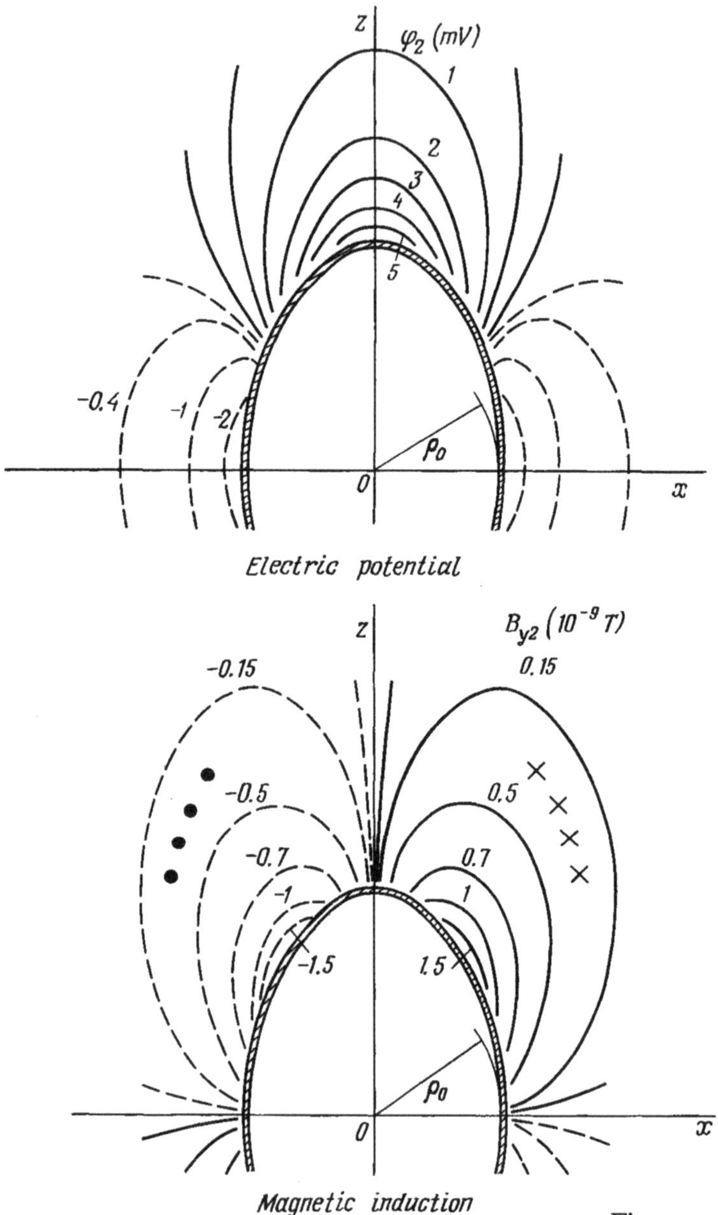

z
φ2 (mV)
1
2
3
4
5
-0.4
-1
-2
ρ0
0
x
Electric potential
z
By2 (10^-9 T)
-0.15
0.15
-0.5
0.5
-0.7
0.7
-1
1
-1.5
1.5
ρ0
0
x
Magnetic induction

Figure

DOES THE "DIPOLAR ELECTROCARDIOGRAPHY" CONTRIBUTE TO THE BETTER UNDERSTANDING OF THE ACTIVATION PATTERN IN RIGHT BUNDLE BRANCH BLOCK AND LEFT VENTRICULAR PACING ?

ZOLTÁN ANTALÓCZY, MD., MIHÁLY MEDVEGY, MD., ÁDÁM BŐHM, MD.

Postgraduate Medical School, 2nd Med. Dpt., XIII. Szabolcs str. 35.
Budapest, 1389 P.O.Box: 112, Hungary

ABSTRACT

Considering the electric activity of the heart as a dipole generator our new method provides a possibility to calculate the magnitude, the direction, the location of the resultant electric dipole; to draw the calculated surface potential map of the resultant dipole and to compute the dipolar index as well as the total energy content. The dipolar index gives information about the relation between the spatial magnitude of the resultant dipole and the total energy content of the heart. To demonstrate the benefit of these parameters we compared two similar activation patterns. The left ventricular pacing and the right bundle branch block are morphologically similar to each other, but the different origin results in some differences of the activation sequence. The knowledge of the location of the dipolar centre and the above mentioned electric parameters helped us in better understanding of the electric events in the examined cases.

INTRODUCTION

The aspect to consider the heart as a dipole generator is not a new one, it occurs in the works of WALLER[1], too. However to determine the origin of the electric resultant dipole is a difficult problem, it requires a modern computer technique. Although in the last few decades the body surface potential mapping has offered the way to compute the dipole position in the heart /GÁBOR and NELSON[2]/, though the method - because of its complexity - has not been widely accepted in the clinical practice. We have tried to determine the dipole by several methods [3, 4].

METHODS

At present we analize the different ECG anomalies by means of two sorts of technique simultaneously. One of them works on the basis of 8 measuring points by a so-called "searching" method[5], the other gives the resultant electric dipole from the 32 leading points of LUX-system by GESELOWITZ' file - decoding method[6]. Both methods provide possibility to draw the so-called "WALLER-type"body surface map calculated from the dipole and to compare this map to real surface one. By the knowledge of the resultant dipole the introduction of a new parameter: the dipolar index /DI/ was possible. According to our view DI would predict a ration of the sums expressing body surface potentials calculated only from the dipole and the potentials measured over the body surface. The calculations can be expressed as follows:

$$DI = \frac{\sum_{i=1}^{8} (U_i^{/calculated/})^2}{\sum_{i=1}^{8} (U_i^{/measured/})^2} \times 100 \quad /\%/$$

There is a connection between the DI, the total energy content /TEC/ and the spatial magnitude of the resultant dipole or the resultant vector /M/ :

$$DI = \frac{M}{TEC} \times 100 \quad /\%/$$

To demonstrate the clinical importance of the DI we show a schematic figure:

1st figure
Interpretation of the dipolar index

Dipolar index /DI/	Resultant dipole	Total energy content	– TEC
100 %	⟶ 1 mV	⟶ +1 mV	1 mV
33 %	⟶ 1 mV	−1 mV ⟵ + ⟶ +2 mV	3 mV

Figure shows us conclusions that can be reached by DI: if values of this parameter are high, lines of forces inducing resultant dipole show the same direction but if they are low, dipole developed as a result of opposite forces.

CASES

By both of our methods we analysed qualitatively 3 cases with left ventricular pacemaker stimulation /LV pacing/ that are morphologically similar to the right bundle branch block /14 cases/.

RESULTS

/See the 2nd figure/

Dipolar analysis of the pacemaker spike itself yielded an interesting result: its growth and direction change quickly and a lot, but its centre unexpectedly is located in a constant point of the heart /in the represented case – LX: 2.5, LY: 7, LZ: -1.5 cm/ and the DI values are low. All the phenomena can be explained by way of running the pacemaker stimulus around the pericardial sac. This running round that is the spike takes about 6 msec.
During about 15 msec after the spike there is no considerable activation. Then the direction of the resultant dipole turns to right, forward, and the DI increases constaneously. In the widest, middle part of the QRS the spatial magnitude shows it highest values, more

2nd figure
Different parameters of the resultant dipole during the QRS

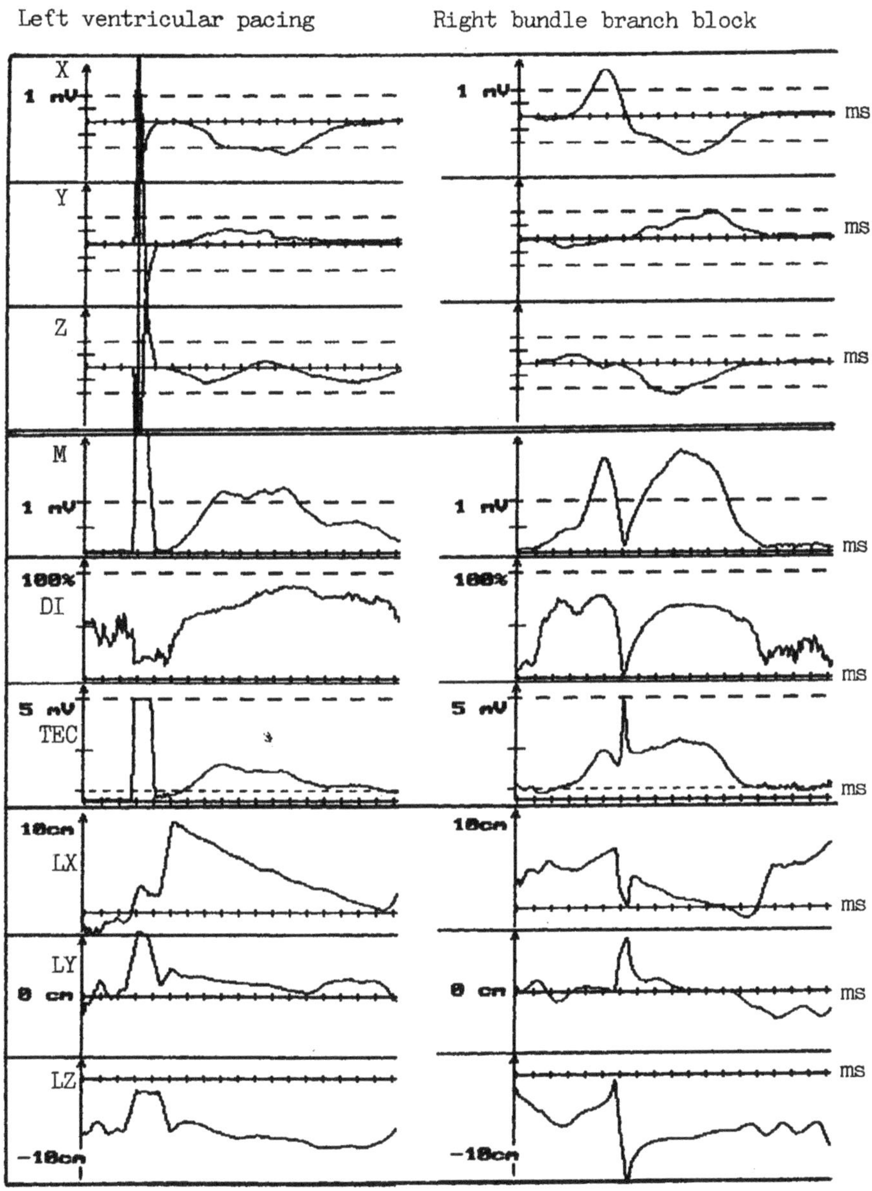

than 1 mV and is directed to the right. In the terminal 40 msec the resultant dipole turns forward. The location of the dipole centre is moving continuously to the right /into the middle of the chest/ during the QRS, while during the ST and T intervals it remains stable /in front, on the left side: LX: 5.5, LY: 0.5, LZ: -5.5 cm/.

The fact that in the greatest part of depolarization the resultant dipole is directed rightward makes the picture similar to the right bundle branch block. On the contrary the left ventricular activation can be well separated in every right bundle branch block.

Also sometimes /in 4 out of 14 cases/ the septal activation is manifested before the left ventricular activation.

Generally /in 12 out of 14 cases/ the DI decreases considerably in right bundle branch block after the first third of the depolarization. It indicates that the decreasing left and the increasing right ventricular activation are equal. The opposite forces result in a low spatial magnitude, but the TEC is high. The DI does not decrease in 2 cases, but the M and TEC show a very low minimum point. By our interpretation the activation of the two ventricles are separated from each other unambigously. In the very instant the polarity of the resultant dipole changes from left to right side within 1-2 msec.

In the largest, terminal part of the QRS the dipole centre is located in front, on the right side of the heart and it is directed definitely to the right, forward.

During the ST - T intervals the location of the dipole centre remains permanently in the heart centre /LX: 4, LY: 0, LZ: -4 cm/.

The aim of our report is to draw the attention on the fact that simultaneous analysis of the resultant dipole and the DI provides a new approach for the better understanding of the heart's electrical activity.

REFERENCES

1. P. M. Rautaharju, Can. J. of Cardiology **3** (1987) p. 362.
2. D. Gábor and C.V. Nelson, J. Appl. Physics **25** (1954) p. 413.
3. Z. Antalóczy, M. Medvegy and G. Endrőczy, Advances in Cardiology /Proc. 16th Int. Congr. ECG/ eds. Z. Antalóczy, I. Préda, E. Kékes (Elsevier, Amsterdam, 1990), p. 19.
4. G. Endrőczy, Z. Antalóczy and M. Medvegy, Advances in Cardiology /Proc. 16th Int. Congr. ECG/, eds. Z. Antalóczy, I. Préda, E. Kékes (Elsevier, Amsterdam,1990), p. 23.
5. M. Medvegy, Z. Antalóczy, Zs.Cserjés and A. Szőke, Proc. of Medicomp'90, eds. T. Asztalos, J. Eller, I. Győri (Szeged, 1990), p. 206.
6. D. B. Geselowitz, Proc IRE. **48** (1960), p. 75.

REQUIRED COMPLEXITY OF INVERSE HEART MODELS IN TERMS OF MULTIPOLAR COMPONENTS: CONCLUSIONS OF A DOG HEART EXPERIMENT

KOZMANN GY., CSERJES ZS.
Dept. Bioelectronics, Central Research Institute for Physics,
1525 Budapest P.O. Box 49, Hungary

and

BARUFFI S., SPAGGIARI S.
Inst. General Physiology, Univ. Parma,
43100 Parma, Viale delle Science, Italy

ABSTRACT

An increasing number of truncated multipolar equivalent sources, estimated from the data of an electrolytic tank dog heart experiment, were used to study the required complexity of heart models when epicardial activation maps (EAMs) are estimated. Results show that the four terms (24 components) considered in this study could guarantee only a correlation coefficient (CC) of 0.71 between the measured and simulated EAMs.

1. Introduction

Multipolar expansion (ME) is a theoretically sound method for characterizing the potential field of cardiac sources with an infinite set of equivalent electrical sources placed in the origin of a suitably chosen coordinate system[1]. The potential field generated by the equivalent sources is convergent outside of a sphere surrounding all the electric sources of the heart. The infinite set of ME terms has only a theoretical importance, in practical simulations only a truncated set of equivalent generators can be estimated. In our study, simulation results gained by truncated ME components up to 4 terms were compared with experimental data to assess the required heart representation complexity of EAM estimations on a "near-epicardial" surface.

2. Methods

Experimental data of this study were provided by a perfused isolated dog heart experiment[2] carried out at the University of Parma, Italy. In our analysis 72 electrodes close to the heart supplied reference data on the epicardial signals, while 108 tank-wall ECGs were used for estimating equivalent multipolar sources throughout the cardiac cycle in each 2 msec. ME was carried out up to 4 terms, i.e. up to 24 components (dipolar,D: 3, quadrupolar, Q: 5, octupolar, O: 7, hexadecapolar, H: 9) by the least-squares truncation method suggested by Geselowitz[1,3]. The origin of ME was placed in the approximate center of gravity of the heart. Reference EAM was computed from the 72 ECG signals taken only a few millimeters from the epicardium, while simulated EAM was estimated on a heart-shape like "near-epicardial" surface 3 cm apart from the epicardium, to ensure that all the points on this surface should be in the region of convergence. The time of activation in an arbitrary electrode location was defined as the instant of the most negative time derivative. Correlation coefficients (CC) of the real EAM and EAM estimated on the "near-epicardial" surface were used to characterize the quality of the simulations.

3. Results

Based on our data gained by the truncated ME up to 4 terms the quality of EAM simulations vs. the number of ME terms was increasing in tendency, but not monotoneously. The best result was gained by considering all the four terms (D+Q+O+H). At this complexity of representation a CC of 0.71 was achieved. In spite of the rather low correlation the general pattern of the activation sequence has been preserved correctly (Fig. 1.). However, considerable differences were observed in the map details especially on the posterior view of the heart. The RMS value of the activation time errors over the heart surface was 3.65 ms, the average mismatch between the correct and the estimated epicardial breakthrough sites was a few cm.

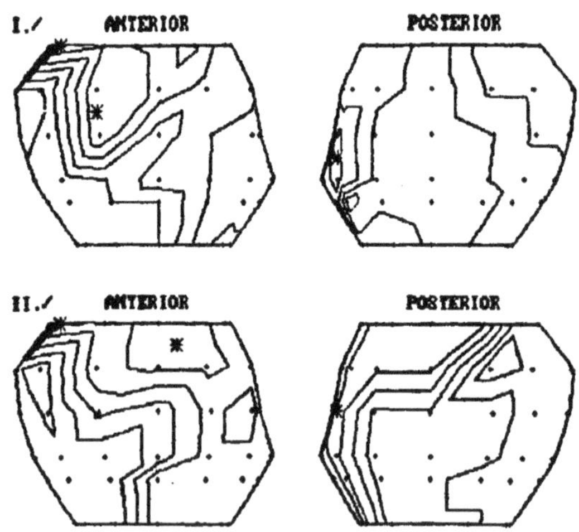

Fig.2. Measured EAM (I) and EAM computed on the "near-epicardial" surface (II) by the use of 4 multipolar terms. (Breakthrough points are marked by asterisks, time increment between subsequent isochrone lines is 5 ms.)

4. Conclusion

On the "near-epicardial" activation map by 4 truncated ME terms a precision of CC = 0.71 could be achieved. Based on the estimation quality (expressed by the CC) vs. the number of ME terms, approximately 2 additional terms (24 components) would be required to achieve a precision of CC = 0.9. However, due to practical reasons the reliable estimation of such a large number of terms is unlikely.

5. Acknowledgements

This study was partly supported by a grant of the National Research Foundation, Budapest.

6. References

1. D.B. Geselowitz, in "The Theoretical Basis of Electrocardiology", eds. C.B. Nelson, D.B. Geselowitz (Oxford Univ. Press, London, 1976) p. 202.
2. B. Taccardi, E. Musso, L. De Ambroggi, in "The Electrical Field of the Heart", P. ed. Rijlant (Presses Academiques Europeennes, Bruxelles, 1972) p. 566.
3. Zs. Cserjes, "Computer-aided models for the investigation of the heart electrical activity", Ph. D. Thesis, Budapest, 1990, Ch. 4.

CORRECTION OF AMPLITUDE DISTORTIONS CAUSED BY EXTRACARDIAC FACTORS INFLUENCE ON BSPD

ZDENEK DRSKA
Institute of Physiological Regulations, Czechoslovak Academy of Sciences, FNsP Bulovka, pav. 11, Prague, Czech and Slovak Federal Republic

and

DAGMAR VALOVA, ANNA MALKOVA, MILENA POLANKOVA
Institute of Physiological Regulations, Czechoslovak Academy of Sciences, FNsP Bulovka, pav. 11, Prague, Czech and Slovak Federal Republic

ABSTRACT

The procedure for extracardiac factors influence correction on BSPD properties taking advantage of relationship between VCG interpretation of EFH and processing of BSPD was developed. This method based on equality of family of unit vectors of orthonormal VCG, is not requiring the time consuming measurement of geometrical coordinates of matrix of points characterizing the chest surface.

1. Introduction

Significance of distance differences of individual surface points from equivalent source of electrical field of the heart (EFH) for the interpretation of BSPD is generally accepted (1,2,3,4).

To contribute to the elimination of discussed deformations of BSPD, we have developed a procedure for extracardiac factors influence correction on BSPD properties (1). This method also permits to reach the non-dipolar residue as a part of electrocardiological signal that is not possible to obtain by VCG (2).

2. Material and methods

Developed procedure for solving this problem is based on equality of family of unit vectors of orthonormal VCG system of axes, end-points of which are creating spherical surface concentric to the equivalent generator of EFH.

To this spherical surface, the unification of transfer coefficients of individual surface leads has been performed using the normalization of appropriate equations determining ECGs of these individual leads in VCG system of axes.

All ECGs (both VCG orthogonal ECGs and matrix of ECGs for mapping) were measured simultaneously and processed by the system for BSPD mapping CARDIAG 128.1 – ZPA Čakovice ČSFR.

The procedure can be described as follows: from VCG orthogonal ECGs matrix of ECGs [VD(ij)] optimally corresponding to ECGs measured in regular grid of surface points [VM(ij)] has been synthesized. This synthesis is done by solving the appropriate linear equation (Eq.1) for every surface ECG using the least squares fit method:

$$VM(ij,t)=D(ij)+A(ij).x(t)+B(ij).y(t)+C(ij).z(t)+e(ij,t) \quad [1]$$

where $e(ij,t)=[VM(ij,t)-VD(ij,t)]$, $VM(ij,t)$ is measured ECG(ij), $VD(ij,t)$ is corresponding synthesized ECG(ij), $x(t)$, $y(t)$, $z(t)$ are orthogonal ECGs of Frank VCG system and $e(ij,t)$ are residual time depending deviations of corresponding pairs of ECG values minimized using the least squares fit method. This way x, y, z components of transfer coefficients A(ij), B(ij), C(ij) are obtained.

By equation normalization (Eq.2), this equation can be transformed as follows:

$$VMk(ij,t)=\frac{D(ij)}{M(ij)}+\frac{A(ij)}{M(ij)}.x(t)+\frac{B(ij)}{M(ij)}.y(t)+\frac{C(ij)}{M(ij)}.z(t)+\frac{e(ij,t)}{M(ij)} \quad [2]$$

where VMk is measured ECG after the amplitude correction,

$M(ij)=\sqrt{A(ij)^2+B(ij)^2+C(ij)^2}$, and for every ECG the

sum of $\frac{A(ij)}{M(ij)}$, $\frac{B(ij)}{M(ij)}$, $\frac{C(ij)}{M(ij)}$ squared is equal to 1.

Ratio D(ij)/M(ij) in the main normalized equation (Eq.2) can be interpreted as a distance of zero potential plane of individual ECGs from the center of the source of EFH (along the normal erected over the center of the source). This normalization can be applied to correct amplitudes of both measured and synthesized ECGs. Amplitudes of corrected ECGs are then corresponding to the unit value of transfer coefficient (spatial orientation and mutual relationships of individual ECGs resting unchanged).

3. Results

Range of this amplitudes correction corresponding to the variability of values of transfer coefficient (i.e. coefficient of amplitude correction) of original surface ECGs was found within the values 0.35 - 2.1.(Fig. 1)

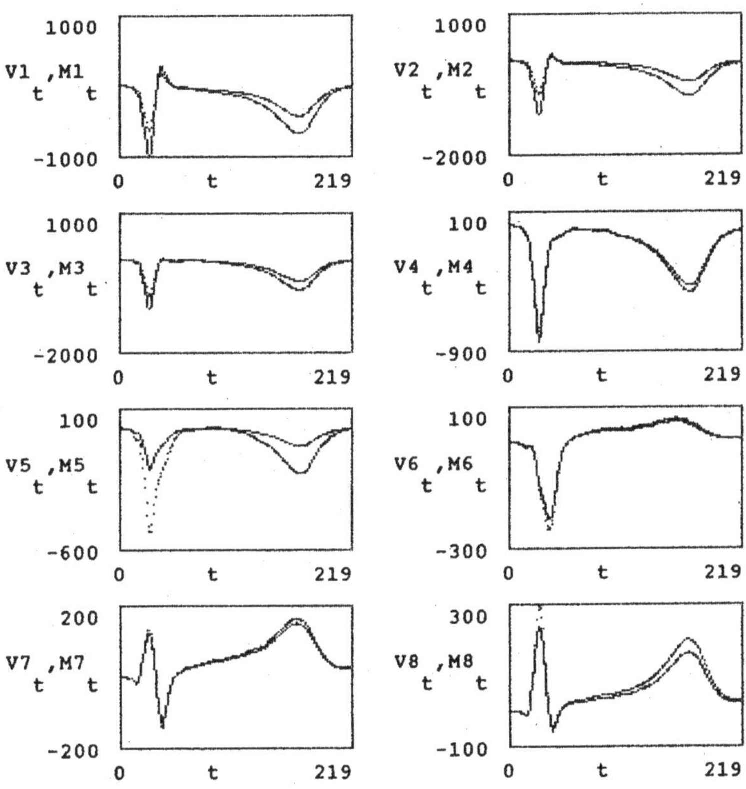

Fig.1: ECGs from anterior chest wall at the level of 2nd intercostal space as a part of ECG matrix of 16 columns and 5 rows measured in regular grid on the thoracic surface. Dotted curves represent original ECGs, full line curves are the same ECGs after the amplitudes correction.

Significance of this amplitudes correction can be also demonstrated by differences between original and corrected isopotential maps (1).

4. Discussion

Discussed amplitude correction covers not only correction of differences in the distances of surface points from the source but unifies also the distortions in BSPD done by electrical inhomogeneity of internal medium of the thorax and those done by boundary conditions. Influence of these extracardiac factors is unified to be corresponding to conditions equal to actual conditions in lead vectors of VCG system of axes. Least squares fit method used for ECG matrix synthesis corresponds to the presumption of global electroneutrality of dipolar component of EFH on equidistant spherical plane. As has been just mentioned, described procedure permits to obtain the non-dipolar residue at individual instants of electrical systole and at individual points of the surface (2).

5. Conclusions

Described procedure of transfer coefficients unification permits the extraction of extracardiac factors influence on the properties of BSPD without necessity of measuring the geometric coordinates of thoracic surface.

Influence of electrical inhomogeneity of internal medium and of boundary conditions in individual leads are equalized with their influence in resulting VCG orthogonal leads.

Significance of described amplitude correction for interpretation of standard 12-leads ECG (criteria being mostly based on amplitudes relations) is also evident.

This procedure leads to significant changes of individual potential values and position of potential peaks in BSPD. The appearance of new peaks in BSPD was also observed.

6. References

1. Z. Drška, D, Valová A. Málková, *Electrocardiology'87* (Akademie Verlag, Berlin, 1988) pp. 185 - 188.
2. Z. Drška, A. Málková, M. Polánková, D. Valová: *Advances in Electrocardiology*, eds. Z. Antaloczy, I. Preda, E. Kekes (Excerpta Medica, Amsterdam - New York - Oxford, 1990) pp. 145 - 148.
3. I. Ruttkay-Nedecky, L. I. Titomir, O. V. Baum, L. Bacharova, *Electrocardiology'87* (Akademie Verlag, Berlin, 1988) pp. 145 - 148.
4. L.I. Titomir, *Elektritcheskoe pole serdca* (Nauka, Moskva, 1988) 371 p.

CONCEPT OF MODEL-BASED VERIFICATION OF INVERSE PROBLEM IN ELECTROCARDIOGRAPHY

PETER KNEPPO, JANA ŠVEHLÍKOVÁ, JANA KUŽMOVÁ, MILAN TYŠLER
Biomeasurements Laboratory, Institute of Measurement Science, Slovak Academy of Sciences
Dúbravská cesta 9, 842 19 Bratislava, Czechoslovakia

ABSTRACT

The equivalent representation of cardiac electrical activity by a multipole series expansion has been studied. The forward problem solution formulated by integral equations was used for computing the potential distribution. The realistic geometry of inhomogeneous torso and heart have been assumed. The heart generator was modeled by a uniform double layer spreading through the cardiac muscle. Two methods for the multipole terms estimation were used: a method based on surface integration of BSPM assuming homogeneous torso model, and a method based on the transfer matrix between torso and generator, which allows to use homogeneous and also inhomogeneous torso model. The electrical field of computed equivalent multipolar generators in relation to the field of the original generator was studied on the surface just around the modeled heart. From the results it implies that the multipolar cardiac generator equivalent in the sense of BSPMs seems not to be sufficient for recovery of the electrical field near the realistic spatially distributed cardiac generator.

1. Introduction

The equivalent representation of cardiac electrical activity by a multipole series expansion is an important theoretical construct of electrocardiography. If a simplified body model without internal heterogeneities is considered, then two versions of the solution may be used. In the first case the forward problem is solved by the transfer coefficients, which are found to relate the potentials at a finite number of the body surface points with a finite number of the equivalent (multipole) generator components. Then a system of such equations for body surface points is solved in a least-squares sense for the generator components. In the second case the method of potential integration over the body surface is used.

In a comparative analysis of these two approaches of determining the multipole components similar results for estimation of the epicardial potential were achieved[1].

2. Method

A further important step towards noninvasive identification of cardiac excitation from the body surface measurements is the development of methods for solving the inverse problem in the strict sense, that is in terms of characteristics of a cardiac equivalent generator, which are subsequently transformed into characteristics having a straightforward electrophysiological meaning.

This inverse method[2,3] seems promising and relatively easy applicable in electrocardiographic diagnostic. But there is an important question of verification of this method on realistic subjects. Because it is difficult to make invasive measurements on the patients, we have used the forward problem simulation in inhomogeneous realistically shaped torso model[4]. The depolarization wave in heart is modeled by the uniform double layer spreading through the cardiac muscle. The volume conductor of human body is modeled as homogeneous, containing four subregions with different conductivity. These are two ventricular cavities with conductivity three-times higher than the basic conductivity and two lungs with five-times lower conductivity. All the surfaces are closed and triangulated. The geometry was measured by MRI technique, the data on the activation sequence were digitized on the closed surface bounding the ventricular walls. By this formulation of the forward problem the simulated body–surface potential maps can be obtained on the realistic torso model and they can simulate ECG in arbitrary point of the torso, too. These are later used as the input information for inverse problem solution which we wanted to verify.

For the inverse problem solution two methods for the multipole terms estimation were used: a method based on surface integration of body-surface potential map which assumes the homogeneous torso model and also a method based on the transfer matrix between torso and generator. This method uses singular value decomposition of the transfer matrix[5] and allows to include the internal inhomogeneities of the torso. The equivalent multipolar generator was computed for each time instant of the modeled depolarization from the reference body surface potential maps simulated on the torso. Then the potential distributions (quasiepicardial maps) were computed on the surface around the modeled heart or on the spherical surface respectively and then compared to the original quasiepicardial maps.

3. Results

At first the effect of the inhomogeneities on the results of forward problem solution was investigated. In forward problem simulation the systematic character of the error was confirmed as it is shown in Fig.1. From this result it implies, that the global character of the maps is very similar, but the amplitudes are different.

In Fig.2 the results of comparison between the reference quasiepicardial map computed from the original heart model and the map computed from multipole

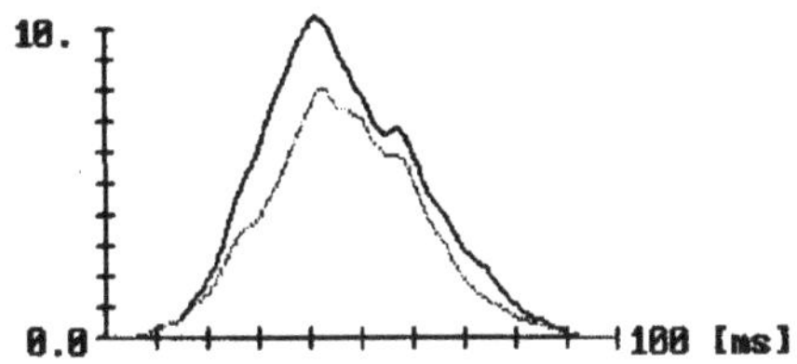

Fig.1a RMS signal in homogeneous (dashed line) and inhomogeneous (solid line) case during modeled depolarization

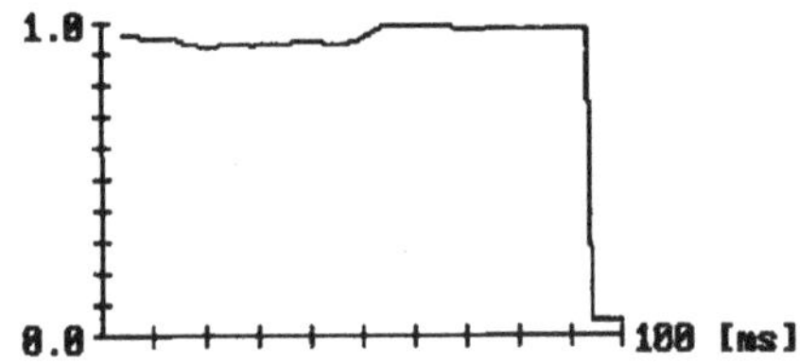

Fig.1b Correlation coefficients between body surface potential maps in homogeneous and inhomogeneous case during modeled depolarization

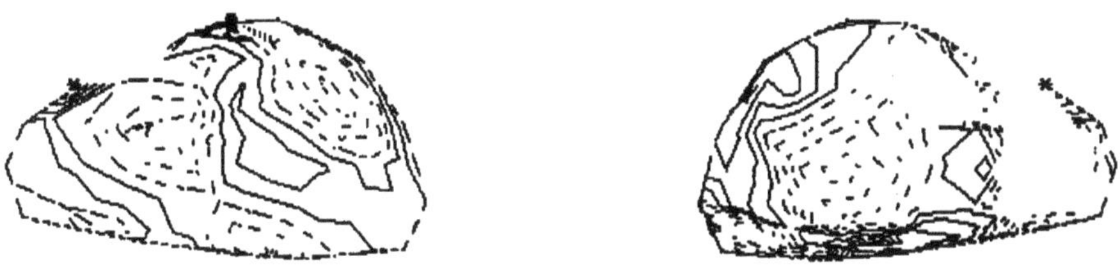

Fig.2a Reference quasiepicardial map

Fig.2b Quasiepicardial map computed from multipole obtain by SI method

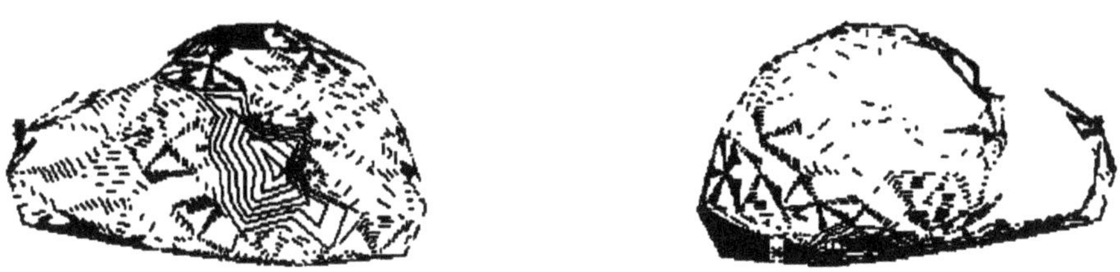

Fig.2c Quasiepicardial map computed from multipole recovered by transfer matrix including the internal inhomogeneities

obtained by surface integration method (assumption of homogeneous torso) and the map computed from multipole recovered by transfer matrix including the internal inhomogeneities for the same time instant (40 ms) are shown. Correlation coefficients for all studied cases are presented in Fig.3.

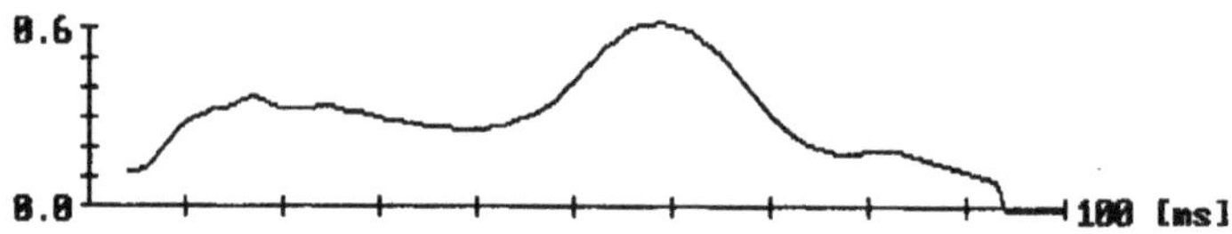

Fig.3a Correlation coefficients between reference quasiepicardial maps and maps computed from multipole obtained by SI method – assumption of homogeneous torso

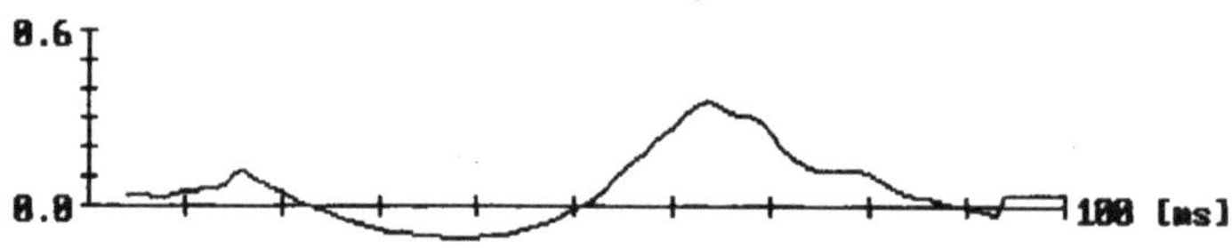

Fig.3b. Correlation coefficients between reference quasiepicardial maps and maps computed from multipole recovered by transfer matrix including the internal inhomogeneities

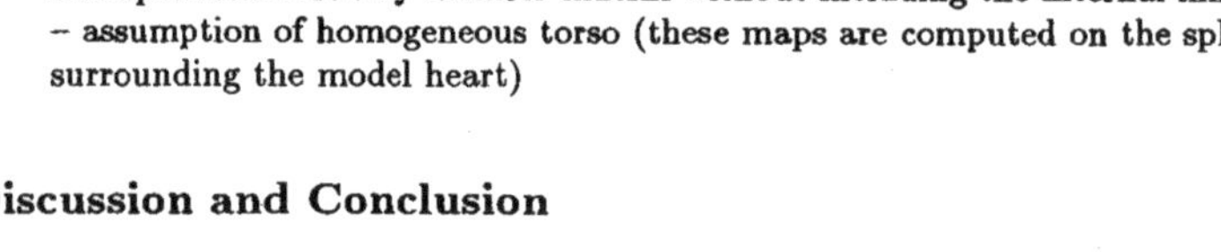

Fig.3c. Correlation coefficients between reference quasiepicardial maps and maps computed from multipole recovered by transfer matrix without including the internal inhomogeneities – assumption of homogeneous torso (these maps are computed on the sphere just surrounding the model heart)

5. Discussion and Conclusion

Assuming that the potential maps constructed from a heart model represent correctly the real situation, there are many factors influencing the maps reconstructed from multipolar generator. One of the most dominant is the absence of inhomogeneities in the inverse problem solution based on surface integration of potential distribution on the torso. The presumption of the inverse problem solution is that the general influence of inhomogeneities has relatively strong systematic character which could be eliminated at diagnostic interpretation. The next important factors having an influence on the reconstructed maps are the position of the center of the sphere, the estimation of the radius of the sphere just surrounding the generator and the estimation of the threshold level representing the dipole moment density on this sphere.

From this reasons it implies, that there is a great variability of possible results in inverse problem solution. The question is, how substantial are the differences among results and whether these results could really represent the cardiac electrical field. From our preliminary results it implies, that

- the obtained differences are significant and interesting for another study,
- substantial in evaluation of the inverse problem is the definition of the equivalent generator (the multipolar generator acceptable in the sense of BSPMs equivalence seems not to be sufficient for recovery of the electrical field near the realistic – spatially distributed cardiac generator),
- neglecting of inhomogeneities causes systematic error in the forward solution and great and non-systematic differences in the inverse estimation of the equivalent multipolar generator,
- the next important factor in multipolar terms reconstruction is the choice of computation technique (we have tried to verify three methods for reconstruction of original - spatially distributed generator from equivalent multipolar generator and from our results it implies, that these methods give unsatisfactory results).

6. Acknowledgement

This research was supported by grant GA-SAV No.319/91 and in part by grant GA-SAV No.242/91 from the Slovak Academy of Sciences.

7. References

1. T. C. Pilkington and M. N. Morrow, *CRC Crit. Rev. Biomed. Eng.* **7** (1982) 175.
2. P. Kneppo and L. I. Titomir, in *Models and Measurements of the Cardiac Electric Field*, ed. E. Schubert (Plenum Press, New York and London, 1982).
3. L. I. Titomir, Automatic Analysis of the Cardiac Electromagnetic Field (Nauka, Moscow, 1984) p.175 (in Russian).
4. A. Oosterom, *PhD-thesis* (University of Amsterdam, Amsterdam 1978) p.181.
5. J. J. M. Cuppen and A. van Oosterom, *IEEE Biomed. Eng.* **BME-31** (1984) 652.

MODEL-BASED COMPARISON OF LIMITED LEAD MAPPING SYSTEMS

MARIE TURZOVÁ, PETER KNEPPO, MILAN TYŠLER, JANA ŠVEHLÍKOVA, VLADIMÍR ROSÍK
Biomeasurements Laboratory, Institute of Measurement Science, Slovak Academy of Sciences, Dúbravská cesta 9, 84219 Bratislava, Czechoslovakia

ABSTRACT

Preliminary study is presented on possibility of using limited lead mapping systems in forward model simulation of heart activation and in analysis of extracardial factors influence. Uniform double layer model of the heart and inhomogeneous realistically shaped torso model was used for the forward simulation of the surface potentials. Three different limited lead systems (LLS) have been studied and compared using surface potential data simulated in full 12×16 mapping grid. Two of the LLS use statistical method for map estimation from 24 leads and from 32 leads, the third one uses adaptive quasimultipole map approximation and 32 lead system. The results show that LLS might give applicable maps for using in model study and allow judgment about the model acceptability: relative approximation error was 2.3% and correlation coefficient 0.99 for Barr's leads, 5.3% and 0.97 for Lux's leads, 8.9% and 0.96 for NEKTAL leads. However, these results are slightly worse than in comparable real measurements (1.1, 2.3, 5.8 % and 0.995, 0.99, 0.97 respectively).

1. Introduction

Investigating the variability of the cardiac electric field we use simulated surface data: computer model of the myocardium activation[1] simulates propagation in ventricular walls with an approximate resolution of 1 cubic mm of the tissue and enables to simulate different conduction velocities in the working myocardium and in the specific conducting system. For computation of body surface potentials a realistic inhomogeneous torso model including intracavitary blood, heart shape, lungs and torso boundary is used[2]. A realistic solution of the forward problem is attempted by combining the two above mentioned models.

In the study we tried to find how the LLSs will perform on simulated data: with what accuracy the generated maps can be estimated and whether this results are comparable with real measurements. This might allow to use the LLS maps for evaluation of model simulations and to compare the maps with available set of clinical data or perhaps also to use existing clinical data for inverse solution studies. Body surface potential mapping using limited number of leads is used in experimental clinic in Bratislava and extensive set of normals and patients is available.

2. Material and methods

The inhomogeneous realistic shaped torso model with geometry of lungs, epicardium and endocardium of both ventricles was used in forward simulation using the method proposed by van Oosterom[2]. The depolarization wave was approximated as spreading uniform double layer and the surface potentials in 12×16 points on the torso were computed.

Limited leads mapping systems estimate surface potentials ϕ in M points of the mapping grid from limited number of measured leads (L<<M) for each time instant using the formula

$$\left\{\hat{\phi}\right\} = W\left\{u\right\}$$

where $\hat{\phi}$ is the vector of M estimated mapped potentials,
u is the vector of L measured potentials,
W is the (L×M) transfer matrix.

There are several approaches how to define transfer matrix W. We compared two LLSs where statistical methods were used to specify number and positions of optimal leads and the transfer matrix W for estimation of full map potentials. Experimental covariance parameters were obtain from large training set of maps. While Barr[3] used principal component analysis and 30 basis patterns (generators) for estimation of potentials in all 10×15 mapped points including 24 irregularly spaced measured leads, Lux[4] used 32 measured leads and least mean-squared error criterion for estimation of potentials in the rest of 12×16 mapped points. The third LLS NEKTAL[5] was used for adaptive quasimultipole approximation of potential where the basis patterns were formed by means of 18 spatial spherical functions. In this method the transfer matrix is dependent on the torso geometry and adapted standard torso geometry is used. The selection of different sets of measuring electrodes as well as approximation of potentials in arbitrary mapping grid is allowed.

In this study we have used Lux's LLS with no electrodes on the back and LLS NEKTAL with 32 electrodes and 12×16 point mapping grid.

Experimental data were measured using PC-based measuring and processing system CardioPC[6] designed for multichannel ECG measurements and for mapping in the three LLS mentioned above. The data were measured in 12×16 grid in 6 synchronized sequences of 32 points. The potentials in 10×15 mapping grid were obtained from the 12×16 grid by linear interpolation. Adapted standard torso geometry[2] (similar to used model torso geometry) which needed only three basic dimension of real torso was used for NEKTAL LLS.

The accuracy of potentials estimated from LLS's with respect to original full grid potentials was specified using root mean square (rms) potential in the map P, root mean square error of the estimated map E, relative power error $e = E^2/P^2$ and correlation ρ between measured and estimated maps.

3. Results

Several map patterns resulting from model simulation and also their estimation from limited number of leads and their statistical parameters are shown in Fig.1. The best results were obtained using 24 leads according Barr and also dependence of the error parameters on the time instant within the ecg cycle (and, in this way, on the map pattern) was smaller. In the LLS according Lux the errors were higher especially at the QRS beginning and end. The results obtained from NEKTAL LLS were less satisfactory, although the statistical parameters of the maps were not very different from the Lux system, the map patterns showed visible differences.

For comparison the same evaluation was made for real measured data. Although the overall error in real data was lower than in simulated data, the performance of the individual LLSs was consistent with the simulated data. Mean values of approximation parameters during the QRS for all three LLS and for both simulated and measured data are summarized in table 1.

Lead system	*rms error* mV	*rms signal* mV	*relat. error* %	*correlation*
BARR–24	.035 (.031)	.240 (.353)	2.3 (1.1)	.989 (.995)
LUX–32	.044 (.040)	.237 (.347)	5.3 (2.3)	.974 (.988)
NEKTAL–32	.075 (.075)	.237 (.347)	8.9 (5.8)	.958 (.971)

Tab.1 Mean parameters of map estimation from LLSs during QRS komplex in simulated and measured (in parenthesis) data

This results corespond with analysis of experimental data of several persons for two of the LLS, BARR-24 and NEKTAL-32 as reported earlier[6].

4. Discussion and conclusions

In Barr's 24-lead system visual comparison of map patterns shows good agreement in shape and there are only slight moves in extremes positions in maps 1, 2, 3 and 6 (fig.1). However, the good results may also be influenced by the smoothing effect of the linear transformation from original 12×16 to 10×15 grid. In Lux's LLS the imperfection of posterior potential estimation is visible in maps 2, 3, 5 and 6, extremes from posterior torso are moved to anterior. This might be due to the lack of electrodes on the back. NEKTAL LLS shows relatively good approximation of amplitude and position of extremes but the overall pattern is visibly changed.

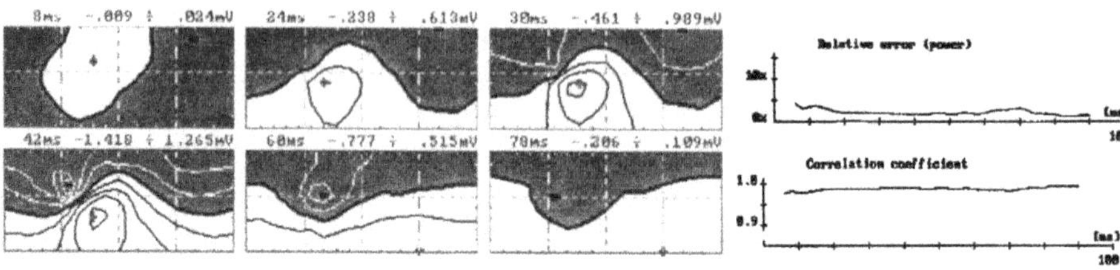

BARR-24 maps

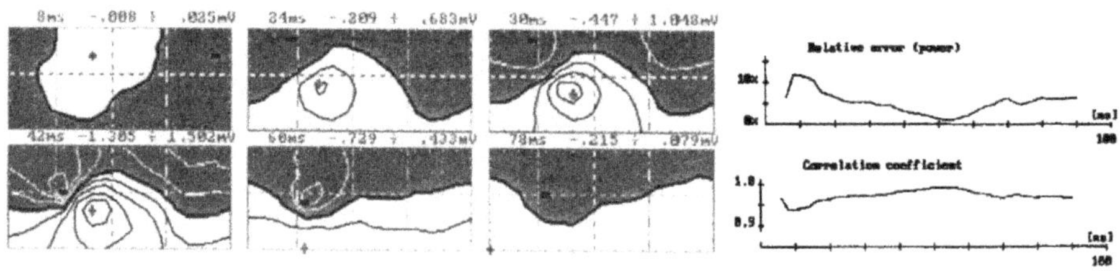

LUX-32 maps

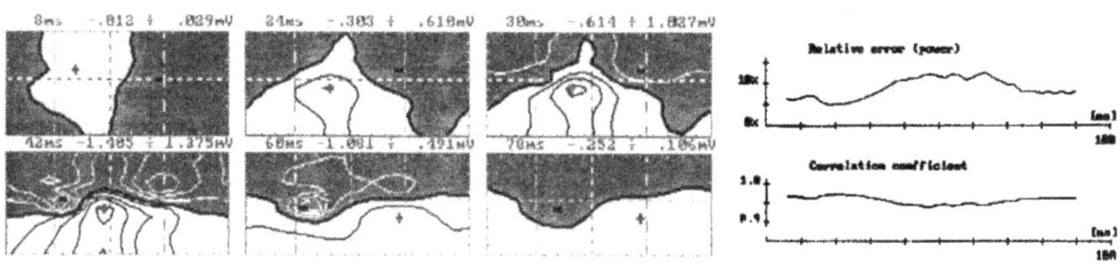

NEKTAL-32 maps

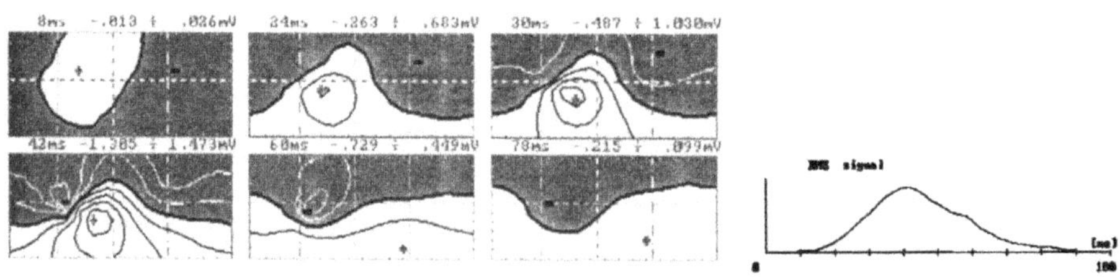

Full grid maps

Fig.1 Model-based simulated data
Map patterns and parameters of LLS estimation during QRS komplex

Although in measured data the map patterns show more variability the estimation error is lower. This might be due to the fact that the estimation methods were derived from real data. In real measurements there is good approximation of posterior extremes positions also in Lux LLS. In NEKTAL LLS the extremes are moved and the patterns are changed again.

The obtained preliminary results indicate that it might be possible to use carefully selected LLS in the model studies for evaluation of extracardial factors influence on the cardiac electric field and, possibly, to use the results for comparing with available real data.

5. Acknowledgments

The authors are grateful to prof. A.van Oosterom for providing them with the data and software for implementing the forward model, prof. R. Barr, prof. R. Lux and prof. L.I. Titomir for providing them with the data for LLS reconstruction algorithms. This research was supported by grant GA-SAV No. 319/91 from the Slovak Academy of Sciences.

6. References

1. I. Ruttkay-Nedecký, A. Drkošová and V. Szathmáry, in *Advances in Electrocardiology,* ed. P. d'Alche (Centre de publications de L'Universite de Caen, 1985).
2. A. Van Oosterom, in *Pediatric and Fundamental Electrocardiography* , ed. J. Liebman, R. Plonsey, and Y. Rudy (Martinus Nijhoff, Boston etc., 1987).
3. R. C. Barr, M. S. Spach and G. S. Herman-Giddens, *IEEE Trans. Biomed. Eng.* **BME-18,** (1971) 125.
4. R. L. Lux, C. R. Smith, R. F. Wyatt and J. A. Abildskov, *IEEE Trans. Biomed. Eng.* **BME-25** (1978) 270.
5. P. Kneppo and L. I. Titomir, *Physics in Medicine and Biology* **33 (Suppl.1),** (1988) 164 .
6. M. Tyšler, V. Rosík, P. Krakovský, M. Turzová, *Cardiac Electrical Field, its Measurement, Modelling and Interpretation* (Symposium Stará Lesná, Czechoslovakia, 1990).

CONTRIBUTION OF BIOELECTRICAL ACTIVITY OF INTRAMURAL MYOCARD LAYERS IN FORMATION OF CARDIOELECTRIC FIELDS ON THE EPICARD AND BODY SURFACE

ROSHCHEVSKY MICHAEL, SHMAKOV DIMITRI, ROSHCHEVSKAYA IRENE

Institute of Physiology of the USSR Acad. Sci., Ural Division, Syktyvkar, USSR

ABSTRACT

It was shown, that the forms of extracellular potentials on the epicardium correlated with different types of ventricle myocard activation. The bioelectrical activity of different heart layers (epicardial, intramural, and endocardial) were projected on the body surface.

Introduction

One of the fundamental problem of the heart electrophysiology is the study of the mechanism of cardioelectric field (CEF) formation. None of the existing hypothesis of informativity of bioelectrical activity of heart layers has not experimental confirmations. The problem of correlation between heart ventricle depolarization sequence and the form of extracellular potentials (EP) of CEF on the epicard and the body surface has not been solved yet.

The comparative - electrophysiological study of excitation in heart with different types of organization have laid the foundation for solution of the problems of CEF genesis.

Methods

The experiments have been carried out in fish, amphybians, reptilians, birds and mammals. The animals were anesthetized with sodium thiopentalum-natrium 30 mg/kg body wt. After intubation a thoracotomy was performed and multipolar intramural electrodes were introduced perpendicular to ventricular surface. For cardioelectric mapping on the body and epicardial surface the 64-channel system of simultaneous computer registration and treatment was used.

Results

In the result of detailed investigation of intamural bioelectrical activity of the heart ventricles several types of activation of myocard in vertebrates were discovered.

In fish in the most parts of myocardium heart excitation is characterized by the distribution of depolarization wave with saw-edged front along the ventricle walls. In amphybians and reptilians depolarization wave consistently spreads from endocard to epicard. In birds and ungulates we discovered frequent changes of movement of depolarization wave in the ventricles . In cornivores subendocard layers are excited almost simultaneously. Then successive movement of depolarization wave to epicard takes place.

Several mechanisms of formation of EP of CEF on the

epicard and body surface were determined of depolarization sequence of intramural myocard layers. It was shown, that the form of EP on the epicardium correlated with different types of ventricle myocard activation.

The "flash" character of depolarization of heart ventricles in birds is similar to that in ungulate animals. The presence of conducting fibres of small diameter in the subendocardial, intramural and subepicardial layers is the structural base for multipolar depolarization of the bird and ungulale heart ventricles. The simularity of sequence of depolarization of heart ventricles in this animals causes the identical negative forms of EP of CEF on the epicard. Their negativity is caused by the presence of foci of primary excitation situated near by the epicard. From them the activation waves move into the depth of myocard.

In amphybians and reptilians the epicardial EP are characterized by biphase and positive form.

In mammalians cornivores in the area of primary excitation of the epicardium the EP had negative deflections. The biphase and positive form potentials are formed in the most parts of ventricle surface. Thus, the CEF on the epicardial surface reflected the activation of underlying layers.

It was determined, that the bioelectrical activity of different heart layers is projected on body surface. The analysis of the experimental data showed that the initial phase of potentials of CEF on body surface is formed by electrical activity of subendocardial layers.Middle and final phases- by electrical potentials of the intramural and subepicardial myocard layers and final parts of potentials reflect the electrical activity of the outer myocard layers.

The foci of primary negativity are electrocardiographically silent, at any rate, when strengthening of electrical potentials is equal to 10-30 mm/mv.

Conclusion

Correlation between the form of epicardial EP and depolarization sequence in intramural layers in the heart of vertebrates was discovered.Animals with the "flash" type of myocardial depolarization in most cases have the negative EP in the greater part of the epicardial ventricular surface. Animals with the consecutive type of myocardial activation - the positive and biphase potentials.

All myocardial layers are electrocardiologically informative. The comparative-physiological analyses of the depolarization of myocard intramural layers showed that the mechanism of formation of the extracellular CEF on the body and myocardium surface is clously connected with the activation process in the heart.

It is necessary to take into account the spatial - time characteristic of excitation waves in the intramural myocard and informativity of bioelectric activity of different layers of heart in theoretical and experimental investigations of biophysical and physical nature of CEF.

EPICARDIAL AND BODY SURFACE MAPPING IN RABBIT

MOSTIVENKO KSENIA, VITYASEV VLADIMIR, KUVETKIN BORIS

Institute of Physiology of the USSR Acad. Sci., Ural Division, Syktyvkar, USSR

ABSTRACT

Correlation between ventricular epicardium depolarization and body surface potential maps was studied in rabbits. In the position on the back process of activation of ventricular epicardium was projected on the body surface earlier than in the position on the belly and was finished respectively earlier.

Introduction

We studied cardiac electrical field of the rabbit as a traditional object of electrocardiology using instantaneous mapping of normal potential distribution over epicardium and body surface. Unipolar ECG were recorded from 64 lead points. The electrodes were located regularly on the thoracic surface in the form of a grid containing 8 columns and 8 rows. The epicardial electrode also had the form of a grid.

Methods

Experiments were performed on 7 adult rabbits anesthetized with 50 mg/kg pentobarbital. The surface cardiac electrical field was recorded in two positions of the animal: on the belly and on the back. The rabbits were ventilated with a pump respirator and chest was opened through a midline sternotomy. The heart was exposed and suspended in pericardial cradle.

Results

On the basis of the instantaneous surface potential maps it was established that at the onset of QRS the positive extremum was formed to the left of the midsternum, with the positive area covering the ventral body surface excluding the clavicular and neck regions, and the negative one covering the dorsal surface. During 10-12 ms magnitude of positive potential reached of the maximal value (1-2 mV). After that, the positive extremum moved to the right and cranially, gradually decreased and disappeared. The negative extremum appeared at 10-12 ms from the QRS onset, below and left from the sternum; approximately in 4-5 ms it reached its maximal magnitude (0,8-1,6 mV). At that moment the negative area covered the inferior hemithorax of the ventral surface, sometimes including the left hemithorax of the dorsal surface. At about the 26-th ms, the negative extremum disappeared. Thus, the duration of the ventricular complex on the body surface of the rabbit is 24-28 ms.

In the position on the back process of activation of ventricles was projected on the body surfase earlier than in the position on the belly and was finished respectively earlier. These variations are essential and statistically significant in first 4 ms and last 6 ms of surfase ventrical complex ($p<0,05$)(Fig.1).

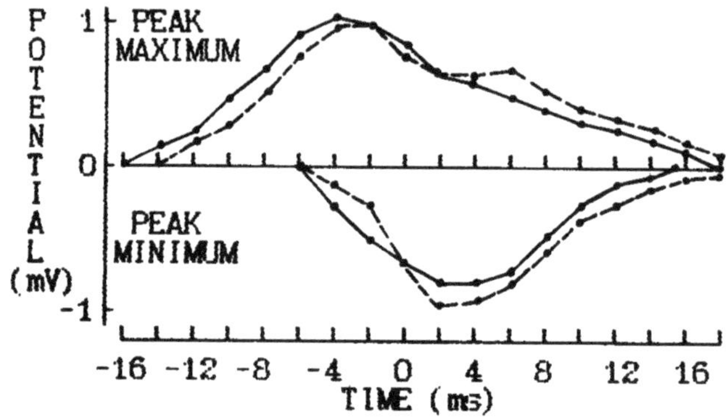

Fig.1. Variation in amplitude of potential maxima and minima at the position of the animal on the back (solid line) and on the belly (dotted line).

The analysis of the activation sequence maps over the epicardium showed that the wave front of depolarisation breacs through in the middle part of the right ventricle.2-3 ms later the basis of the right ventricle was excited; then the process of activation, spreading laterally, dorsally and toward the basis of left ventricle, completely depolarized the epicardium of both ventricles. The duration of the depolarization process of the ventricular epicardium is 7-8 ms. Last was excited the section in the septal basis and a bordering area of the left ventricle.

<u>Conclusion</u>

On the whole surface electrical cardiac field of a rabbit was characterized by some originality, which can be explained by special disposition of heart in the chest. Because of narrow anterior portion of the chest the heart fills in most of it. The apex of heart is directed to below and slightly to the left. With regards to the spine, heart is directed into 45 angle and lies flat on the sternum.

Surface electrical cardiac field depend on the type of electrical activity of the heart, the geometric relationship between the recording electrodes and the position of the heart. It is apparent that changing the position of the animals torso causes the displacement of heart position, which leads to variations in the surface potential.

VECTORCARDIOGRAPHIC FEATURES OF LEFT VENTRICULAR ENLARGEMENT. A MODEL STUDY.

VAVRINEC SZATHMÁRY, IVAN RUTTKAY-NEDECKÝ, RÓBERT OSVALD
Institute of Normal and Pathological Physiology,
Slovak Academy of Sciences, Sienkiewiczova 1, Bratislava,
Czech and Slovak Federative Republic

ABSTRACT

Three types of left ventricular enlargement were simulated by a computer model of ventricular activation propagation. In eccentric hypertrophy, the magnitude of instantaneous cardiac vectors increased only during the last two thirds of ventricular activation time. The loop become prolonged posteriorly with a leftward shift of terminal vectors. Concentric hypertrophy resulted in a decrease of vector magnitudes during the first half of ventricular activation followed by their slight increase. In dilatation the simulated cardiac vectors were increased from the beginning of activation and the configurational changes of the loop resembled those seen in eccentric hypertrophy.

1. Introduction

Left ventricular enlargement is due to increase of wall thickness and/or diastolic chamber volume. Both factors play a role with not yet fully understood proportions in determining the vectorcardiographic features in this condition. In this study computer simulation of ventricular activation propagation under gradually changed ventricular wall and chamber dimensions was used to demonstrate their relative role played in the shaping of vectorcardiogram.

2. Method

The computer model of the propagation of ventricular activation[1] was effectuated by a hypothetical three-dimensional grid of elements. The left ventricle was demarcated by segments of two half ellipsoids and the right ventricle by segments of two quarter ellipsoids. Since the shape of ventricles was determined analytically, their dimensions as well as the thicknesses of their walls could be easily changed.

The sequence of activation propagation was realized according to the Huygen's principle of wavefront propagation. The wavefronts may be characterized by two parameters - the size of their surface by the number of activated elements (unit dipoles) and by the vectorial sum of these elements determining the simulated instantaneous heart vector. The time course of the end point of heart vectors - the vectorcardiogram - may be computed either in the coordinate system of the heart model, or after its transformation into the coordinate system of the body.

The geometry of the model heart was determined in agreement with published anatomical dimensions of human hearts[2]. The ventricular walls consisted of 149017 elements, so that the resolution of the model is about 1 mm^3. The velocity of activation propagation on the endocardial surface was three times higher than in the residual myocardium. The localization of starting elements and the delay of their activation, with respect to earliest activation, were derived from human data published in Durrer et al[3]. The localization of 5 starting elements was following: (i) in the central part of the left septal surface (earliest activation); (ii) in the left ventricular free wall, posteriorly one third of distance from apex to base (delay 1 t.u.); (iii) in the upper part of the anterior free wall on an area corresponding to the attachment of the mitral valve (delay 2 t.u.); (iv) on the anterior apical right ventricular wall (delay 6 t.u.); (v) in the middle part of the anterior free wall of the right ventricle (delay 9 t.u.).

The following types of left ventricular enlargement were simulated: (i) eccentric hypertrophy with unchanged end-diastolic volume, realized by a gradual increase of the thickness of the left ventricular wall, including the septum, until it reached one and half of its original value (Fig.1a).(ii) concentric hypertrophy by gradual increase of the thickness of left ventricular wall up to 150% of its original one (since this increase was concentric the diastolic chamber size decreased) (Fig.1b).(iii) dilatation by gradual increase of the end-diastolic volume, while the thickness of wall was held constant (Fig.1c). The external dimension of the left ventricle was increased by a value corresponding to 50% of normal wall thickness.

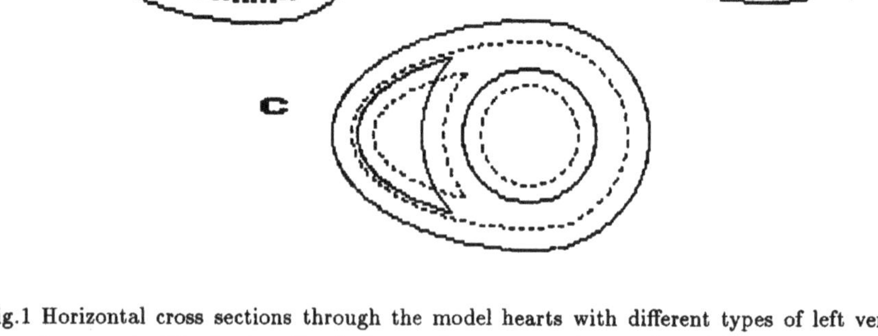

Fig.1 Horizontal cross sections through the model hearts with different types of left ventricular enlargement. The broken line indicates the contour of normal model heart. a - eccentric hypertrophy with unchanged end-diastolic volume, b - concentric hypertrophy, c - left ventricular dilatation.

3. Results

The resulting heart vector, determined at any instant of ventricular activation, was used for the evaluation of changes in cardiac electric field effectuated by different types and degrees of simulated enlargements. The changes of its spatial magnitude and orientation were more pronounced in the horizontal plane projection.

In eccentric hypertrophy with unchanged end-diastolic volume, the spatial magnitudes of heart vectors increased during the last two thirds of activation time, proportionally to the degree of simulated hypertrophy (Fig.2a). The characteristic changes of loop configuration were the increase of the magnitude of posteriorly oriented vectors and a leftward shift of terminal QRS vectors. The duration of activation was slightly prolonged.

The increase of wall thickness in simulated concentric hypertrophy led to a decrease of spatial magnitude of heart vectors during the first half of activation, while the magnitudes of the terminal vectors were slightly increased. The whole vectorcardiographic loop was shifted posteriorly (Fig.2b).

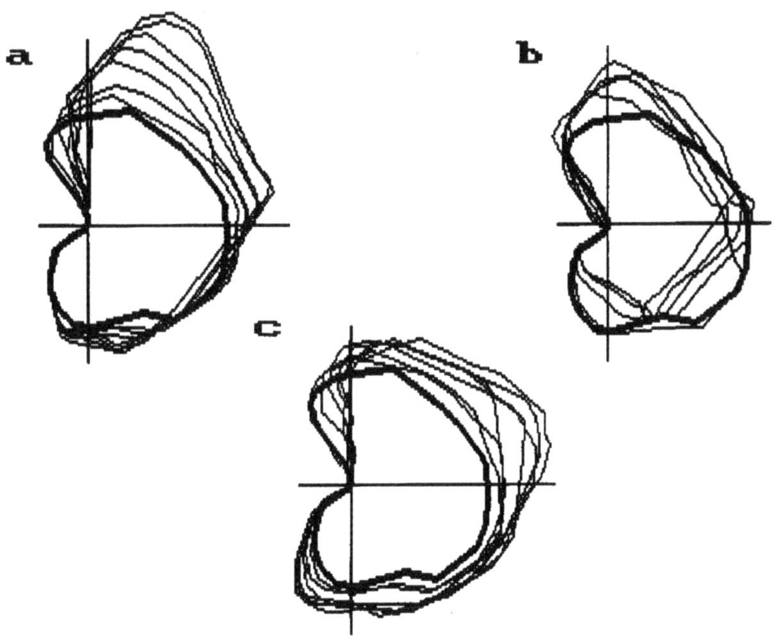

Fig.2 Horizontal plane vectorcardiographic loops for three simulated types of left ventricular enlargement. The series of loops correspond to gradually increased degree of enlargement. The loop of the normal heart is indicated by heavy line. a - eccentric hypertrophy with unchanged end-diastolic volume, b - concentric hypetrophy, c - left ventricular dilatation.

The vectorcardiographic pattern of the left ventricular dilatation was similar to that of eccentric hypertrophy. The difference was only in the increase of magnitudes of heart vectors already from the beginning of the activation process (Fig.2c).Again, the characteristic changes of the horizontal plane VCG were an increase of to the left and posteriorly oriented vectors and the leftward shifting of terminal vectors.

4. Discussion

The correlations of electrocardiographic signs of left ventricular hypertrophy with parameters characterizing the geometry of ventricle (e.g. left ventricular end-diastolic volume or diameter, posterior wall thickness, interventricular septal thickness) were not always conclusive[4,5]. This fact used to be explained by the presence of extracardiac factors (e.g. the proximity effect, the Brody effect) influencing the cardiac electric field. Our computer simulation of left ventricular enlargement showed that the increase of ventricular wall thickness does not necessarily result in the increase of heart vector magnitudes. In concentric hypertrophy the increase of wall thickness led to a decrease of instantaneous heart vector magnitude during the first half of ventricular activation time, while during the second half the magnitudes did not change significantly. If the wall thickness was increased to 150% of the original value, the magnitude of maximal heart vector increased only by about 10%.

5. References

1. I. Ruttkay-Nedecký, A. Drkošová, V. Szathmáry, in *Advances in Electrocardiology*, ed. P. d' Alché (Publications de l' Université de Caen, 1985).
2. G.M. Hutchins, B.H. Bukley, G.W. Moore, M.A. Piasion, F.V. Lohr, *Am.J. of Cardiology* **41** (1978) 646.
3. D. Durrer, R. Th. van Dam, G.E. Freud, M.J. Jause, F.L. Meijler, R.C. Azbaecher, *Circulation* **41** (1970) 899.
4. M. Dolgin, V.J. Fisher, A. Shah, B. Fisher, *Am.J.Med.Sci.* **273** (1977) 301.
5. D.H. Bennett, D.W. Evans, *Br. Heart J.* **36** (1974) 981.

ELECTROCARDIOGRAPHIC MANIFESTATION OF EXPERIMENTAL LEFT VENTRICULAR HYPERTROPHY

LJUBA BACHAROVA
Research Institute of Medical Bionics
Jedľová 6, 833 08 Bratislava
Czech and Slovak Federative Republic

and

MARIAN BERNADIC, ALZBETA FIZELOVA
Institute of Patophysiology, Faculty of Medicine
Comenius university, 812 35 Bratislava
Czech and Slovak Federative Republic

ABSTRACT

Changes of cardioelectric field were studied in the course of development of experimental left ventricular hypertrophy and compared with left ventricular size. The experimental model of volume overload in rabbits was used. Frank orthogonal electrocardiograms were recorded and related to the left ventricular mass and area. A new parameter - the specific potential - was calculated as a ratio of maximum spatial QRS vector magnitude (QRSmax.) to left ventricular mass. After a transient decrease of QRSmax. in the early postoperative period its increase was observed in the stage of developed hypertrophy. Values of the specific potential were decreased during the entire followed-up period, they did not reach the initial values, not even at the stage of developed hypertrophy, when the maximal increase of QRSmax. was observed. Changes of cardioelectric field during LVH development are not proportional to the LV mass increase. The suggested new parameter - the specific potential - enables the quantification of this relationship.

1. Introduction

The discrepancies between ECG findings and corresponding left ventricular mass (LVM) in left ventricular hypertrophy (LVH) diagnostics is chronically known. We try to describe and quantify the relation between left ventricular mass and maximum spatial QRS vector magnitude ($QRS_{max.}$) by introducing the index "specific potential" (SP) in our previous works[1,2]. The aim of this study was to evaluate the changes of cardioelectric field in relation to the left ventricular mass during the development of experimental left ventricular hypertrophy using SP as a parameter of these changes.

2. Material and methods

The data of the experimental model of the volume overload of the left ventricle in rabbits were used[3,4]. The volume overload of the left ventricle was induced by perforating the aortal valves[5]. Frank orthogonal electrocardiograms were recorded in 25 healthy rabbits before the operation. The post-operative changes of ECG were recorded in 12 rabbits in following intervals[4]: the early postoperative period (the 3rd day), the stage of developing hypertrophy (the 7th and 30th days), the stage of developed hypertrophy (the 150th and 200th days) and in the stage of developing heart failure (the 250th day).

The maximum spatial QRS vector magnitude was calculated from R amplitudes of X, Y, Z electrocardiograms using the equation:

$$QRS_{max}=\sqrt{x^2+y^2+z^2} \qquad (1)$$

Left ventricular mass and area were measured post mortem in corresponding groups of rabbits [3]. Left ventricular mass was indexed to the body weight. Left ventricular area was measured planimetrically after dissecting the heart to the left ventricle, right ventricle and interventricular septum.

A new parameter - specific potential - was calculated as a ratio of maximum spatial QRS vector magnitude and left ventricular mass:

$$SP=\frac{QRS_{max}}{LVM} \qquad (2)$$

3. Results

Results are presented in Figure 1. LVM increased gradually from 0.729 g/kg before operation to 1.691 g/kg in the stage of developed hypertrophy representing the increase of LVM by 110%. The spontaneous regression of LVM was observed during the developing heart failure. Maximum increase of $QRS_{max.}$ was observed in the 150th postoperative day in the stage of developed hypertrophy. The early postoperative period was characterized by considerable decrease of $QRS_{max.}$ (-60% at the 7th postoperative day). Values of the specific potential were decreased during the whole follow-up period. They did not reach the initial values, not even at the stage of developed hypertrophy, when the maximum increase of $QRS_{max.}$ values was observed The maximum decrease was observed at the 7th day (- 58 %) during the early

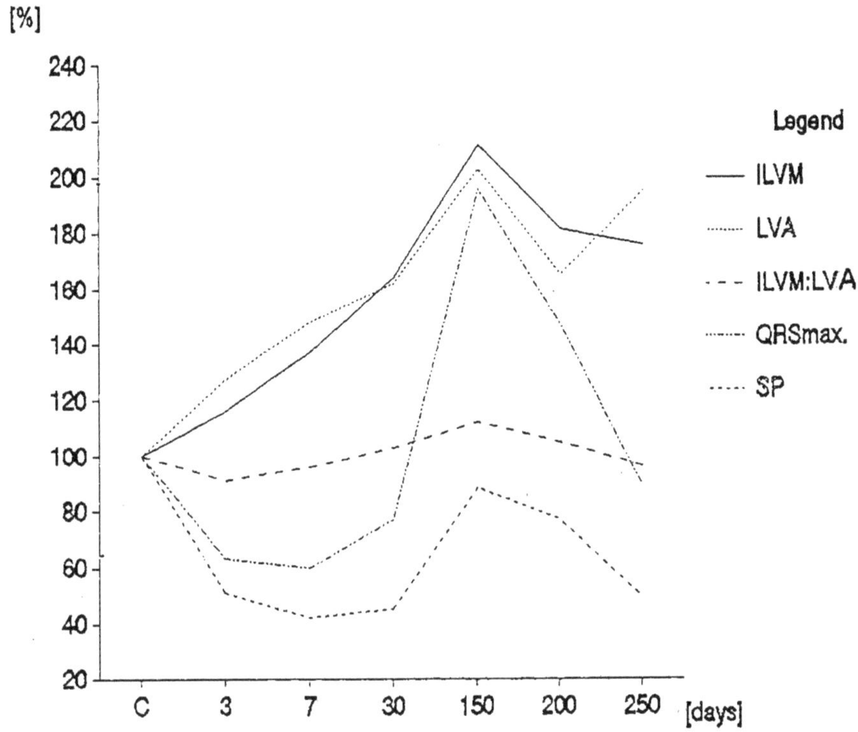

Figure 1
Changes of ILVM, LVA, ILVM to LVA ratio, QRSmax. and SP during the course o experimental left ventricular hypertrophy. Relative values are presented (control values = 100%).

postoperative period. Maximum values of SP during the postoperative period were found at the 150th day at the stage of developed hypertrophy, still they were about 13 % lower than control values.Changes of left ventricular area followed the behaviour of LVM values - the gradual increase to the maximum at the 150th day at the stage of developed hypertrophy. The ratio of left ventricular mass to left ventricular area decreased about 9 % in the early postoperative period, about 4 % at the 7th postoperative day.It increased by about 3 % at the 30th day and by 12 % at the 150th day - (the stage of developed hypertrophy), it was within the limits -9% to +12%.

4. Discussion

The difference in information content of ECG and methods of LVM assessment is obvious and accepted. But paradoxically, the discrepancies between these two approaches in diagnostics lead to stressing the prior particular methods. In the case of echocardiography, it is the good correlation mortem findings and echocardiography is considered to be a "golden stand clinical LVH studies. Non-electrocardiological arguments are often used in t of ECG: financial, the low time consumption of ECG examination, or relati number of non-echogenic patients[6].

Without stressing priorities, we try to combine both information in order to obtain a parameter for describing the fact that a small sized heart can produce a strong cardioelectric field, and on the opposite - a large mass of LV can be a less efficient generator of cardioelectric field.

We introduced an index "specific potential" as a ratio of $QRS_{max.}$ to LVM or left ventricular cross-sectional area, respectively. SP represents the potential contribution of a myocardial unit to the total cardioelectric field.

The results of our pilot clinical studies[1,2] were interesting:

* SP values decreased with the increasing values of LVM,
* SP values were lower in hypertensive patients compared to healthy persons on the contrary to higher values of $QRS_{max.}$ recorded in hypertensive patients

With the aim to analyze the SP,we reevaluated available experimental data which allowed one to study the process and development of LVH in defined stages[7] under defined experimental model conditions. Conclusions of this reevaluation:

* Changes of cardioelectric field during the development of left ventricular hypertrophy were not proportional to the left ventricular mass increase.
* Maximum discrepancies between $QRS_{max.}$ and left ventricular mass were observed during the stages of developing hypertrophy and developing heart failure. These discrepancies could not be explained by simple interpretation of the Brody efect.
* The suggested new parameter - specific potential - enables the quantification of this relationship.

5. References

1. L.Bachárová, J.Melotová, K.Sedláková, K.Hrušovská, in *Electrocardiology* 1988, ed. H.Abel (Elsevier, Excerpta Medica, Amsterdam, 1989)

2. L.Bachárová, F.U.Gadžaeva,J.Melotová, in *Teorija i praktika avtomatizaci kardiologičeskich issledovanij,* ed. J.Blužas (Spindulio, Kaunas, 199O)

3. A.Fízeľ, *The adaptation of the heart to the work overload* (Commenius University, Bratislava 1977) p.394.

4. M.Bernadič, A.Fízeľ, A.Fízeľová, M.Bakosová, E.Sapáková, *1 Bratisl.lek.Listy* **84** (1985) 683

5. A.Fízeľ and A.Fízeľová, *Z. Kreisl.-Forsch.* **58** (1969), 1115

6. H.K.Wolf, G.W.Burggraf, E.Cuddy, J.A.Milliken, P.M.Rautaharju E.R.Smith, J.W.Warren, *J Electrocardiology* **24** (1991) 121

7. F.Z. Meerson, *Circ Res,* **Suppl.2** (1969) 1

REAPPRAISAL OF THE COUPLING INTERVAL OF PREMATURE VENTRICULAR BEATS AS AN INDEX OF ECTOPIC MECHANISMS

YUJI MURAKAWA, MD, HIROSHI INOUE, MD, and TSUNEAKI SUGIMOTO, MD
Second Department of Internal Medicine,
Tokyo University Hospital,
Tokyo, Japan

ABSTRACT

A mathematical model of modulated ventricular parasystole was developed in an attempt to distinguish parasystolic automaticity from other mechanisms based on the relationship between the coupling interval (CI) of premature ventricular complex (PVC) and the preceding R-R interval. The CI vs. R-R diagrams obtained from simulation with various modulation modes showed that the diagonal dot-free space was unique to the parasystolic mechanism, while a consistently linear accumulation seemed to indicate a non-parasystolic mechanism.

1. Aim

To know the likely and unlikely relationships between coupling interval (CI) and preceding R-R interval for parasystolic premature ventricular complex (PVC), we developed a mathematical model of modulated ventricular parasystole.

2. Methods

Mathematical model

Sinus cycle length was set from 400 ms to 1150 ms in 50 ms steps, and was shortened or lengthened up to 20 ms. Either fixed (2 seconds) or variable parasystolic cycle length was used. Modulation of parasystolic cycle length by the sinus beat followed the biphasic phase-response curve (PRC) which had been proposed in earlier biological and clinical studies (1-3).

CI of each parasystolic beat was plotted against the preceding R-R interval.

Analysis of clinical observation

Sixty consecutive 24-hour ambulatory ECG recordings with frequent PVCs were selected. Based on the observations from the mathematical model, possibility of parasystolic or non-parasystolic mechanism was graded in each patient.

Diagnosis of parasystolic automaticity was made by intrinsic periodicity in the appearance of PVCs. Frequency histograms of the interectopic intervals were constructed for every 200 ms. To elucidate periodicity, the autocorrelation function was also calculated.

3. Results

Observations in the mathematical model

The CI vs. R-R diagrams usually had one or more diagonal dot-free spaces in common that divided the dots into two or more clusters. Even when such a dot-free space was not apparent, the irregular indented contour suggested heterogeneous, discontinuous accumulation of dots. A straight, linear accumulation over a wide range of R-R with a smooth contour never occurred.

Clinical observations

Type 1: When a diagonal dot-free space or a bizarre contour that suggested an overshadowed dot-free space was seen in the CI vs. R-R diagram, PVCs were considered parasystole (n=15). In 14 of these 15, intrinsic periodicity of PVCs, which is suggestive of parasystolic automaticity, was observed.

Type 2: If a consistently linear accumulation of dots over wide range of R-R existed, PVCs were considered due to non-parasystolic mechanisms (n=17). Intrinsic periodicity was never observed in this group.

Type 3: PVCs in 28 patients other than Types 1 and 2 made the third group. Parasystolic mechanism was likely in 11 of this group.

4. Conclusion

Neither the relation between CI and R-R nor the measurement of interectopic interval provide a definite diagnosis of ectopic mechanisms. However, since the two methods led to almost the same conclusion in more than half the patients, the relation between CI and R-R may prove parasystolic and non-parasystolic mechanisms with an excellent degree of accuracy in selected patients in whom Type 1 or Type 2 patterns was obtained.

References

1) J. Jalife, G.K. Moe, Circ Res 39 (1976) 801

2) G.K. Moe, J. Jalife, W.J. Mueller, B. Moe, Circulation 56 (1977) 968

3) Jalife J, Moe GK. A biological model of parasystole. Am J Cardiol 43 (1979) 761

RECOGNITION OF MYOCARDIAL INFARCTION USING NON-INVASIVE ELECTROPHYSIOLOGICAL MAPPING OF THE HEART (A MODEL STUDY)

V.G.Trunov and L.I.Titomir

Institute for Problems of Information Transmission, Acad. Sci. USSR
Ermolovoy 19, 101447 Moscow, USSR

Non-invasive determination of localization and size of necrotic areas in the ventricles from body surface multilead measurements is proposed and investigated, using MULTECARTO technique presented at the preceding International Congress on Electrocardiology. The real set of measured body surface potential distributions for a typical normal subject was used for computer modelling of the method proposed. From these data the instantaneous quasiepicardial potential distributions and heart excitation maps were calculated. A necrotic zone was simulated as unexcitable area with given shape, size and localization in the ventricles. For corresponding pathological depolarization fronts the forward, and then inverse electrodynamical problem was solved. Resulting pathological quasiepicardial potentials and heart excitation maps give a useful pictorial representation of the non-invasively observed dynamics of the ventricular depolarization, revealing straightforwardly the infarctional zone on the proper sites of the ventricular surface projection.

A technique has been developed for non-invasive mapping of the most significant electrophysiological characterisics of cardiac excitation. This technique abbreviated as MULTECARTO (MULTipolar ElectroCARdioTOpography) provides for solving the inverse electrodynamical problem based upon rather simplified thin-wall model of ventricles, and obtaining quasiepicardial potential distribution and a set of so called maps of heart excitation. The instantaneous maps of excitation represent the distribution of three main states of the heart wall, namely the resting state R, activation state (presence of the depolarization front) A, and completely excited (depolarized) state E, all the characteristics being projected onto the heart surface. Also the summary maps of excitation include the isochronous maps (endocardial as well as epicardial), activation duration map, showing temporial duration of the activation state, and recovery acceleration map reflecting the change of the action potential duration across the heart wall. The main purpose is to visualize pictorially the excitation process under investigation, and to represent straightforwardly and explicitly normal as well as pathological states and properties of the heart. In this particular work we demostrate abilities of this technique to help in recognition of old myocardial infartion, or zones of necrotic myocardial tissue in the ventricles.

To perform computer modelling, we first of all chose a typical normal subject. Then aforementioned instantaneous maps of quasiepicardial potential and maps of excitation were calculated from his body surface mapping data (the 1st and 2nd culumns in the Figure). The depolarization front obtained was considered as a model, or template for the normal excitation process.

The infarcted zone was simulated as an unexcitable area with given shape, size and localization in the ventricles (the 3rd column in the Figure). For the resulting pathological depolarization front, that is front with removed unexcitable regions, the forward electrodynamical problem was solved and the body surface potential found. This potential was then used for an inverse solution to calculate the epicardial potential and heart excitation maps (the 4th and 5th columns in the Figure). Thus non-invasively observed, or apparent depolarization front in artificially infarcted ventricles was obtained and compared with normal front as well as with initially given true pathological front. Similar comparisons may be performed between the potential distributions on the quasiepicardium as well as body sur face.

The results demonstrated show that in spite of some smoothing and distortion of the pathological zone, it is quite explicitly distiguishible on the inspected pictures obtained by means of the inverse solution based upon MULTECARTO technique. It is concluded that proposed method in principle ensures straightforward visual identification of pathologically unexcitable, or infarcted regions in the heart. Certainly, the method needs thorough further quantitative estimation and experimental verification.

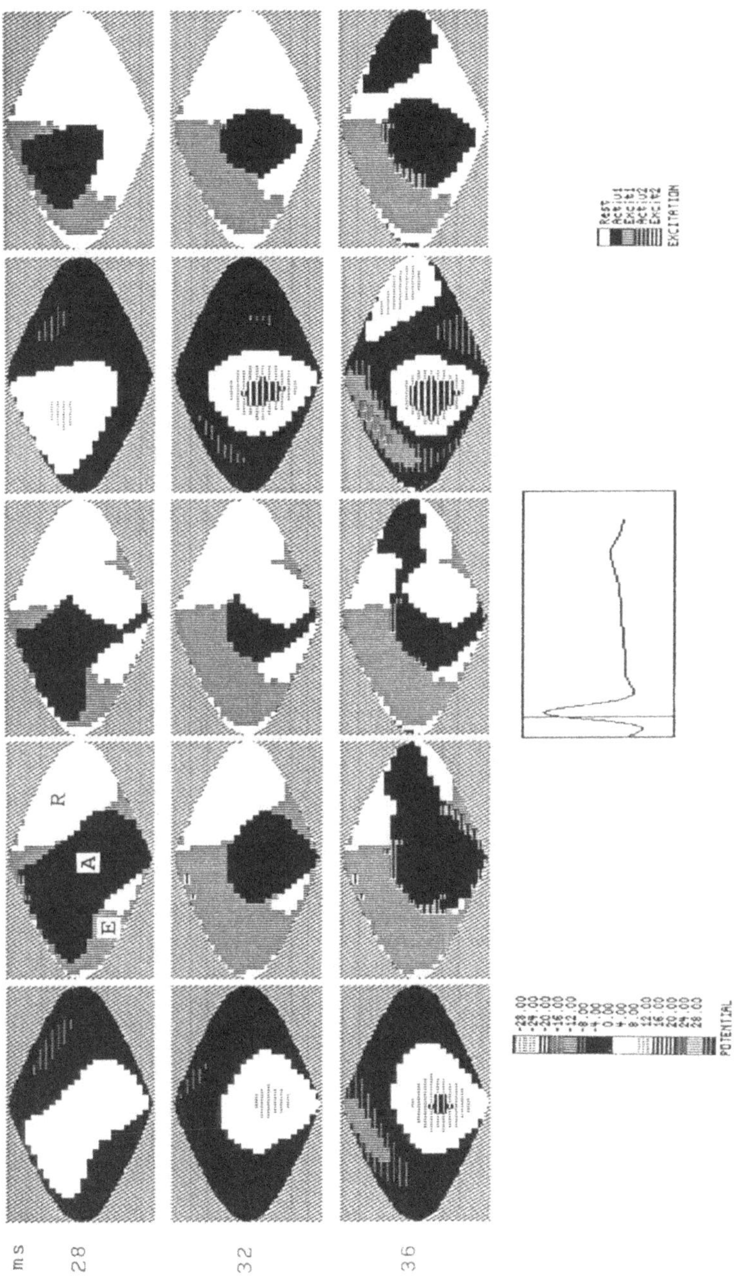
ms
28
32
36
R
A
E
-28.00
-24.00
-20.00
-16.00
-12.00
-8.00
-4.00
0.00
4.00
8.00
12.00
16.00
20.00
24.00
28.00
POTENTIAL
Rest
Activ1
Excit1
Activ2
Excit2
EXCITATION

Figure

Ischemic ST Patterns Induced by Changing the Duration of Action Potential on Computer Heart Model

Osamu Okazaki
Nakano National Chest Hospital,
3-14-20 Egota, Nakano-ku, Tokyo 165 Japan

and

Daming Wei*, Masafumi Kasama**, Takeshi Tsutsumi**,
Tetsuo Michihata, Toshihiko Hara, Masaaki Iio,
Hiroshi Tsunakawa**, Saburo Mashima** and Kenichi Harumi***

*Nihon Koden Corporation, Tokyo 161 Japan
**Showa University Fujigaoka Hosp., Yokohama 227 Japan
***Director of Nakano National Chest Hospital

Introduction

The possible contribution of the action potential duration (APD) on the pattern of ST was studied by computer simulation. There have been three proposed mechanisms causing ST deviation of conventional electrocardiogram. One is about the phase 3 of action potential, second is injury current and the other is solid angle. The purpose of this study is to clarify the influential factors of ST depression on a three dimensional cardiac model.

Method

An electrocardiographic simulation system (Cardiomaster, Nihon Koden Co.) was implemented on Sun-4 workstation. A 3-dimensional heart model for ECG was composed of 50,000 discrete units with spatial resolution of 1.5mm in diameter and mounted in a human torso model. (Fig.1) Cross sections of the human heart were collected from the Durrer's human data(1). There were in direct contact with adjacent 12 cells, and the function of Sinus Node(SN), Atrium(ATR), AV Node(AVN), His, Bundle Blanch(BB), Purkinje(PKJ), Ventricle(VTR) and ventricular gradient of 5msec by layer were included. Body surface potential was calculated by means of the boundary element. The calculated body surface potentials, ECG and especially VCG were closely similar to the average normal human electrocardiograms (2). Ischemic zones were made on this model with reference of PET images of the patients with ischemic heart disease during exercise.(Fig.2) Electrophysiological parameters were set on the assumption of ischemic changes with keeping the resting potentials. Alterations of phase 2 or 3 of the APD and delay of conduction velocity(CV) were applied to the localized ischemic area and the shape of ST was calculated from simulated ECGs as shown on the underline of Table.

(Table 1) **Electrophysiological Setting Parameters**

	SN	ATR	AVN	HIS	BB	PKJ	VTR
(APD) (msec)							
Time of phase 0	30	1	2	0	0	0	0
Time of phase 1	0	1	0	1	3	3	5
Time of phase 2	0	2	20	30	80	80	(72-)80
Time of phase 3	175	120	175	175	175	175	(155-)175
Abs. Rec. Period	200	140	200	200	200	200	200
Full Rec. Time	245	164	237	246	298	298	300
Resting Pot.	-50	-65	-70	-80	-90	-90	-90
Action Pot.	10	15	20	20	25	30	30
Plateau Pot.	10	5	20	10	15	20	20
Gradient of APD	250	0	0	0	0	0	5
(Conduction)							
CV (m/sec)	0.5	1.0	0.1	2.5	2.5	2.5	(0.1-)0.5

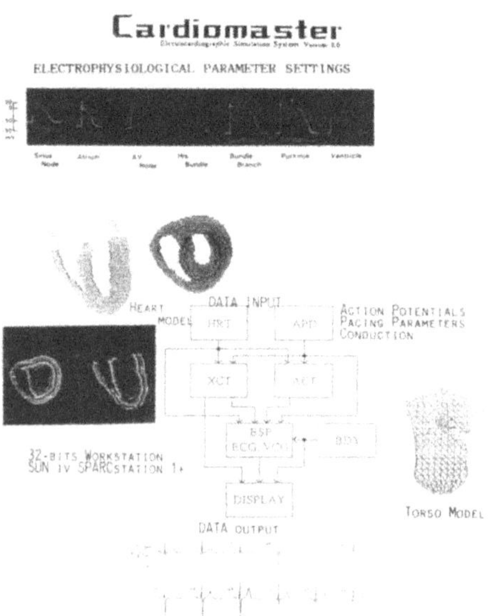

(Fig.1)
Flow Chart of Cardiomaster.

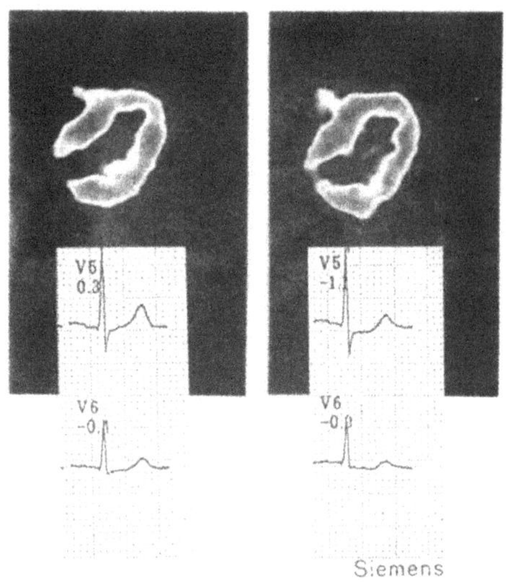

at rest during exercise
(Fig.2) (25W x 5min)
PET images and simultaneous
recording ECG.

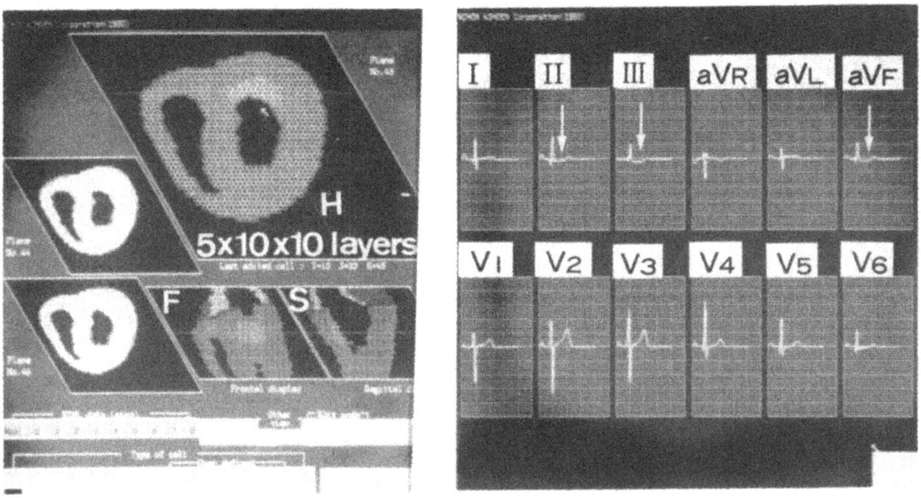

(Fig.3)
The model of posterior endocardial ischemia showed on the left panel. The minimum size of ischemic on zone with 7.5x15mm by 10 layers was obtained with ST depression of 0.05 to 0.1mV in II, III, aVF leads.

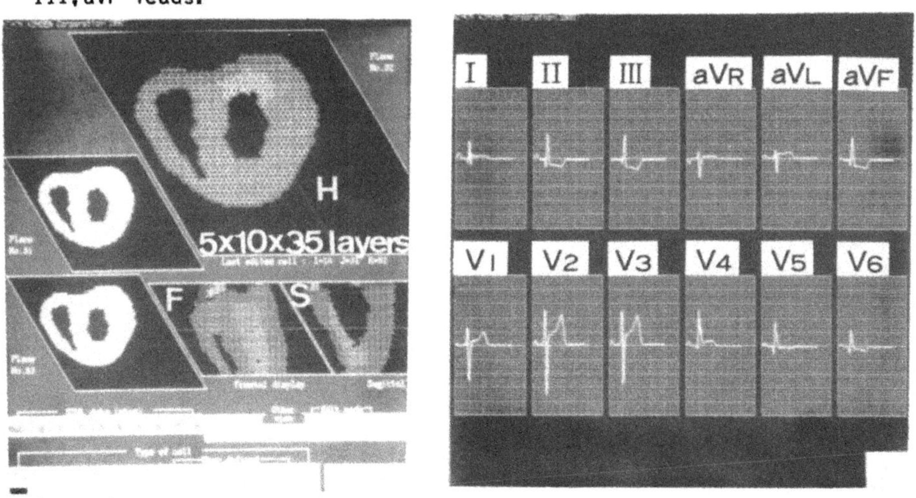

(Fig.4)
The ischemic region was extended to apex until 35 layers. The degree of sagging pattern of ST depression in II, III, aVF and ST elevation in I, aVL, V1-4 was increased as reciprocal changes.

Results

1) Under the alteration of APD at the phase 2 without the delay of CV, there was no significant change of ST segment. Simulated ECGs with ST changes were made in good agreement to the clinically obtained with the PET by changing the value of the APD and the CV. The shape of horizontal ST depression was mainly affected by the extents of the shortening at least 10% in the phase 3 of the APD and in the delay CV, while the sagging features of the ST depression were mainly affected by the duration of phase 2. 2) The smallest size of ischemic zone on this model was 7.5x15x15mm3 (Fig.3). 3) The ST depression became deeper as the region of ischemic zone was extended towards to the apex (Fig.4). The ischemic region was extended to apex until 35 layers. The degree of sagging pattern of ST depression in II,III, aVF and ST elevation in I,aVL,V1-4 was increased as reciprocal changes.

Discussion

We measured regional myocardial blood flow using 13-NH3 PET at rest and during exercise in order to estimate endocardial ischemia on a patient with coronary artery disease. ECG showed horizontal ST depression in V5 simultaneously. These changes may have been associated with a shortening refractory period and a prolongation of the QT interval(3). However it is difficult to distinguish APD shortening from injury current etc. Simulation studies are widely used so that it is convenient for this model to testify the contribution of APD shortening to ST depression. Our previous investigation concluded that ST segmental depression in myocardial ischemia was determined both by the site of ischemia and the action potential wave form (4). These results suggested that these combined factors might be necessary for ST depression as a mechanism of endocardial ischemia.

Conclusion

The three-dimensional cardiac computer model can simulate ST depression under certain physiologic parameters, especially with the conduction delay and shortening of phase 3 of APD on the regional ischemic zone. One of the implications of the ischemic ST abnormalities on three dimensional computer heart model, by referencing PET images, might suggest that the shortening of APD and reduction of conduction velocity may play an important role on ischemic ST changes.

(REFERENCES)

1. Durrar D, et al.: Total excitation of the heart. Circ. 41:899-912,1970

2. Harumi K, et al.: Clinical Application of Electrocardiographic Computer Model. J Electrocardiol 22(supple)54-63,1989

3. Harumi K, et al.: Ventricular recovery time changes during and after temporary coronary occlusion. Am J Cardiol 25:26, 1970

4. Kasama M, et al.: Computer Simulation of ST Segment Depression due to Myocardial Ischemia. Jap Circ J. 55(supple)(1991)in press

Determination of infarct size using QRST isointegral maps in canine hearts

Yoshio Ichihara, MD., Hiroshi Hayashi, MD., Yasushi Tomita, MD., Masayoshi Adachi, MD., Akira Suzuki, MD., Makoto Hirai, MD.

Division of Cardiology, First Department of Internal Medicine, Nagoya University, School of Medicine

65 Tsurumai-cho, Showa-ku, Nagoya 466 JAPAN
Phone 81-52-741-2111 Fax 81-52-741-1612

Summary: We examined the feasibility of estimating infarct size using QRST isointegral mapping (I_{QRST} mapping) in dogs. Myocardial infarction was produced by embolizing the left coronary anterior descending branch with glass beads in eight dogs. One week later body surface ECGs were recorded by 87-unipolar-lead system. In each lead QRST integral value was calculated to construct I_{QRST} map, and these values were summed up to get QRST index. After recording ECGs, hearts were excised and cut into slices to determine infarct by planimetry. QRST index was correlated to the infarct size. Infarct size varied 9% to 44%. QRST indices showed inverse correlation to infarct size.($r=-0.89$, $p<0.005$) These findings suggested the feasibility of estimating the infarct size from body surface ECGs.

Introduction: It is usually observed that patients with large anteroseptal myocardial infarction show larger negative area in the I_{QRST} map, while in those with localized infarction the map show almost normal pattern. On the other hand it is experimentally shown that QRST integral values are dependent on the spread and severity of the change in myocardial recovery property.[1] Thus it is suggested that I_{QRST} map can represent the size of infarction. The purpose of this study was to examine the feasibility of estimating infarct size during abnormal ventricular activation using the I_{QRST} mapping.

Methods: Eight mongrel dogs were anesthesized by intravenous pentobarbital. All procedures handling animals comforted with the Guideline Manual of the Institute for Experimental Animal Research (Nagoya University School of Medicine, Nagoya Japan). Myocardial infarction was produced by embolizing the left coronary artery with glass beads, using catheter technique under fluoroscopy. One week later body surface electrocardiography (ECG) was recorded using 87-unipolar-lead mapping system. I_{QRST} maps were constructed from these ECGs, and QRST integral value of each lead was summed to calculate an index (QRST index).

After recording ECGs each heart was excised and sliced in 1 cm thick. Infarct size was measured by planimetry, and expressed in percent(%), and they were correlated to the QRST index by polynomial regression.

Results: A representative example of the I_{QRST} map was shown in Figure 1. Each I_{QRST} map obtained from the eight animals reflected infarction by its negative area and the decreased peak value. The infarct size varied from 9.7% to 43.7%. The QRST index derived from the I_{QRST} map distributed between -179.1 mVmsec and 1071.0 mVmsec (Table). This index showed significant inverse correlation to the infarct size. The correlation coefficient between the QRST index and the infarct size was r=-0.89 (p<0.005). The correlation distribution was shown in Figure 2.

Figure 1 QRST isointegral map of a dog with myocardial infarction

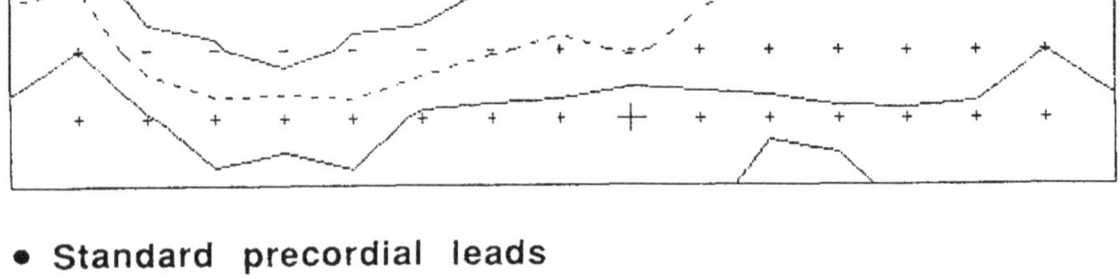

• Standard precordial leads

Increment=10 mVmsec

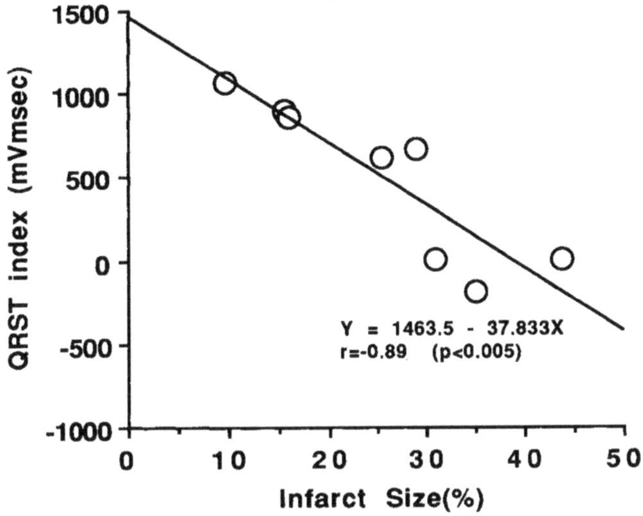

Figure 2; Correlation between QRST indices and Infarct size

Table ; QRST index (mVmsec), infarct size (%) and correlation coefficient

Dog No	QRST index (mVmsec)	Infarct Size (%)
1	674.2	28.8
2	4.5	43.7
3	866.2	16.0
4	901.7	15.5
5	1071.0	9.7
6	-179.1	34.9
7	618.5	25.4
8	2.5	30.8

r=-0.89 (p<0.005)

Discussion: The QRST index was shown to be inversely correlated to the infarct size significantly. Since Abildskov introduced QRST isointegral mapping as a representation of ventricular gradient,[2] many authors have documented utility and usefulness of isointegral map: detecting myocardial infarction complicated by abnormal activation sequences. However no one referred to the infarct size using the I_{QRST} map. There have been reports concerning the infarct size and ECG findings. Selvester et al made QRS scoring system.[3] We have introduced a new index and correlated it directly to infarct size. This index largely represented the myocardial electrical activity. These findings imply a new application of QRST isointegral mapping for not only detecting infarction but also estimating infarct size in the presence of abnormal ventricular activation.

References

1 Burgess MJ et al: The relation of localized myocardial warming to change in cardiac surface electrograms in dogs. *Circ Res* 1978; 43: 899-907

2 Abildskov JA et al: Body surface distribution of QRST area. *Adv Cardiol* 1978; 21: 59-64

3 Wagner GS et al: Evaluation of QRS scoring system for estimating myocardial infarct size. 1. Specificity and observer agreement. *Circulation* 1982; 65: 342-347

EXCITATION OF THE ATRIA IN VERTEBRATES

SHMAKOV DIMITRI, ROSHCHEVSKY MICHAEL

Institute of Physiology of the USSR Acad. Sci., Ural Division, Syktyvkar, USSR

ABSTRACT

The sequence of the atria depolarization was studied by epicardial and intramural multipolar techniques in vertebrates. Similarity of topography of atrial activation process was discovered in mammals which were characterized by different types of heart ventricles depolarization

Introduction

In the plan of future development of the problems of evolutional electrocardiology[1] the comparative - physiological experimental research of the excitation of the atria was carried out in fish, amphibians, reptilians and mammals.

Methods

Animals were anesthetized with sodium thiopentalum-natrium 30-50 mg/kg body wt. After intubation a thoracotomy was performed. Epicardial external potentials were recorded from atrial surface by means of multipolar electrodes. Along with epicardial activity the external electrical potentials were recorded from the intramural myocardial layers in mammals.

Results

In the fish auricle excitation begins in the region situated near by venous sinus. From initial foci excitation the electrical activity spreads along the caudodorsal wall in all derections. During 9-18 ms from the begining of activation the excitation wave (EW) at first reaches the right lateral wall and then left auricle lateral wall. Next it spread from the right to the left and to the auricle apex. The activation of the caudoventral wall is caused by the movement of the EW from the apex to the base of the auricle mainly and simultaneously from the left to the right. And at last the regions near the atrioventricular orifice are depolarized. In grailings the time of auricle depolarization is equal to 55-73 ms, in pikes - 63-86 ms.

In reptilians earliest activation is always present on the right atrium epicard, very close to venous sinus. From there the EW spreads over the atrial surface in all directions. At first the ventral surface of the right atrium is depolarized by movement of EW from right to left. Then the EW envelopes a ventral part of left atrium. The dorsal area of the left atrium is activated late.

In birds activation of atria begins in the region of the sinus node. From this area the EW spreads over atrial surface according to more or less radially. The isochrone lines involve simultaneously the ventral and dorsal areas of the right atrial wall. A more rapid spread of EW occurs in a craniocaudal direction and from right to the left. The latest activated area is the dorsal part of the left atrium.

Mammals. Cornivores. In the most zones of the dog's atrial myocard we observed the spread of the EW with the different pattern of the atrial EW front along walls. The perpendicular spread of the atrial EW front to the epicard and endocard is recorded in the some regions. Simultaneous depolarization of all walls thickness occurs in the lateral parts of the left atrium. The angle spread of the EW front arises for instance,for activation of the zones of the middle third of the lateral region of the right atrium. In sother regions the analogous angle spread of the EW front arises when depolarization of the subepicardial region forestalls of the excitation of the subendocardial zones.

The process of the dog atrial depolarization lasted from 54 to 82 ms but the sequence of the EW is constant in the thickness of the atrial free walls and the atrial appendixices.The earliest depolarization is recorded in the myocardial thickness of the cranioventral region of the right atrium. From there the EW with a saw-edged front spreads along the thickness of the atria.

Ungulates. The similarity in the succession of intramural and epicardial activation of atrial myocard in the ungulates and cornivores is found. In sheeps the EW moves from sinoatrial node along the atrial walls, captures the whole of their thickness and alsow as in dog's atria has various patterns of the EW front.

There are differences in the duration of the excitation process in dog and sheep atria. In dogs the atrial depolarization lasted to 66+4ms, in sheeps - to 54+5 ms.The chronotopography of the intramural EW front shows a more complicated picture of the atrial excitation than a simply radial one. Apparently it is connected with the presense of the atrial conduction system.The morphological investigation of the atrial conduction system[2] can explain this irregularity and acceleration in the spread of the EW in a number of atrial regions.

Conclusion

Similarity in the succession of epicardial activation of atria was found in vertebrates. First,by the radial spread of EW the regions near venous sinus in fish and reptilians and about sinoatrial node in other vertebrates are excited.Then the radial movement of EW is dusturbed and the common character of the excitation does not correspond to the radial spread of activation.

Thus, the simular topography of atrial excitation was discovered in mammals which were characterized by different types of heart ventricles activation.

References

1.M.P.Roshchevsky, Evolutional electrocardiology (L: Nayka, 1972), 252 p.

2.T.N.James and L.Sherf, Amer. J. Cardiol.(1971),p.414.

THE CLUSTEROUS STRUCTURE OF MYOCARDIUM AND HEART ARRHYTHMIAS

V.I.Cobrin and E.D.Ignatova

The 2 Medical Institute, Moscow, USSR

With the help of the microelectrode technology the fragmentation of an electric activity of cardiomyocites of intact heart was registred during the on-clusters fibrillation measuring 0.5-1.0 mm. The cluster myocardial structure model was worked out.

The key words: cluster, fibrillation, myocardial, transmembrane potential.

Modern theories of fibrillation are based on the conception of "functional syntitium" /1,2/. In this work one tried to consider the process of heart ventricles fibrillation from the view of "cluster" structure of myocardium.

METHODS

65 experiments were done on quinea pigs, 25 on rats, 10 on rabbits, 25 on pigeons, 20 on chickens. The electric activity of cardiomyocytes registred by "swimming microelectrodes". At the same time activity of the paired cells, luing on different distances from each othes (0.5-4 mm) was registred. Fibrillation of the heart caused ventricls was by using electrical stimullation or application aconitine.

RESULTS

Stimulation of the heart caused typical reaction: depolarisation of cell membrane by 25-35mv was caused on the phone of which synchronic and asynchronic potentials of different configuration and amplitude were formed. As a rule cells were excited synchronically of the distance between them does not increase more than 1mm. If the distance between them was more than 1.5mm , full disagreement of excitation of cardiomyocytes was seen. This fragmented excitation was seen in every animal under supervision. During this zone of common excitation had complicated configuration. The inipartant factor here is the close relation the between dinamic of fibrillatory process by the parametres of transmembrane potentials during fibrillation and morphological characteristics of cellular structures in the heart of different living beings. In quinea pigs, rabbits and rats, the fibrillation, as a rule, was noticed as spontaneously reversible and in pigeons and chickens as spontaneously irreversible /4/. Most of the scientist noticed few and miniature intercellular contacts in the myocard of birds and a large number of highly differenciated contacts in the heart of mammals /5/. Different cells of myocard form groups or "clusters" surrounded by a common basal membrane. According to different authors these clusters consist of 5 to 10 cells, and the diametre of the cells varies from 6 to 70 mkm and their length from 100 to 150 mkm /5,6/. The morphological size of the clusters may vary from 100 mkm to 1.5 mm. In fig.1 the schematic representation of the areas of contracted myocard of the ventricles formed of is given clusters. Practically cells A and B which belong to the same cluster reach the excited state simultaneously and possess similar parametres of transmembranal potentials.

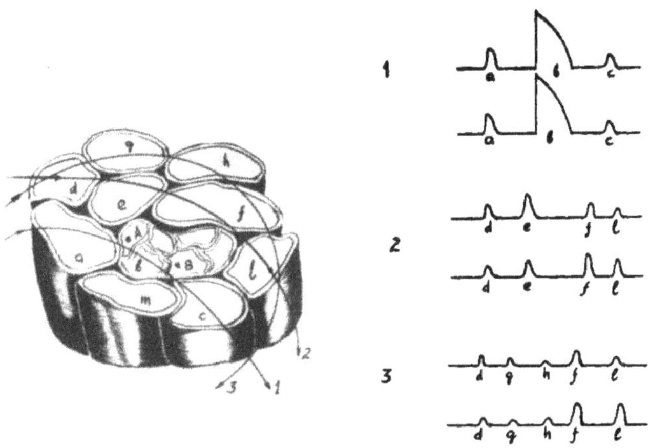

Fig.1 The scheme of the myocardium's cluster structure, spreding of the excitation waves 1,2,3 and the origin of the low amplitude potentials.

Asynchronic action for example electric current or aconitine depolarises the cell membrane and inactived the fast Na canals /3/. During such conditions the velocity of conduction of excitation througn heart is decreased /7/. A block is formad on the site of contact of Purkinje's fibres with the contractile myocard and circulation of excitation tabes place in the contractile myocard.

The conduction of the wave 1 through clusters 'a' causes low amplitudinal potential in the cells A and B due to electrical interaction between clusters 'a' and 'b'. Meanwhile due to different position of A and B cells with respect to clusters "a" the value of amplitude potential wile remain different. After that the wave of excitation catches the cluster 'b' carring to the cells action poential with the same amplitude and configuration. Further conduction of wave of excitation with the shift to cluster 'c'again causes low amplitude potentials. During the conduction of wave 2 or 3 only low amplitude potentials may occur. In the real myocard the movement of wave of excitation may be noticed in different directions which causes interaction of electrotonic potentials with each other giving rise to potentials with different configuration and amplitude.Depending upon the expressing power of intercellular contacts there is difference in the electric activity of the cells of myocardium of mammals and birds. Practically the heart of birds has less number of contacts, which results in low number of lowamplitude potentials.

During this in the heart of birds the excitation may circulate in the net of Purkinje's fibres with the release of clusters of cells of contractile myocard. Meanwile during fibrillation of ventricles in the heart of mammals the excitation may circulate through contractile myocardium. It's evident, that in the last case there is more probability of synchronic excitation and spontaneous cessation of fibrillation.

References

1.Weidmann S. Ann.Rev.Physiol.1974,36:p.155
2.Rosensthrauck L.V. In:Heart Phys.(L),1980,p.118
3.Cobrin V.I.e.a Cardiol.(USSR),1981,21:N10,p.67

4.Cobrin V.I.e.a. In:Comp.Electrocar.1981,p.102
5.Dewey M.M. In:Comp.Physiol.Heart 1969,p.10
6.Legato M.J. Circul.1973,47:,N1,p.178
7.Wit A.L.,Rosen M.R Amer.Heart J.1983,106:p.798

PART II
Applications of Computing in Electrocardiography

Computerized ECG-based Time-Insensitive Predictive Instrument (TIPI): Integration of the Q Wave, ST Segment and T Wave in Patient History for the Diagnosis of Acute Myocardial Infarction by the Computerized Electrocardiogram

Michael M. Laks, M.D.,* Charles B. Cairns, M.D.**
James T. Niemann, M.D.,*** Harry P. Selker, M.D.****

* Cardiology Division, Department of Medicine, Harbor-UCLA Medical Center, Torrance, CA
** Department of Emergency Medicine, University of Colorado, Denver, Colorado
*** Department of Emergency Medicine, Harbor-UCLA Medical Center, Torrance, California
**** TIPI Project, New England Medical Center, Boston, Massachusetts

1. Introduction

I formally wish to thank the organization committee of the International Congress on Electrocardiography and particularly Professor Peter Macfarlane for inviting board members of the International Society for Computerized Electrocardiography, called ISCE, to present this symposium on current research in electrocardiology. We are most honored. I hope we can invoke the spirit of ISCE, as shown, dedicated to catalyze communication among individuals from the university, industry and the users by encouraging open discussion at this conference. Thank you for the invitation!

For years, the electrocardiographer has been forced to use solely the individual ECG waveforms - Q waves, R wave diminution, ST segment and T wave changes to make the diagnosis of acute myocardial infarction (AMI). Although physicians have been maintaining that the patient's history is important for the improvement of clinical diagnosis by the ECG, no organized integration of the ECG and the clinical history has been reported in the diagnosis of AMI. In fact in most hospitals the accurate reliable completion of the ECG requisition is rarely carried out. In spite of the electrocardiographers' insistence of the value of the demographics and history in the ECG diagnosis, doctors have been recalcitrant to comply. This study will give the important rationale to expedite compliance!

In the United States about 1.5 million patients with chest pain are annually admitted to the intensive care unit for the presumptive diagnosis of AMI. This costs over $ 5 billion annually. A considerable savings of money would occur if one were merely to decrease the number of patients admitted to the hospital. However, if this increase in specificity results in low sensitivity, it could result in an unacceptable number of patients sent home with an undiagnosed AMI. The resolution of the major conflict of whether to admit or not to admit could result in an enormous shift in resource allocation. In 1984, Pozen et al. [1] published in the New England Journal of Medicine a landmark paper demonstrating that the integration of the patient's history with the ECG waveform resulted in a significant decrease in the false positive diagnosis of an acute cardiac ischemia (ACI). Consequently, a 30% reduction in the admission of patients would occur in ICUs without a reduction in the number of true positive diagnoses of ACI. Shortly after this 1984 paper, the Harbor-UCLA (HUCLA) Medical Center group started to work with the New England Medical Center (NEMC) group that had developed the original predictive instrument. Part of the task of the NEMC group was to develop the time-insensitive predictive instrument (TIPI) * that could be programmed into a computer by the HUCLA group to expedite the rapid diagnosis of ACI.

* The TIPI study was done prospectively and retrospectively and consequently can be used in the future both prospectively and retrospectively, hence, the name, "T"ime-"I"nsensitive "P"redictive "I"nstrument (TIPI).

The purposes of this study were:

1. To develop a computer program to link TIPI with a computerized interpretation for real-time use as a function of conventional computerized electrocardiography in the emergency department (ED).
2. To assess the utility of this TIPI program to predict not only ischemia but also AMI in patients presenting with chest pain.
3. To compare the efficacy of the TIPI computer program with ED physicians' assessment of patients for the diagnosis of AMI.

2. The Development of the TIPI Program

The following review of the development of the TIPI program **highlights** the importance for the need to pursue intimate details in order to make a computer program work in the real world of medicine! Initially, we developed a computer program using the Pozen et al. variables and equation for the original predictive instrument for ACI [2-4]. The following clinical inputs were integrated into the computerized ECG program: chest pain or left arm pain which was considered to be secondary, or chest pain or left arm pain which was considered to be the chief complaint of the patient coming into the ED. Other inputs were a history of a heart attack and nitroglycerin use. Specific waveforms on the ECG were integrated such as ST segment elevation and depression. In the original predictive instrument ST segment straightening was one of the variables needed for the computation of the probability of ACI. The following scenario is a testimony to the power of the computer in forcing the investigator to ask important specific questions. Since the computer requires quantitative information, the following were critical questions posed related to programming ST segment straightening: How many milliseconds (msec) should the ST segment be at the baseline? 100 msec? 150 msec? How much change from this baseline would be the variance of normal to indicate "straightening?" At what specific point would the ST segment begin to elevate into the T wave? The answer to these questions was that no specific time-dependent quantitative data existed for the ST segment in the normal and the ischemic heart. Consequently, we had to delete the ST segment straightening parameter. The other important questions posed were: How reliable are the histories in the ED required for the original predictive instrument, namely, a patient's telling the physician that they had a heart attack, or that they have been taking nitroglycerin? To avoid inaccuracy and intrusiveness, we decided to rewrite the computer program with more specific reproducible criteria. Dr. Selker and colleagues went back to their predictive instrument equation with a more easily defined variable: the TIPI [4]. The TIPI is expressed by the following probability formula [1,3]:

Predictive Instrument Equation:

$$p = 100 \times [1 + \exp(B_o + \sum_{i=1}^{n} B_i X_i)]^{-1}$$

where **exp** represents **e**, the base of the natural logarithm. The following variables were inserted into the above equation:

As shown below (Table 1), both age and sex were integrated into the new TIPI equation [3-4]. The major historical input was chest pain and whether chest pain or discomfort was a secondary or a chief complaint. If the patient came to the ED primarily because of chest pain, it would be categorized as a chief complaint and would be given a higher coefficient. If the chest pain was present, but not the chief reason for coming to the ED, the chest pain would be categorized as secondary. Instead of a history of MI, the presence of abnormal Q waves, a more objective and verifiable variable, was integrated into the computer program. The ST and T wave elevation and depression variables were given more detail. Of note, the less easily defined variables of ST segment straightening, history of MI, and history of nitroglycerin use were eliminated.

TABLE 1

B0 CONSTANT
B1 (A40) AGE ≤ 40
B2 (A51) ≥ 51
B3 (M) SEX = MALE
B4 (MA51) AGE ≥ 51 AND SEX = MALE
B5 (SCP) SECONDARY COMPLAINT CHEST OR LEFT ARM PAIN
B6 (CCP) CHIEF COMPLAINT CHEST OR LEFT ARM PAIN
B7 (Q) SIGNIFICANT Q WAVES IN AT LEAST 2 LEADS
B8 (SE) ST ELEVATION IN AT LEAST 2 LEADS
B9 (SD) ST DEPRESSION IN AT LEAST 2 LEADS
B10 (TE) T ELEV IN AT LEAST 2 LEADS
B11 (TD) T INVERSION IN AT LEAST 2 LEADS
B12 (STD) ST DEP AND T INV IN 2 LEADS

In order to integrate the history into the ECG computer-generated waveforms we developed at Harbor-UCLA Medical Center an expanded computer program in which we could link 9,999 history statements or codes into the ECG language developed by Hewlett-Packard (ECL)[5]. This ECL language has allowed us to program all the waveform measurements and the clinical history variables needed for the TIPI into an integrated final statement, thereby the electrocardiogram would automatically have computed and printed out the TIPI's predicted probability of ACI.

3. The Computer Program

Figure 1 is an example of the TIPI analysis of our computerized ECG program. Based upon the following evidence the probability of ACI is 22%. Below this TIPI percent are presented the factors responsible for this percentage. At the upper right quadrant is the history code input, CC for chief complaint of chest pain. The next statement is that the inferior T waves are flat or slightly inverted. The specific criteria are presented on the right side. The advantage of this program is that one can visually confirm that T waves are flat or specifically less than 0.1 Mv. The reader can thereby document the specific measurement used by the computer in the decision making. The advantage of this format is that it reveals to the doctor the step-by-step components from whence the TIPI score evolved and thereby makes the program user-friendly.

The computer statements below are from the actual program in ECL:

```
PRINT #PTEI1   NS
"INF T FLAT OR SLIGHTLY INVERTED"
"T 0.1 O -0.09 mV IN 2 OF 2, 3, F, V6"
IF (T : AMPLITUDE SLE 0.1 OR T':
AMPLITUDE SLE 0.1) AND (T : AMPLITUDE
+ T' : AMPLITUDE SLE 0.1 AND T :
MEASURED)) IN 2 OF L2 L3 aVF V6
```

```
PRINT #PTI1   NS
"INFERIOR T WAVES INVERTED" "T -0.1 mV
IN 2 OF 2, 3, F, V6"
IF (T : AMPLITUDE SLE -0.01 OR T'
: AMPLITUDE
SLE -0.01) IN 2 OF L2, L3, aVF, V6
```

The above statements illustrate the simplicity of the ECL computer program. With minimal training, one can easily learn to read it. The following is a translation of this ECL program: Print a statement if the T absolute is SLE, "S" stands for "sign considered by the computer program" (positive or negative); in this case the sign is positive; **LE** means "less than or equal to" 0.1 or that the T prime is less than or equal to 0.1. Most importantly, the computer reminds us to appreciate that there are frequently T primes. At the bottom line it states that this change must occur in 2 of lead II, lead III, AVF or V6. All 4 leads are considered inferior or apical leads. If the T waves are less than or equal to -0.1 Mv, the next statement, inferior T wave inverted, would be printed out.

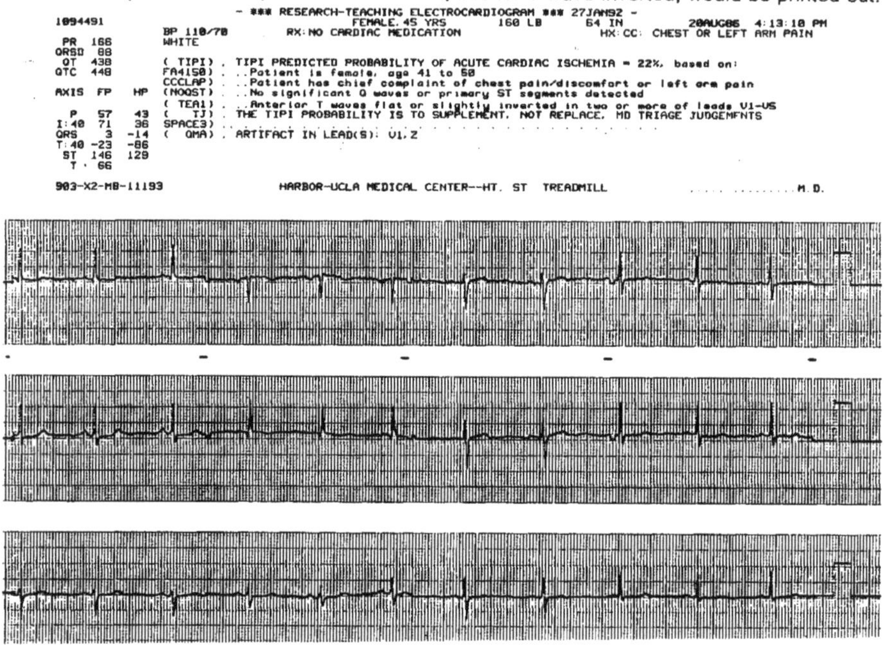

Figure 1: TIPI Predictive Probability of Acute Cardiac Ischemia

4. Methods

A preliminary 3-month prospective single-blind and consecutive ECG study of patients with chest pain was performed. Emergency Department (ED) patients over the age of 35 were enrolled with the complaint of chest pain but no history of thoracic trauma or chest x-ray evidence of primary pulmonary disease. A 12-lead ECG was obtained and a TIPI-predicted probability of ACI disease was generated by the computer. The ED physicians were blinded to the TIPI score. The ED physicians were mainly residents in training supervised by the ED staff physicians. Patient deposition was based upon the clinical assessment. Additionally, the physicians recorded their own probability of ACI.

5. Results

During the 3-month period 189 patients were entered into the study. Of the 101 patients admitted, 17 were sent to the ward, 38 sent to telemetry and 46 to the ICU. Eighty-eight patients were discharged. The TIPI scores related to the physicians' disposition. Patients with lower scores (25 ± 3; mean ± SEM) were sent to the wards and those with higher scores were sent to telemetry (41 ± 4) and the ICU (52 ± 3). Complications were defined as patients having ventricular fibrillation, ventricular tachycardia, congestive heart failure or patients requiring continuous IV medications such as nipride for hypertension or IV NTG for ongoing chest pain. The TIPI score appropriately predicted the complications. Patients with no complications had scores of 21 ± 4 while patients with complications had higher scores.

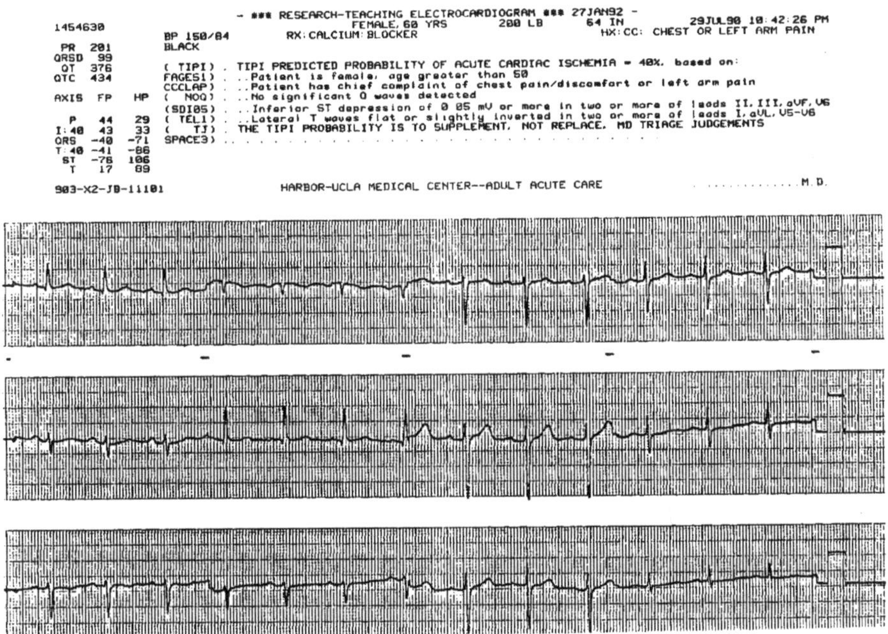

Figure 2: TIPI Predictive Probability of Acute Cardiac Ischemia. An example of an ECG with the prediction of a non-Q wave myocardial infarction.

The following is an ECG analysis of the TIPI computer score. Fig. 2 , above, illustrates a case with a computer-generated TIPI ECG probability score of ACI of 40%. This score is based upon the patient's being female, aged greater than or equal to 50 and a chief complaint of chest pain or left arm pain. The computer did not find significant Q waves. The ST segments were recorded to be depressed greater than 0.05 Mv in 2 or more of leads II, III AVF and V6. Furthermore, lateral T waves were flat or slightly inverted in 2 or more of leads I, AVL, V5 or V6. Most ED physicians and cardiologists would call this a nonspecific change. This patient had an AMI with no complications. In our study a TIPI score greater than or equal to 38% was the breaking point for the diagnosis of AMI. This ECG with a low but abnormal TIPI score of 40% is an example of a TIPI-diagnosed non-Q-wave infarction generated by demographic data and a history of chest pain.

Figure 3 shows a receiver-operating characteristic (ROC) curve which summarizes the 3-month study of the 101 patients admitted to the hospital with chest pain. The ROC curves have the advantage to the user of the capability to select any specific sensitivity and specificity for an entire range of probabilities. Of importance, as the sensitivity of the test is increased in order to detect all the cases of AMI, the specificity is decreased. An ideal test would be one with a 100% sensitivity and 100% specificity. The horizontal scale is plotted as 1 minus the specificity in order to have all the data plotted positively. The patient in Fig. 2 with a TIPI score of 40% would have a sensitivity of 95% and a specificity of 65%. We decided that in our ED the best compromise for diagnosing an AMI was a TIPI score greater than or equal to 38% which would give us optimal decision for admission of a patient with minimal false negatives with a sensitivity of 95%. This set very high sensitivity meets the mission of the ED by establishing a high probability of not sending a patient home with an AMI. The ED physicians' generated ROC curve was to the right and downward to the TIPI curve (Fig. 3B).

6. Discussion

The TIPI score appears to be a reliable method for predicting which patients with chest pain are at risk for AMI, AIHD or the complications thereof when integrated into a computerized electrocardiograph. Indeed, the findings of this study suggest that a computer-based TIPI program is as good as, and may be better than, the physician's estimate of the likelihood of AMI. A computerized TIPI score ≥ 38% appeared to be more accurate than ED physicians in predicting which patients would have AMI and complications of AMI. The area under the TIPI curve was 0.85 and greater than under the area of the physician's curve of 0.71. The physician's estimated probability curve was lower and to the right

Figure 3A

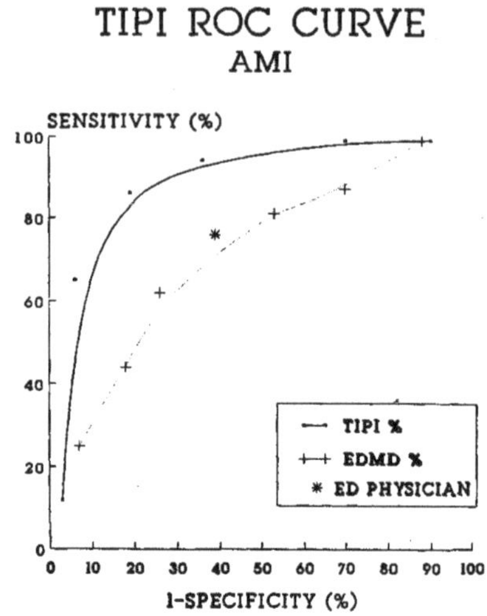

AMI- CK-MB ≥8%

Figure 3B

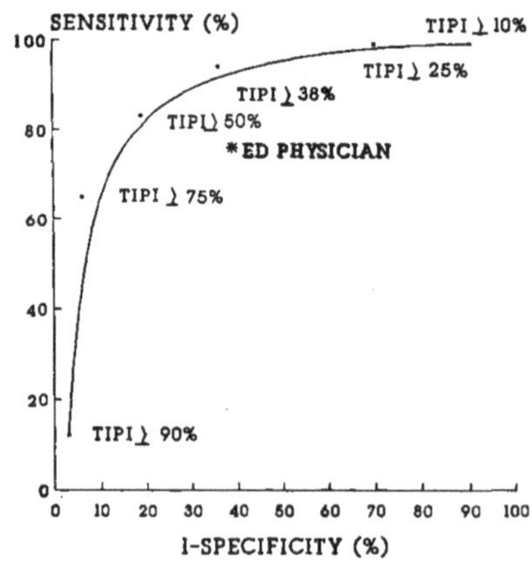

Figure 3: TIPI Receiver Operational Characteristic (ROC) Curve. Note (3A) that the ED physician's ROC curve is to the right of the TIPI curve. The TIPI probabilities are inserted into TIPI 3B.

and therefore less sensitive and less specific than TIPI. At the same specificity of 65% for the diagnosis of AMI, the TIPI computer program was more sensitive (95%) than the physician (77%). In summary, the computerized electrocardiograph incorporating the TIPI was probably better.

An important finding suggested by this study is that one may be able to make the diagnosis of non-Q-wave infarctions by incorporating the TIPI formula with its integration of the patient's demographics and chest pain history along with a detailed, quantitative analysis of the Q, ST and T waveforms on the patient's ECG. This study demonstrates that one can not only predict ACI but also make a diagnosis of AMI if one integrates the patient's demographics and history into a computer program. This study highlights the important role that the computer plays in the use of ECG-based decision aids for clinical decision making. Because the computer demands specific and reproducible data, the original predictive instrument for ACI was modified, leading to a new predictive instrument that takes better advantage of the computerized ECG: the TIPI. The beginning of a new era in computerized electrocardiography is marked by this study which demonstrates that the history and demographics integrated into the ECG waveforms optimizes the diagnosis of an AMI. It is appropriate that I, the President of the International Society for Computerized Electrocardiography, acknowledge the pioneering work of your senior and honorary member, Dr. Hubert Pipberger, for his development of the first computer integration of demographics into ECG databases and clinical decisions. I am most pleased to continue his work. Thank you for the opportunity to present our research to you.

7. Conclusion

1. TIPI and ECG interpretation have been linked into a user-friendly program.
2. TIPI is more sensitive and specific in predicting AMI or complications in ED patients admitted for chest pain.
3. TIPI may be better than physicians in making ED triage decisions of AMI.

8. References

1. M.W. Pozen, R.B. D'Agostino, H.P. Selker et al.: A predictive instrument to improve coronary care unit admission practices in acute ischemic heart disease: A prospective multicenter trial. N. Engl. J. Med. **310** (1984) 1273-1278.

2. H.P. Selker, R.B. D'Agostino and M.M. Laks: A predictive instrument for acute ischemic heart disease to improve coronary care unit admission practices: A potential on-line tool in a computerized electrocardiograph. J. Electrocardiol. **21** (1988) (Suppl) 11-17.

3. M.M. Laks, C.B. Cairns and H.P. Selker: An on-line computerized ECG program for the prediction of acute ischemic heart disease. Computers in Cardiology **1989** (1989) 505-508.

4. H.P. Selker, J.L. Griffith and R.B. D'Agostino: A tool for judging coronary care unit admission appropriateness, valid for both real-time and retrospective use: A time-insensitive predictive instrument (TIPI) for acute cardiac ischemia. Medical Care **29** (7) (1991) 610-627.

5. M.M. Laks and J.T. Niemann: Computer linkage of the clinical history to electrocardiographic language (ECL) permitting the use of Bayes' theorem. Computers in Cardiology **1986** (1986) 537-540.

NEURAL NETWORKS FOR THE DIAGNOSIS OF LEFT VENTRICULAR STRAIN

P.W. Macfarlane, B. Devine,
University Department of Medical Cardiology,
Royal Infirmary,
Glasgow,
Scotland.

ABSTRACT

A neural network was trained to differentiate the ST-T pattern of LV strain from other ST-T configurations. The results showed a lower sensitivity but higher specificity compared to conventional criteria.

In 1974, one of us suggested that electrocardiography was a playground for mathematical games(1). In some senses this has remained true and at present there is to be found a widespread range of advanced mathematical techniques being used in electrocardiography. It is only necessary to consider time series analysis in the study of RR interval variation, non linear mathematics (chaos theory) in the study of arrhythmias and myocardial ischaemia, Fourier analysis for the study of the signal averaged ECG (late potentials) etc. Despite these advanced methods being available, the 12-lead electrocardiogram still remains the most popular form of ECG recording in widespread use at the present time. For this reason, in our laboratory every attempt is still being made to enhance the diagnostic usefulness of computer assisted ECG interpretation. One relatively recently introduced method for classification of patterns has been the science of neural networks. Although the basic approach was introduced over 20 years ago, it has only been within the last 5 years that significant advances have been made in allowing neural networks to be implemented in the form of software that can be readily used by the non-specialist.

A neural network allows the association between a set of input measurements and a set of outputs or diagnostic classifications in the case of the electrocardiogram. It was therefore thought to be of interest to assess the usefulness of a neural network in a simple task such as in differentiating a particular type of ST-T abnormality (left ventricular strain) from other forms of T wave morphology. In this way the value of the technique could be assessed in a very straightforward manner as a starting point in a study of the application of neural networks to ECG interpretation.

MATERIALS AND METHODS

In order to function, a neural network has to be trained with a known set of patterns i.e. in this case those which are typical of left ventricular strain and those which do not resemble left ventricular strain whether they be normal or abnormal ST-T segments. To this end, a series of 356 ECG wave forms was visually classified by an experienced electrocardiographer as exhibiting LV strain or otherwise. These leads were selected from a database of ECGs which existed in our laboratory and which could easily be processed by computer. 14 measurements from each QRST complex were obtained by computer for each waveform. These consisted of the 8 time normalised amplitudes in the ST-T segment, the 7/8th QRS amplitude, the S wave amplitude, the T+, T- amplitudes as well as the ST junction amplitude and the ST-T slope. For each ECG lead in the training set, these 14 measurements were input to a neural net together with the associated diagnosis. Ultimately the net successfully classified all patterns in the training set.

In order to accomplish the above, software was written locally that enabled neural networks to be studied. The language used was C++ which was compatible with the different operating systems and languages used for other work in connection with ECG analysis by computer. The neural net package allowed the number of input measurements and diagnoses to be selected as well as the number of hidden layers and corresponding neurons. It was found that a net with 14 input neurons, one hidden layer with 24 neurons, and one output diagnosis (LV strain) performed best.

A test set of 132 ECG leads from 33 ECGs was then studied. All of the leads (I, aVL, V5, V6) were visually classified as exhibiting left-ventricular strain or otherwise. For each of these leads, 14 measurements were input to the network for classification.

In order to have some type of comparison with conventional criteria, the existing logic for diagnosing left ventricular strain in the Glasgow analysis program was also used with the ECG leads in the test set. Individual results from the lateral leads analysed by the neural net were then grouped to form an overall ECG interpretation of LV strain or otherwise, i.e. if any of leads I, aVL, V5, V6 were classed as LV strain by the neural net, the ECG as a whole was regarded as being categorised as showing LV strain by the neural net.

RESULTS

Table 1 (a) shows that the neural network had a sensitivity of 90% and a specificity of 94% when individual leads were considered. Table 1 (b) shows that when the leads were grouped into ECGs as described above, the neural net sensitivity was 83% with a specificity of 90%. This has to be compared against conventional criteria with 100% sensitivity but 33% specificity (Table 1(c)).

TABLE 1

a) Results of classifying leads I, aVL, V5, V6 individually, using a neural network.

		Cardiologist		
		LV Strain	Not LV Strain	Unclassified
Neural Network (per lead)	LV Strain	28	6	-
	Not LV Strain	3	94	1

Sensitivity 90% Specificity 93%

b) Results of classifying ECGs using a neural network.

		Cardiologist	
		LV Strain	Not LV Strain
Neural Network (per ECG)	LV Strain	10	2
	Not LV Strain	2	19

Sensitivity 83% Specificity 90%

c) Results of classifying ECGs using conventional criteria.

		Cardiologist	
		LV Strain	Not LV Strain
Conventional Criteria (per ECG)	LV Strain	12	13
	Not LV Strain	0	8

Sensitivity 100% Specificity 33%

DISCUSSION

A cardiologist essentially interprets an ECG using a pattern recognition process, however subconsciously. Only very rarely would he measure the amplitude or duration of a particular wave or complex in order to make an interpretation. Thus it was thought more likely to be the case that a neural network could improve on the more conventional approach to ECG interpretation using deterministic criteria.

As a result of an earlier study of LV strain from this laboratory(2), however, it was felt that the specificity of the neural network could be improved upon. In that study, only 12 measurements from the ST-T segment had been used while in the present study, two additional measurements, namely the S wave and the 7/8th QRS amplitude were added in an attempt to improve the situation. The classical pattern of left ventricular strain is one in which there is no S wave. With the 12 measurement approach, it was found that the ST-T configuration could resemble left ventricular strain and could be reported as such by the neural network even if there were a preceding S wave. With the 14 measurement approach, and proper training of the network such false positive interpretations should and did not arise.

On the other hand, the classical LV strain deterministic criteria used by the Glasgow program do not make reference to the amplitude of the S wave. This is possibly why the specificity of the conventional criteria are somewhat lower than might be expected in this study, as the electrocardiographer (the gold standard) considered LV strain to be present only if an S wave were absent in the same lead.

A major problem with deterministic criteria is that whenever a threshold is crossed, there is a change in interpretation. Thus if a T wave is 200 microvolts on one occasion and 199 on a subsequent occasion left ventricular strain might be reported in the former and not in the latter. It is hoped that the use of neural networks will avoid such problems. This remains to be tested on the basis of studying a series of repeat ECG recordings.

In conclusion, this small study which nevertheless was time consuming in view of the need to write a complete neural network software package, has proved illuminating in demonstrating that as far as training a network is concerned, the diagnostic classifications must be selected with great care while on the other hand it can be seen that the neural network can have difficulties in classifying patterns which might however have presented difficulties to a cardiologist also.

REFERENCES

1. D. Krikler and P.W. Macfarlane, *Standards for Electrocardiographs,* Br. Heart J. 36 (1974) 945-47.

2. B. Devine, *Neural Networks in Electrocardiography,*M. Sc. Dissertation, University of Glasgow, 1990.

INFORMATION AND DECISION THEORY FOR ASSESSING DIAGNOSTIC ECG INTERPRETATION RESULTS OBTAINED BY COMPUTERS AND CARDIOLOGISTS

JOS L.WILLEMS, CSE Project Leader

CSE Coordinating Center, University of Leuven, 49 Herestraat,
Leuven 3000, Belgium

ABSTRACT

Information and decision theory were applied to assess the interpretation results of 15 computer programs (9 ECG and 6 VCG) and 9 cardiologists (8 ECG and 5 VCG) who analysed 1220 clinically validated cases. The study shows that information content and utility indices by providing a comprehensive view on diagnostic performance, can enhance the insight given by the more classic measures.

1. Introduction

Several methods and measures exist for the assessment of diagnostic ECG results with the true condition as reference. Sensivity, specificity, ROC curves, positive and negative predictive test results, as well as total accuracy are most often used [1]. Less well known are the comprehensive measures derived from information and decision theory [2-3]. The application of information analysis to diagnostic testing derives from the recognition that all clinical tests are imperfect. This imperfection introduces uncertainty or noise into the interpretation. Decision theory and utility functions take into account the clinical value and relevance of the diagnostic test results. Both approaches have been applied in the CSE Project "Common Standards for Quantitative Electrocardiography", in the analysis of results derived from 1220 cases, validated by ECG independent means.

2. Methods

2.1. Patient Material and ECG Processing

Details on the patient material and data analysis by the classic evaluation methods have been published recently [4-5]. The following diagnostic groups were included in the CSE diagnostic study : normals (NL; N=382); left (LVH; N=183), right (RVH; N=55) and biventricular (BVH; N=53) hypertrophy ; anterior (AMI; N=170), inferior (IMI; N=273) and combined (MIX; N=73) myocardial infarction; combined infarction and hypertrophy (N=31).The case selection was entirely based on ECG clinical information and was verified by 3 cardiologists. All standard ECG leads, and the orthogonal X,Y and Z leads, were recorded simultaneously with a sampling rate of 500 Hz. Those with major conduction defects or poor technical quality were excluded. That was the only reason why the ECG's were screened.

The ECG's were analysed by 8 cardiologists from 7 European countries and by 9 ECG computer programs. The VCG's were independently read by 5 cardiologists and by 6 programs. The ECG programs were the following : Marquette(2), Hannover(4), Hewlett-Packard(5), Medis(7), Nagoya(8), Glasgow(11), Padova(13), Means(15) and Leuven(16). The VCG programs were Vecto-Louvain(3), Hannover(6), Lyon(9), AVA-

Pipberger(10), Porto(2) and Means(14). The numbers refer to the program identifiers used in this paper. Programs 4, 6, 10 and 16 use a statistical approach to classification. All other apply heuristic or deterministic methods. Only age and sex were given as prior information to all programs and the cardiologists, except for program 10 which was given a code indicating one of 3 conditions to adjust prior probabilities . In addition to the individual results, combined results were calculated by means of weighted averaging for all programs (ECG,VCG and all combined) and similarly for the cardiologists [6].

2.2. Statistical Analysis

Programs and cardiologist results were compared with the true disease category obtained from the independent clinical data. Program results were also compared with the results of the average individual cardiologist and with the combined cardiologist results, i.e. the group opinion [4-5]. Only comparative results with the clinical evidence, i.e. the "golden reference" will be reported in this paper. Different classification matrices were calculated : first in a bigroup analysis, i.e. normal vs abnormal, LVH vs non-LVH, etc; next in a 3-by-3 matrix, i.e. normal vs infarct vs hypertrophy; then in a 5-by-5 matrix, where hypertrophy was split into its 3 respective subgroups (LVH, RVH and BVH); and finally in a full 7-by-7 classification matrix.

The Information Content (I) results have been derived from the 2-by-2 classification matrices, and plotted for various prevalence values in incremental steps of 5 %, according to the formula described by Diamond et al [3] , whereby

$$I = \sum_j [ap \log_2 (ap) + bq \log_2 (bq) - (ap + bq) \log_2 (ap + bq)] - \sum_i p_i \log_2 p_i$$

where
$a = p(T_j / D+)$ = true positive rate
$b = p(T_j / D-)$ = false positive rate
$p = p(D+)$ = prevalence of disease
$q = p(D-) = 1 - p$ = prevalence of non-disease
and p was varied in increments of 0.05

The area under the resulting curve represents the average information content. An ideal test should have an I-value, expressed in bits, of 1 at 50 % disease prevalence and a maximal average of 0.72.

Utilities have been derived by weighting the observed frequencies of the classification matrix, according to the clinical relevance of the different correct and incorrect classifications and summing up the results into one overall utility figure for a specific clinical environment, e.g.hospital vs ambulatory care. The overall *utility* figures were derived from the 7-by-7 misclassification results, whereby the number of predicted diagnoses are multiplied with the "utility scores" awarded for each of the cells and summed up according to the formula : $SUM_{ij} (u_{ij} * n_{ij})$, whereby u_{ij} = utility for each respective prediction and n_{ij} = number of cases in the respective cells.

The applied utility or cost factor for each prediction are arbitrary and depend on the user and the environment in which the program is to be applied. Thus, utilities for health screening will not be the same as for an acute hospital care environment. Results presented in this paper have been derived for the latter setting. During the CSE Workshop of Dec. 1989 [4] 13 participants (7 cardiologists and 6 non-cardiologists) gave their personal utility or respective cost estimates for each of the cells of the 7-by-7 classification matrix, using scores from +10 to -10. They filled in the same form a second time at home. There was a high correlation between their first and second round estimates (r^2=0.88; N=72). Median estimates obtained from the first round have been used in the present paper.

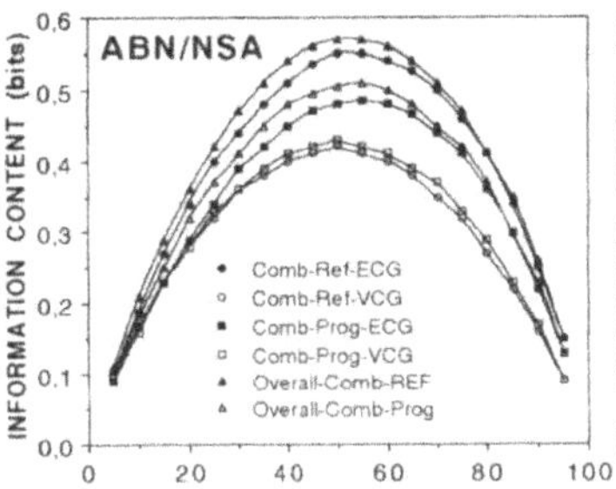

Figure 1

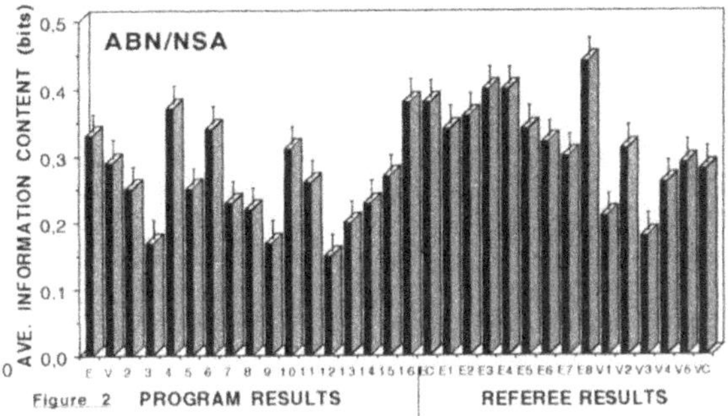

Figure 2

3. Results

3.1. Information Content Results

An information content curve, depicting the classification results of normal vs. abnormal, is shown in Figure 1 for the combined results of the ECG, VCG and overall results (N=15 programs and N=13 human readings). From these curves it is apparent that ECG interpretation was superior over VCG interpretation, both for programs and cardiologists. Figure 1 also shows that combined programs results were almost as good as those of the cardiologists . Figure 2 depicts individual, average information results for the classification of normal vs. abnormal. Note that "Abnormal" means classification into one of the 6 other disease categories. It is apparent that results of the various programs differ widely. The performance of the 4 statistical programs was significantly better than that of the other programs. Their results were almost as good as those of the best cardiologists, when tested against the clinical evidence. The results of the VCG readers, labelled V1 to V5, were significantly inferior to those of the ECG readers, labelled E1 to E8. This is mainly due to the lower specificity of VCG analysis. Median results and ranges of Information Content data for the other groups are presented in Table 1. The highest discrimination was found for the infarction categories, followed by LVH. Results for RVH and BVH were significantly lower. Combined ECG program results are labelled with E in Figures 2 and 3, combined VCG program results with V, combined ECG results of the cardiologists with EC and combined VCG cardiologist results with VC. Overall combined program results are labelled with P.

3.2. Utillity Results

Overall utility results derived from the 7-by-7 misclassification matrices are depicted in Fig.3. Utility results correlated highly with total accuracy. The determination coëfficient (r^2) was respectively 0.896 for the cardiologists and 0.865 for the programs. However, the slope of the curves was steeper for the programs than the cardiologists. Utility scores for the combined- and the statistical program-results were almost as high as those of the best cardiologists. Figure 3 also shows that some programs had a significantly lower performance. The VCG programs and the VCG readers showed in general lower utility scores as well as lower total accuracies, than the ECG programs and the ECG readers. Total accuracy varied between 62.0 % and 77.3 % (median 69.7 % for the 9 ECG programs) and between 64.3 % and 76.2% (median 68.2 %) for the 6 VCG programs. Corresponding results were 72.6 % - 81.0 % (median 76.3 %) for the 8 ECG readers and 66.3 % - 74.4 % (median 70.3 %) for the 5 VCG readers.

Table 1 : Average information content (in bits*100) for the main diagnostic categories.

Average information content (bits*100)		Combined ECG		Combined VCG		Individual Programs	Individual Cardiologists
		Prog.	Card.	Prog.	Card.		
NL	vs Abnormal	33 ±3	38 ±3***	29 ±3	28 ±3	25 (38-15)	32 (44-18)
LVH	vs not-LVH	27 ±3	27 ±3	27 ±3	24 ±3**	20 (33-13)	24 (28-17)
RVH	vs not-RVH	16 ±4	20 ±4**	21 ±4	21 ±4	11 (28- 5)	18 (22-16)
BVH	vs not-BVH	20 ±4	18 ±4	18 ±4	17 ±4	12 (31-10)	15 (30- 7)
AMI	vs not-AMI	38 ±3	46 ±4***	36 ±3	34 ±3*	33 (35-19)	41 (46-26)
IMI	vs not-IMI	30 ±3	36 ±3***	35 ±3	31 ±3**	25 (39-14)	30 (41-22)
MIX	vs not-MIX	30 ±4	35 ±5***	34 ±5	36 ±5*	24 (34-17)	30 (36-24)

Differences between programs and cardiologists : *** = $p<0.001$; ** = $P < 0.01$; * = $p < 0.05$
Average of 19 discrete values computed at prevalence increments of 5%, i.e. from 5 % to 95 %, and standard deviations are given for the combined results; medians and ranges are given for the individual program (N=15) and cardiologist results (N=13).

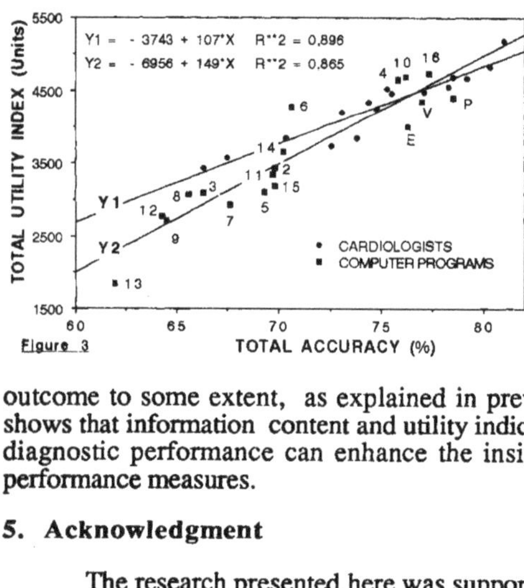

Figure 3

4. Conclusion

In the CSE diagnostic study we have demonstrated that several standard ECG computer programs perform almost at equal level as cardiologists in the classification of 7 main diagnostic categories. However, the results also demonstrate that all the programs can still be improved and that some require overall improvement. The 4 programs which used statistical methods had a higher diagnostic accuracy than the deterministic programs. However, the study design may have favored this outcome to some extent, as explained in previous publications [4-5]. The present study shows that information content and utility indices, by providing a comprehensive view on diagnostic performance can enhance the insight given by the more classic statistical performance measures.

5. Acknowledgment

The research presented here was supported by DG XII of the EC within the frame of its 3rd an 4th Medical and Public Health Research Programmes.

6. References

1. J.Michaelis, S.Wellek, J.L.Willems, *Meth. Inform. Med.* **29** (1990) 289-96.
2. Ph.Smets, J.L.Willems et al., *Biometrie Praximetrie* **15** (1975) 3-35.
3. G.A.Diamond et al., *Circulation* **63** (1981) 915-21.
4. J.L.Willems, *10th and Final CSE Progress Report "Common Standards for Quantitative Electrocardiography"* , Acco Publ., Leuven, 1990 p.1-384.
5. J.L.Willems et al., *New.Engl.J.Med.* (in press December 18,1991).
6. J.L.Willems et al , *Eur.Heart J.*, 9 (1988) 1348-55.

An Ischemia Index for Identifying Candidates for Surgical Enhancing Myocardial Blood Flow

Galen S. Wagner, M.D.

Duke University Medical Center, Durham, North Carolina

An index of left ventricular function such as global ejection fraction is often used in the evaluation of candidates for either coronary artery bypass grafts or coronary angioplasty. When the ejection fraction is low, the clinician may assume that the risk of the procedure is so high that it outweighs the potential benefit. However, the left ventricular dysfunction could be produced by either infarcted or ischemic myocardium. The differentation between these two conditions is of obvious clinical importance because in the later instance the procedure might result in marked improvement in left ventricular function and thereby a low rather than high associated risk.

One might hypothesize that if low ventricular function is associated with infarcted myocardium, there will be a large number of abnormal Q waves on the standard 12 lead electrocardiogram and, conversely, when the decreased function is due only to ischemia that no such QRS changes would present. The Selvester QRS scoring system was developed to estimate the quantity of infarcted left ventricle with each of its 32 points being equivalent to 3% of the left ventricle. A previous study has shown a good correlation between the Selvester QRS score and the global left ventricular ejection fraction in patients immediately following their initial acute myocardial infarction (1). This relationship was used to develop the formula: left ventricular ejection fraction = 60 - QRS score. If, for a given patient who presents for consideration of revasculization, the measured ejection fraction is similar to that predicted from the ejection fraction estimated by QRS changes, one may assume that the majority of the malfunctioning myocardium is indeed infarcted and therefore unable to regain function following the procedure. If, however there is a gap between the electrocardiographic estimated and the directly measured left ventricular ejection fraction, the extent of that gap might be considered as an "ischemia index", that is, the amount of left ventricular function which might be expected to improve following successful restoration of coronary blood flow to the ischemic myocardium.

In a study reported by Hinoharo et al (2) this hypothesis was tested. All patients considered for coronary artery bypass grafting who had a contrast left ventricular ejection fraction of less than 40% received a radionuclide ventriculogram the following day. If this study confirmed the low global ejection fraction, the patients were entered into the study. The QRS estimated ejection fraction from a standard 12-lead ECG obtained on the same day was compared with that obtained from the radionuclide study. The ischemia index was determined by subtracting the measured ejection fraction from that estimated by electrocardiogram.

Patients were then recalled 6 weeks following their coronary artery bypass grafting to repeat the radionuclide ventriculogram.

As seen from the figure, patients could be divided into those with a 0 or negative value for ischemia index, a +1% to +10% index, and a >+10% index. The former showed a mean decrease of 7% in left ventricular ejection fraction, in the second group there was no significant change, and the third group had a mean increase of 4%. Indeed, there was correlation of R = 0.64 when the ischemia index was compared to the change in global left ventricular ejection fraction between the pre- to post-operative studies.

This study indicates the potential value of the ischemia index in the evaluation of patients for possible revasculization. Further studies are needed to confirm these results. It would also be important that a similar study be performed in patients undergoing PTCA and other catheter based interventional therapies. It would also be helpful to compare this ischemia index with that obtained using various imaging techniques. Patients with a high ischemic index might not only be candidates for reperfusion but might benefit from receiving this on an emergent basis. It is likely that the myocardium is quite seriously iscehmic if it is disfunctioning so markedly that global left ventricular function is diminished. In this unstable condition which has been termed "hibernating myocardium", it is important to intervene before the damage becomes irreversible.

References

1. Palmeri ST, Harrison DG, Cobb FR, Morris KG, Harrell FE, Ideker RE, Selvester RH, Wagner GS. A QRS scoring system for assessing left ventricular function after myocardial infarction. *N Engl Med* 1982;306:4-9.

2. Hinohora T, Wagner NB, Cobb FR, Coleman ER, Pope JE, Haisty WK, Wagner GS. An ischemic index from the electrocardiogram to select patients with low left ventricular ejection fraction for coronary artery bypass grafting. *Am J Cardiol* 1988;61:288-291.

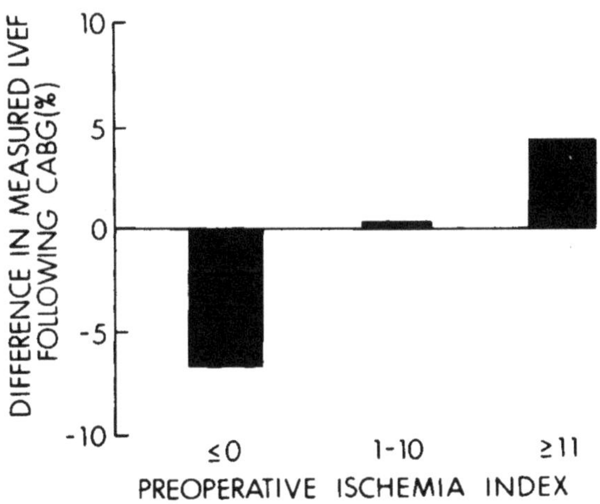

A NEURAL NETWORK SYSTEM BASED ON A MEDICAL QUESTIONNAIRE FOR THE EARLY DIAGNOSIS OF HEART DISEASE

Zeping Shen, Malcolm Clarke, Russell W Jones, Thea Alberti

Department of Electrical Engineering, Brunel University
Uxbridge, Middlesex, UB8 3PH, U.K.

Abstract

A neural network applied to self-applied medical questionnaire data has been investigated for the early diagnosis of heart disease. The data from 28 patients, 14 with confirmed heart disease, and 14 without were chosen as training and test patterns. An encouraging result was obtained when the network was tested using the "leave-1-out" technique and gave confidence to use the trained network on data from a further 50 patients. In this group, 12 people were detected high risk, of which 3, on closer examination, were found to have heart disease.

1. Introduction

Heart disease is a major killer which causes 30% of deaths each year in the U.K. Many of these might be preventable if the disease could be diagnosed early enough. Our work seeks to determine if data obtained by self-applied questionnaire can be used to diagnose the presence of heart disease and perhaps predict those at high risk of developing the disease.

Two prediction methods have received considerable attention: Bayesian analysis, which is based on conditional probability; and expert systems, which are based on rules. Bayesian analysis computes the relative likelihood of different diagnoses using the conditional probability of individual items of patients information. This form of analysis requires a large database of patient information and assumes information to be statistically independent, which is not the case, as symptoms often arise from the same underlying cause[1]. Expert systems are rule-based systems dependant on human experts. However, in practice, these systems are found to be deficient, as the rules may be incorrect, though most often the problem is identifying the rules which describe expert intuition, and the systems are unable to cope with diverse exceptions[2].

Neural networks have properties that overcome the problems associated with Bayesian analysis and expert systems, they learn by example (no rules are required), can work on incomplete data, (a case not handled well by the other two methods), and can make intuitive decisions using patterns of data not previously encountered (thus handling exceptions well). These are ideal qualities for processing medical data, which are often subjective, imprecise and incomplete.

Neural networks have been used in a number of medical areas, for example, recognition of abnormal electrocardiograms and recognition of cause of abdominal pain. However, these studies have all been based on clinical data or clinically derived data. For our study, we have used data from a self-applied questionnaire, which seeks to assess the complete state of health of a patient, including life style, family history of disease, stress, and working conditions. The aim is to assess the current state of health of the individual, and then make a prediction of that person's risk of having the disease, or of developing the disease. The patient may then be offered appropriate instruction and treatment or be referred for further investigation.

Our work has been based on data from a self-applied questionnaire, comprising 360 questions, covering 12 areas (13 for woman) of medical interest. There were 78 participants included in the study, 14 of whom had confirmed heart disease (HD) at the start of the study, the remainder had no medical history of the disease (NHD). From those, 14 NHD patterns were selected to match the 14 HD patterns. These 28 patterns were later used for network training and test. The accuracy of the system was determined by the leave-1-out test, and the jack-knife test. Early results proved promising, and the trained network was then applied to the remaining 50 patients data who had no heart disease according to information given in the questionnaires.

2. An Application of a Back Propagation Network

For initial study, we have chosen a back propagation neural network with three layers (see Fig.1). A data set of the 12 most relevant questions pertinent to heart disease were assembled using a selection criterion designed to maximise the discriminative properties of the set. These were the 12 input nodes. The output layer had one node, which indicated the presence or absence of heart disease with a value of 1 or 0 respectively.

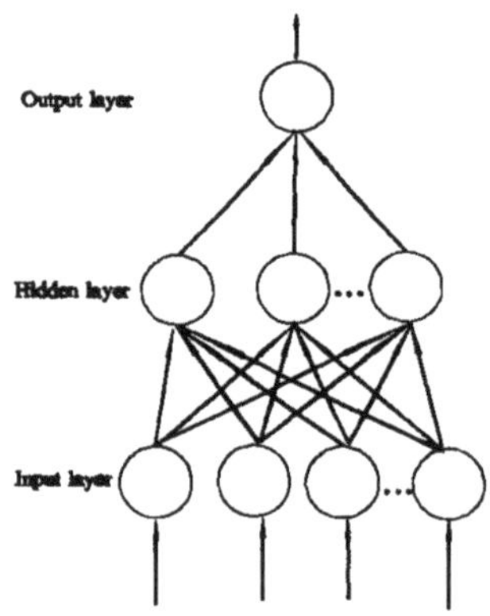

Fig.1 A basic structure of BP network

The number of hidden nodes in a neural network is critical, too few and the network is inaccurate, too many and training time becomes excessive. The behaviour of 2, 4, 6, 8, 10, and 12 hidden nodes was investigated using a ROC (Relative Operating Characteristic) study[3] with the threshold (learning criterion) set to 0.3. A network with 8 hidden nodes was found to be optimum, being the fastest to reach the criterion (see Fig.2) and gave the largest area under the ROC curve (see Fig.3). This also happened to give the largest area obtainable with the test patterns even with continued learning to a smaller threshold. Networks with greater than 8 hidden nodes required significantly more learning iterations to obtain the same size ROC area. However since the verification test only indicates the quality of learning after a specific number of learning iterations, it cannot measure the accuracy of an exhaustively trained network, because a fully trained network can always classify correctly the entire training set. It is more instructive to measure the accuracy of a trained network on unseen data.

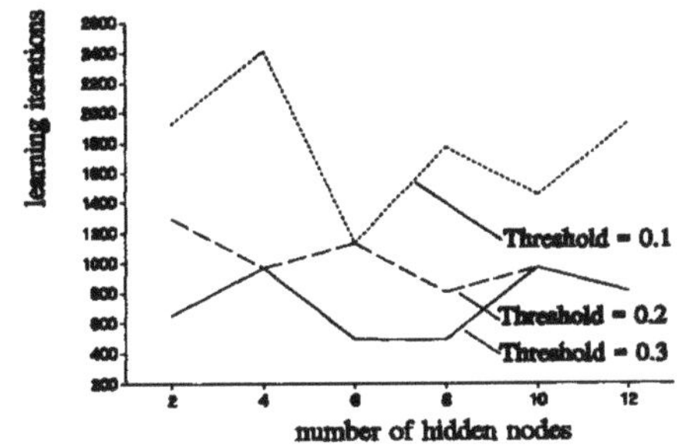

Fig.2 Learning speed with different hidden nodes

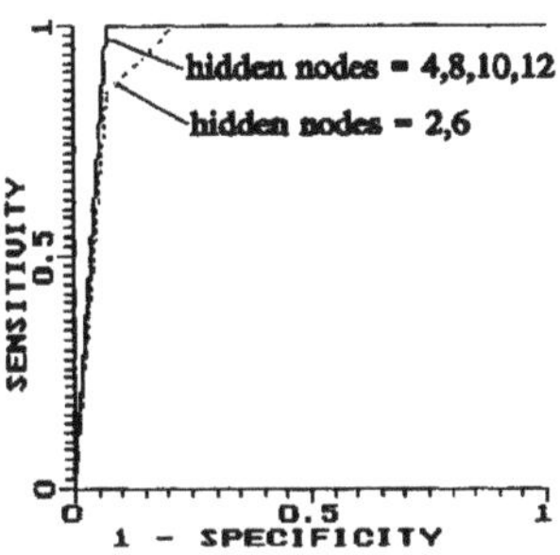

Fig.3 ROC curves for different number of hidden nodes in one hidden layer convergence criterion = 0.3

A network with 12 input nodes, 1 output node and 8 hidden nodes was trained, and was tested using two methods, "leave-1-out" and "jack-knife". The former is useful when there is a lack of training patterns, as in our case. The latter is more useful for comparative tests. For the "leave-1-out" method, the network was trained using randomly ordered patterns from 26 out of the 28 training subjects (13 HD and 13 NHD). When trained, the network was tested using the remaining 1 pair subjects (1 HD and 1 NHD). This procedure could be repeated using every combination of 1 HD patients and 1 NHD patients, but we restricted it to only 14 example cases, which was found to be sufficient to give a measure of the accuracy of the training. For the second method, the 28 patterns were split into two equally sized groups (containing 7 HD and 7 NHD). The network was then trained using one group, and the other was used as test patterns. This is the "jack-knife-test".

Delta learning rule and sigmoid transfer function[4] were employed during training.

3. Results

ROC curves for comparison of the two methods are shown in figure 4. The leave-1-out method gives better performance since it is trained on more patterns.

We applied the trained networks with leave-1-out method to the remaining 50 patients to evaluate their risk factor. Using a threshold of 0.5, above being considered high risk, and below as low risk, 12 people were found to be at high risk of having heart disease. On closer examination, 3 of these were found to have completed the questionnaire incorrectly, and although had answered that they did not have heart disease, were in fact known to have the disease. Of the other 9 patients, closer examination of an exercise ecg stress test, and a 24 hour ambulatory ecg recording, showed that 8 of them had significant ST segment changes, suggestive of heart disease, though at present all are asymptomatic and must remain classified as having no disease. The remaining 1 had normal test results.

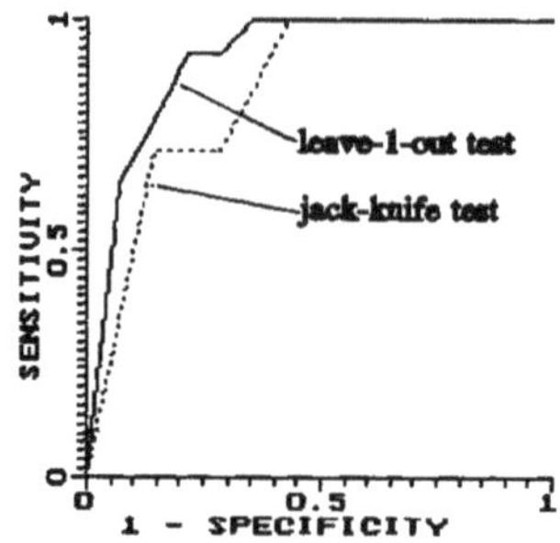

Fig.4 ROC curves for "leave-1-out" test and "jack-knife" test
convergence criterion = 0.05
hidden nodes = 8

4. Conclusions

Neural networks show considerable promise for early diagnosis of heart disease. Self-applied questionnaires have been shown to be a useful way to obtain medical data for the further study of certain kinds of disease. However, we are unable to make conclusions on the accuracy of the system at this stage, and the patients will have to be followed for a number of years within the practice population for cardiac episodes. Having sufficient training patterns is one of the crucial factors for ensuring the performance of the network and gaining more confidence before applying the network in practice.

5. References

1. D.G.Bounds, P.J.Lloyd and B.G.Mathew, *A Comparison of Neural Networks and Other Pattern Recognition Approaches to the Diagnosis of Low Back Disorders*, Neural Network (1990) p.583-591.
2. R.Poli, S.Cagnoni, R.Livi, G.Coppini and G.Valli, *A Neural Network Expert System for Diagnosing and Treating Hypertension*, IEEE Computer (1991).
3. N.Asada, K.Doi H.MacMahon and S.Montner, *Neural network approach for diagnosis of interstitial lung disease*, SPIE **Vol.1233** Medical Imaging IV:Image Processing (1990) p45.
4. Neuralware,Inc., *Reference Guide, NeuralWorks Professional II/plus and NeuralWorks Explorer* (1991) p.184 and p.195.
5. P.K.Simpson, *Artificial Neural Systems*, Pergamon Press Inc. (1990).
6. A.J.Maren, C.T.Harston and R.M.Pap, *Handbook of Neural Computing Applications*, Academic Press Inc. (1990).
7. J.L. McClelland and D.E.Rumelhart, *Explorations in Parallel Distributed Processing (A Handbook of Models, Programs and Exercises)*, The MIT Press (1988).
8. K.Saito and R.Nakano, *Medical Diagnosis Expert System Based on PDP Model*, IEEE International Conference on Neural Networks (1988).

HIGH RESOLUTION ECGs

Edward J. Berbari, Ph.D.
Department of Medicine
University of Oklahoma Health Sciences Center
921 Northeast 13th Street
Oklahoma City, Oklahoma 73104, USA

Paul Lander, Ph.D.
Department of Medicine
University of Oklahoma Health Sciences Center
921 Northeast 13th Street
Oklahoma City, Oklahoma 73104, USA

ABSTRACT

The high resolution ECG is used primarily to record cardiac late potentials. The methodology is heavily dependent upon computerized processing including signal averaging, digital filtering, and automatic detection algorithm. Examples of changes in late potentials as a function of lead and bandwidth are shown. Statistically monitoring the averaging process can also provide a means of quality control which is often lacking in signal averaged studies. The noise function calculated from the signal variance can be used as a tool to ensure that the estimate provided by the signal average is reliable.

INTRODUCTION

High resolution electrocardiography (HRECG) implies an enhanced view of the electrical activity of the heart when compared to the standard ECG. In order to maintain perspective this requires an increased resolution for both the time and voltage axis. In the case of the latter an increased recording gain will also increase the noise into the system. Signal averaging has been used for almost 20 years in electrocardiography as a means of improving the signal to noise ration (SNR) for the purpose of recording low level signals[1,2]. Applications of this technology have included recordings of His-Purkinje potentials[1-3], AV node potentials[4], and cardiac late potentials[5-8]. The latter are, of course, the most common application of the signal averaged HRECG and will be the focus of this paper.

There are two major concerns in using the HRECG. The first is a proper understanding of the technology and the second is the proper application of the technology in the clinical setting. This paper will concentrate on the first aspect because without a technically good HRECG study it will be clinically useless. Finally, there is a discussion about the current problems and future directions of the HRECG.

METHODS

This paper will review the typical approach for obtaining a high resolution ECG and critically examine these methods in light of recent work. A detailed review of methodology can be found in a recent publication[9]. Specifically, this report will concentrate on leads, the vector magnitude transformation, filters, and noise measurements. Most HRECG approaches for identifying late potentials rely on using anatomically orthogenal bipolar XYZ leads. Initially this may have been due to limitations of both hardware and software. Additionally, these leads are often combined into a vector magnitude defined as $(X^2 + Y^2 + Z^2)^{1/2}$. The XYZ lead is spatially limited as the use of such leads have only theoretical advantages in a noiseless recording environment and when the cardiac generator could be considered a true dipole. In practice neither of these conditions are true and both theoretical and practical results have demonstrated that the QRS duration (including late potentials) will be significantly underestimated in the vector magnitude[10]. Thus, it is best to measure late potential parameters from the individual XYZ leads rather than the vector magnitude. This raises another important point: Are three leads adequate for recording all late potential information from the body surface? Several studies have shown that a signal averaged array of body surface leads will reveal late potentials distributed over the body surface[11-12]. In some cases the QRS duration is longest in leads other than the XYZ leads. The role of high pass frequency seems to be less important than the method of implementation. For example, the work of Simpson[6] demonstrated that certain reverse time filters improved the identification of the end of the late potential signals by minimizing the filter artifacts which distort the late potentials. Other filters, such as spectral shaping filters or finite impulse response filters are also valuable in limiting this distortion while also minimizing artifactual distortion in the central portion of the QRS[13-14].

In addition to these approaches for obtaining the HRECG and its analysis, it is important to evaluate the signal averaging method itself in order to ensure the validity of the average[15]. The aim of signal averaging is to increase the signal to noise ratio by reducing noise. As such, it is possible to measure the degree of noise reduction during averaging and use this result as a means of providing a quality control tool for an otherwise statistical estimation procedure.

EXAMPLES

The effects of different high pass filters on both the vector magnitude and the individual XYZ leads are shown in figure 1 which has 6 panels. Panels A, B and C show the vector magnitude filtered at 25, 40 and 80 Hz respectively. Panels D, E and F show the XYZ leads filtered at these same frequencies. The QRS offset in panel A is 5 msec shorter than that seen in the Z lead of panel D. This demonstrates again the shorter QRS duration inherent in the vector magnitude. Panel B obtained after 40 Hz filtering indicates a total loss of late potential identification in the vector while they are still seen in the Z lead in panel E. This demonstrates the loss of late potentials due to the vector transformation. At 80 Hz (panels C and F) the late potentials are lost in both presentations and is due to the excessive filtering.

Figure 2 is a noise curve calculated by a previously described method[15]. It is based on the calculation of the signal variance at the same time the signal average is calculated. When the square root of the variance is taken and divided by the number of beats one arrives at an estimate of the noise in the average. After about 30-50 beats this estimate should approach the $1/\sqrt{n}$ reduction expected by signal averaging. If a non-stationary event occurs, e.g., the patient moves or coughs, the noise curve will reflect this. The subject was asked to move briefly during the data acquisition and is seen in figure 5. The abrupt change at about beat 200 indicates this minor positional change and demonstrates the value of noise estimation during signal averaging.

CONCLUSION

The high resolution ECG has proven to be a powerful tool for identifying reentrant substrates and hence those patients most prone to ventricular tachycardia and sudden death following a myocardial infarction.

Several factors can influence the quality of a signal averaged ECG. No study has established an optimal lead set. The XYZ leads spatially undersample the late potential information as demonstrated by body surface mapping studies. The vector magnitude transformation causes a reduction in the signal to noise ratio and should be used in conjunction with individual XYZ lead analysis. Digital high pass filters which minimally distort the QRS onset and offset as well as central portions of the QRS are preferred. Analog filters will unduly distort the end of the QRS complex. Finally, the on-line measurement of noise based upon the signal averaging process will provide the best estimates of noise. Calculating the noise function can optimize the averaging process and provide a quality control tool for the average itself. Future studies should aim to determine the dynamic character of late potentials, the measurement of ECG indices in diseases other than coronary artery disease, and the natural history of late potentials.

REFERENCES

1. E.J. Berbari, R. Lazzara, P. Samet, and B.J. Scherlag, *Circulation* **48** (1973) 1005.
2. N.C. Flowers, R.C. Hand, P.C. Orander, C.B. Miller, M.O. Walen, and L.G. Horan, *Am. J. Cardiol.* **32** (1974) 384.
3. E.J. Berbari, B. J. Scherlag, N. El-Sherif, B. Befeler, J.M. Aranda, and R. Lazzara, *Circulation* **54** (1976) 219.
4. E.J. Berbari, B.J. Scherlag, and R. Lazzara, *Am. J. Physiol.* **235** (1978) H110.
5. E.J. Berbari, B.J. Scherlag, R.R. Hope, and R. Lazzara, *Am. J. Cardiol.* **41** (1978) 697.
6. M.B. Simson, *Circulation* **64** (1981) 235.
7. J.J. Rozanski, D. Mortara, R.J. Myerburg, and A. Castellanos, *Circulation* **63** (1981) 1172.
8. G. Breithardt, R. Becker, L. Seipel, R.R. Abendroth, and J. Ostermeyer, *Eur. Heart J.* **2** (1981) 1.
9. E.J. Berbari, *CRC Critical Reviews in Biomedical Engineering* **16** (1988) 67.
10. P. Lander, R.B. Deal, E.J. Berbari, *IEEE Trans. Biomed. Engr.* **35** (1988) 629.
11. E.J. Berbari, L. Ozinga, and D. Albert, in *Computers in Cardiology*, (IEEE Computer Society Press, Los Angeles, 1986).
12. K. Nakai, M. Syobuzawa, C. Itoh, T. Miyakawa, M. Kato, T. Onishi, H. Kasanuki, and S. Hosoda, *Angiology* **41** (1990) 639.
13. E.J. Berbari, W.M. Jackman, K.J. Friday, *Circulation* **74** (1986) II-52.
14. P. Lander, E.J. Berbari, *J. Electrocard.* **22(suppl)** (1989) 7.
15. E.J. Berbari, S.M. Collins, R. Arzbaecher, *IEEE Trans. Biomed. Engr.* **33** (1986) 922.

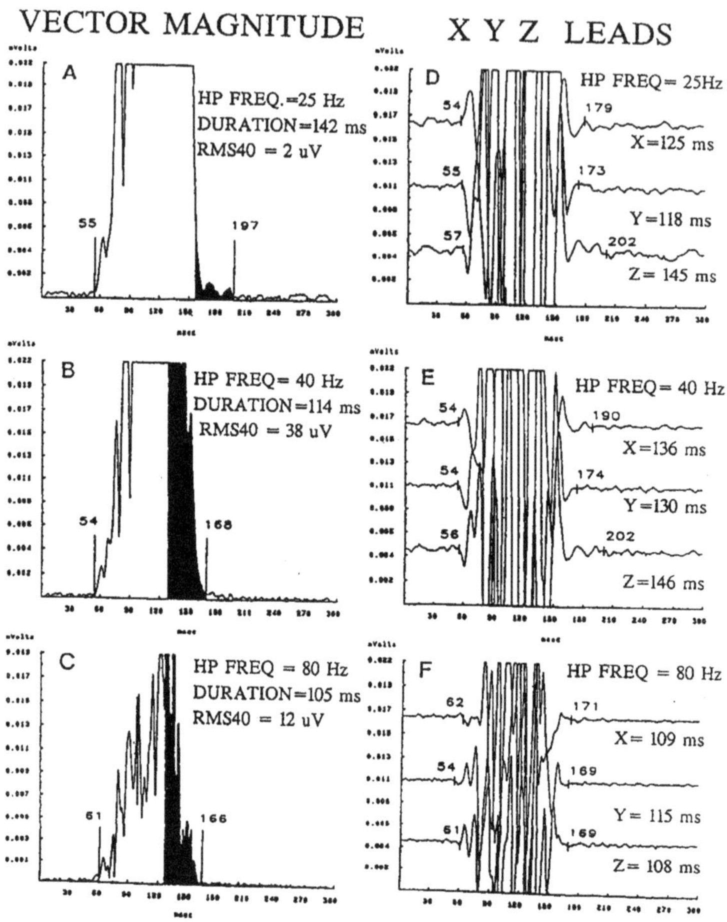

FIGURE 1

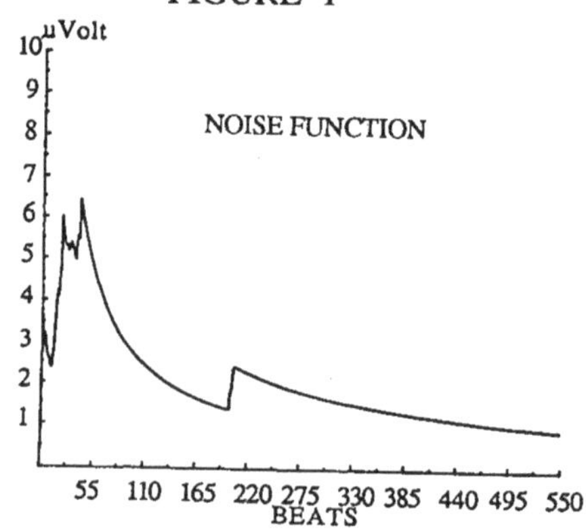

FIGURE 2

KALMAN FILTERING FOR AVERAGING OF ECG SIGNAL

JACEK ŁĘSKI
MEDEA Corp., Kormoranow 17/4, 44-100 Gliwice, Poland.

ABSTRACT

Signal averaging is a very common method for noise reduction in ECG signal processing. The stationarity of noise is usually assumed but for example muscle noise and motion artifacts are not stationary. This results in rather bad performance of the averaging process. Our new method based on the Kalman filter theory provides variance of noise in averaged beat that is less than in the traditional method always when the noise is not stationary. The method is especially suitable for noisy ECG signal such as from exercise tests, from monitoring and for late potentials and His bundle activation potentials processing.

1. INTRODUCTION

Noise reduction is a first step in every ECG signal processing system. Accuracy of all later measurements depends on the quality of noise reduction algorithms. This is why the improvement of the noise reduction part of a signal processing system is of practical importance. ECG signal is quasiperiodical and therefore an averaging in time domain is used very often. The signal averaging in time domain leads to noise reduction factor not better than $\sqrt{N}$, where N is the number of averaged beats. The assumption is that the noise is white, stationary and not correlated with the signal. In fact most kinds of noise are not stationary [2].

2. METHOD PRESENTATION

We employ the following model of the ECG signal

$$\begin{cases} \underline{x}(k+1) = \underline{x}(k) & \text{message model} \quad (1) \\ \underline{z}(k) = \underline{x}(k)+\underline{v}(k) & \text{observation model} \quad (2) \end{cases}$$

where: $\underline{v}(k)$ - random noise disturbing the k-th ECG beat

$\underline{z}(k)$ - measurable ECG signal of the k-th beat

$$\underline{x}(k)=\begin{bmatrix} x_1(k) \\ x_2(k) \\ \cdot \\ x_c(k) \\ \cdot \\ x_j(k) \end{bmatrix}$$ - noise free ECG signal of the k-th beat (nonrandom value)

$\underline{x}(k)$ is the state vector for the k-th beat.

$x_1(k),\ldots,x_j(k)$ are the subsequent samples of the signal which belong to the k-th beat.

$x_c(k)$ is the sample where the FP was found.

We assume that all beats belong to the same class of normal beats - aberrant beats are excluded, signal does not change from cycle to cycle and signal is corrupted with the zero mean and uncorrelated in subsequent beats noise.

$$E\,[\underline{v}(k)] = \underline{0} \quad (3)$$

$$E\,[\underline{v}^T(k)\underline{v}(l)] = I\;R(k)\;\delta_{k,l} \quad (4)$$

$\delta_{k,l}$ denotes the Kronecker symbol

Now we can employ the known Kalman filter equations [1]:

$$\hat{x}(k+1/k+1) = \hat{x}(k/k) + K(k+1)\tilde{z}(k+1) \quad (5)$$

estimate of the k+1-th beat

$$\tilde{z}(k+1) = z(k+1) - \hat{x}(k/k) \qquad \text{innovation process} \quad (6)$$

$$K(k+1) = \frac{P(k/k)}{P(k/k) + R(k+1)} \qquad \text{the gain of the Kalman filter} \quad (7)$$

$$P(k+1/k+1) = [1- K(k+1)]\;P(k/k) \qquad \text{variance of the estimation error} \quad (8)$$

$$V_{\tilde{z}}(k+1) = P(k/k) + R(k+1) \qquad \text{variance of the innovation proces} \quad (9)$$

For simplicity and without loss of generality we

consider one sample of the k-th beat only. This means that we deal with one sample from each beat, i.e. samples equally apart from the appropriate FPs. This is why we use scalar values instead of vector ones in equations (5) to (9).

Since we are going to compare the new averaging method with the conventional one we must present both of them.

According to the conventional averaging the estimate $\hat{x}(k)$ equals:

$$\hat{x}(k+1) = \frac{1}{k+2} \sum_{i=0}^{k+1} z(i) = \frac{1}{k+2} \left[\sum_{i=0}^{k} z(i) + z(k+1) \right] \tag{10}$$

Since

$$\hat{x}(k) = \frac{1}{k+1} \sum_{i=0}^{k} z(i) \qquad \text{so:}$$

$$\hat{x}(k+1) = \frac{1}{k+2} \left[(k+1)\,\hat{x}(k) + z(k+1)\right] = \left(1 - \frac{1}{k+2}\right)\hat{x}(k) + \frac{1}{k+2}\, z(k+1) = \hat{x}(k) + \frac{1}{k+2}\left[z(k+1) - \hat{x}(k)\right] \tag{11}$$

If we compare equations (5) and (6) with (11) we can find that conventional averaging can be seen as a special case of the Kalman filter applied to the signal modeled with the equations (1) and (2) when the gain $K(k+1)$ of the Kalman filter equals $1/(k+2)$. The $K(k+1)$ is the weighting factor for the k+1-th beat in estimate $\hat{x}(k+1/k+1)$ by the new method. This is also the weighting factor for all beats in conventional averaging.

Using equations (5) to (9) one can obtain optimal estimate of the signal $x(k)$ in the sense of minimum estimation variance. This method is always better than the conventional one when the noise is not stationary. The weighting factors are optimal on condition that the actual variances of noise in beats are known. It is impossible to measure them. So, estimate of that variance is of great importance. We find $\hat{R}(k+1)$ using variance of the innovation process [3]:

$$V_{\tilde{z}}(k+1) = \frac{1}{j} \sum_{i=1}^{j} [\tilde{z}_i(k+1)]^2 \qquad (12)$$

where $\tilde{z}_i(k)$ is the i-th sample of the k-th beat of the innovation process.

We use all the samples from the beat to compute the estimate of the innovation process in that beat. We assume that the baseline drift is removed. From equation (9) we obtain:

$$\hat{R}(k+1) = V_{\tilde{z}}(k+1) - P(k/k) \qquad (13)$$

3. CONCLUDING REMARKS

The just presented method of signal averaging offers significant improvement of ECG signal quality, especially when applied to exercise systems where noise is not stationary. It is not sensitive, in contrary to the conventional method, to artifacts that affect signal morphology. The unbiased estimator guarantees that the signal is not distorted.

When the noise has non Gaussian distribution our estimate is not optimal but it is still the best from all linear estimators [1].

The method was successfully applied in our new commercial Medea Stress Testing System and Medea Late, Early and P-wave μpotentials analysis system.

4. REFERENCES

1.B.D.O.Anderson,J.B.MOORE, Optimal Filtering,(Prentice-Hall, Inc.London,1979).

2.O.Y.De Vel,R-Wave Detection in the Presence of Muscle Artifacts, IEEE Trans. Bio. Eng.,Vol BME-31, no.11.(1984)

3.K.A.Mayers,B.D.Tapley, Adaptive sequential estimation with unknown noise statistics, IEEE Trans.Autom. Con., Vol. AC-21, No.4. (1976).

UTILIZATION OF PROBABILISTIC EXPERT SYSTEM FOR VCG DATA CLASSIFICATION

DAGMAR VALOVA
Institute of Physiological Regulations, Czechoslovak Academy of Sciences, FNsP Bulovka, pavilon 11, Prague Czech and Slovak Federal Republic

and

ZDENEK DRSKA, ANNA MALKOVA
Institute of Physiological Regulations, Czechoslovak Academy of Sciences, FNsP Bulovka, pavilon 11, Prague Czech and Slovak Federal Republic

ABSTRACT
This paper deal with our experiences with utilization of probabilistic expert system for VCG classification. Correct classification of studied groups was found equal to 84.2 %, 79.5 %, 83.3 % in data recorded at early recovery period after exercise test.

1. Introduction

In practice mubh of the information obtained from experts as well as data provided by users are not known with certainty. The exact processing of uncertain information is the important assumption of successful expert system application, especially in medicine where a great number of less informative parameters is necessary to evaluate.

For solution of VCG signal interpretation problem the probabilistic expert system was chosen. It enables to express the uncertainty by probability distribution, the resultant diagnoses admit more possibilities with different weights.

2. Material and methods

Probabilistic expert system can be viewed as a memoryless information channel with noise. The aim of a probabilistic expert system is to derive the marginal probabilities of goals from a given knowledge base and marginal probabilities of questions.(4,5)

This expert system exhibits followed suitable properties:

1. Uncertainty is expressed by probabilistic distribution in the histogram form which could be estimated from data files or suggested heuristically.
2. Knowledge base is represented by a set of conditional distributions having the form of finite mixtures of product components.
3. The evaluating procedure is possible to use on incomplete data file.
4. The variables may be continuous, discrete or logical.
5. Probabilistic expert system can be realized on PC XT/AT computers.

For testing this probabilistic expert system as model study in electrocardiology the application for three group classification was used. A group of 76 healthy subjects, a group of 161 patients with old myocardial infarction and a group of 36 patients with angina pectoris without old myocardial infarction were investigated. The VCG data of all these three groups were recorded at rest and at early recovery period after exercise test. The VCG data were measured by Frank lead system.

Many years ago a program Kardio for quantitative evaluation of VCG signal has been developed in our institute(1). By this program the original set of 106 parameters is obtained. Characteristic points on module, curvature and velocity curve, time and space characteristics of VCG loops are represented by these parameters. The set of these parameters could be subdivided into two groups :

1. Local characteristic of VCG
2. Interval characteristic of VCG

Thousands of patient's records supplied with results of cardiological investigation has been studied that's why we have decided to use VCG data for clasiffication.

The method for selection of the best predictors utilizes followed criteria:

1. maximal frequency for correct classification
2. maximal share between correct component frequency and the frequency of the others.

This method leads to reduction of the input space dimension on its half, so 53 parameters were used.

The classification was made by statistical jackknifed method - it means that evaluated patient was not included in knowledge base.

3. Results

Correct classification for healthy subjects was found equal to 57.9 %, for patients with old myocardial infarction equal to 81.4 % and for patients with angina pectoris to 88.8 % in data recorded at rest and respectively 84.2 %, 79.5 %, 83.3 % in data recorded at early recovery period after exercise test. Complete classification results are summarized in the table I./a,b/

Table I.:
Summary of VCG classification by probabilistic expert system (in %)

	H	I	A
B	0.0	0.0	2.8
H	57.9	1.2	2.8
I	7.9	81.4	5.6
A	34.2	17.4	88.8

a) values for the data obtained at rest

	H	I	A
B	0.0	0.0	5.6
H	84.2	6.8	0.0
I	1.3	79.5	11.1
A	14.5	13.7	83.3

b) values for the data obtained at early recovery period after exercise test

B = common background (subject belong to this group when the probabilistic expert system is not able to decided for classification to any other group - its knowledge base is given as a mean of all other groups knowledge bases)
H = healthy subjects
I = subjects with old myocardial infarction
A = subjects with angina pectoris

4. Conclusion

Results of three groups classification using probabilistic expert system were significantly better then results obtained by multiple discriminant analysis (2,3). It was then proved, that chosen probabilistic expert system is suitable for VCG interpretation problem solution and the significant contribution to other cardiology interpretation problem could be expected.

5. References

1. Z. Drska, V. Kral, V. Novak: *Neue Ergebnisse der Electrocardiologie II*. (Gustav Fischer Verlag, Jena 1974), pp. 263-265.
2. Z. Drska, M. Polankova, D. Drozen, V. Kral: *Annales de Cardiologie et d'Ángiologie*, 1990, 30, 4, p. 199-201.
3. Z. Drska, M. Polankova, A. Malkova, D. Drozen: *Abstracts of XVIIth Internat. Congress on Electrocardiology*, Florence, 1990, p. 161.
4. J. Grim: *Pocitace a umela inteligence*. (1988)
5. A. Perez: *Natiowide Scientifical Congress of Biomedical Engineering BMI'83*, Marianske lazne 1983.

THE DISCRIMINATION PARAMETERS OF THE MULTIPOLAR COMPONENTS IN LAHB AND LBBB

BARBARA NOWAK
and
JÓZEF JAGIELSKI

Department of Pathophysiology, Medical Academy
Marcinkowskiego 1, 50-368 Wrocław, Poland

ABSTRACT

In this study electric activity of human heart is represented by multipole expansion. The multipole investigations aim at settling upon the parameters which can be made use of in clinical practice. The multipolar components were represented as a time function corresponding to the QRS complex and the ST section of a conventional electrocardiogram. The revealed differences in LBBB and LAHB in comparison with HS, referring to the curves of the multipolar components (dipolar and quadrupolar), enabled to determine the measurable variables defining the components. The most useful were: the wave surface measurement, the wave duration time and the amplitude.

1. Introduction

The aim of multipolar investigations is to create a set of parameters useful in clinical diagnosis in ventricular conduction abnormalities. For this set of parameters a discriminant function is constructed, which is a linear combination of variables. The function describes diagnostic groups with different levels of conduction disturbance.

2. Materials and Methods

The examination concerned 15 patients with left bundle branch block (LBBB) at the age of 49-72 years and 25 patients with left anterior hemiblock (LAHB) in age range 37-72. The control group included 30 healthy subjects (HS) (age 20-30).

The following procedure was employed to establish diagnostic parameters of the multipolar components [1]:

A. Visual assessment of the curves of multipolar components.
B. Defining the measurable multipolar variables useful in computer analysis.
C. Variables selection criteria
   1) the mean values of selected variables in groups showed statistically significant differences,
   2) the value of the correlation coefficient $r(Y,X_i)$ of the discriminant function Y and each of the variables X_i is statistically significant.
D. Differentiation or separation of the groups examined is based on the value of the discriminant function.

3. Results

A. The results of visual assessment of multipolar curves. The curves of appropriate components of groups LBBB, LAHB and HS were drawn and compared. In each curve, in the QRS complex, two waves can be seen: positive and negative, marked as II and III.
Figure 1 shows three dipolar components.

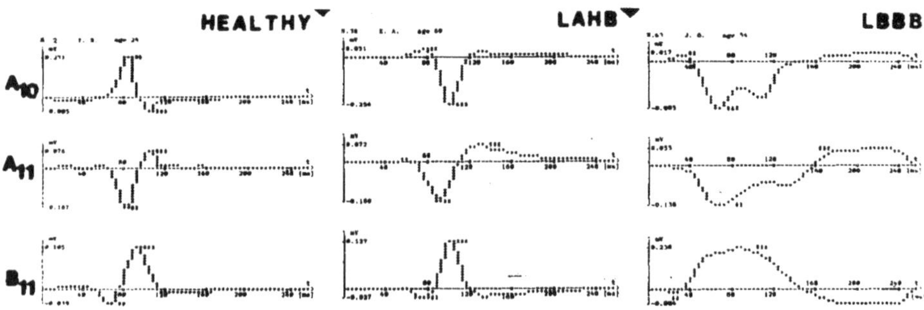

Figure 1. The three dipolar components: A_{10}, A_{11}, and B_{11} in three groups: healthy, left anterior hemiblock and left bundle branch block.

All the three dipolar components A_{10}, A_{11}, and B_{11} display differences in the shape and the sequence of electropositivity and electronegativity of the waves. The most discriminatory dipolar component is A_{10}. Components A_{11} and B_{11} are much less useful in group discrimination. Similarly, the quadrupolar components may distinguish HS from those suffering from LAHB and LBBB. The most discriminatory is A_{20}.

B. Defining measurable variables of multipolar curves.
In the mathematical analysis of the multipolar curves the following variables characterized the waves used (Table 1): duration time, surface, amplitude (parameters 1,2,3,4,5) and their relationships (parameters 6,7).

Table 1. Variables employed for the description of wave II and wave III of multipolar curves, submitted to discriminant analysis.

1. t_{II}, t_{III}	:	duration time of waves II and III respectively.
2. $\sum A_{II}$, $\sum A_{III}$	:	the sum of the curve value of waves II and III (wave surfaces).
3. $\max A_{II}$, $\max A_{III}$	:	wave amplitudes.
4. $\frac{\sum A_{II}}{\max A_{II}}$, $\frac{\sum A_{III}}{\max A_{III}}$	:	wave widths.
5. tA_{II}, tA_{III}	:	duration time of the wave part of the value higher then 1/3 of the amplitude.
6. $\frac{\sum A_{III}}{\sum A_{II}}$	:	absolute value of both surfaces.
7. $\frac{\max A_{III}}{\max A_{II}}$	:	absolute value of both amplitudes.

C,D. Variables selection criteria and group discrimination.
After selecting appropriate variables, described in point C, a special vector composed of 21 variables for each person was established. The discriminant function constructed on the basis of multipolar variables of this vector, differenciates adequately the examined groups. Group discrimination on the basis of values of this function is presented in Figure 2. The horizontal axis represents the persons examined, the vertical axis represents

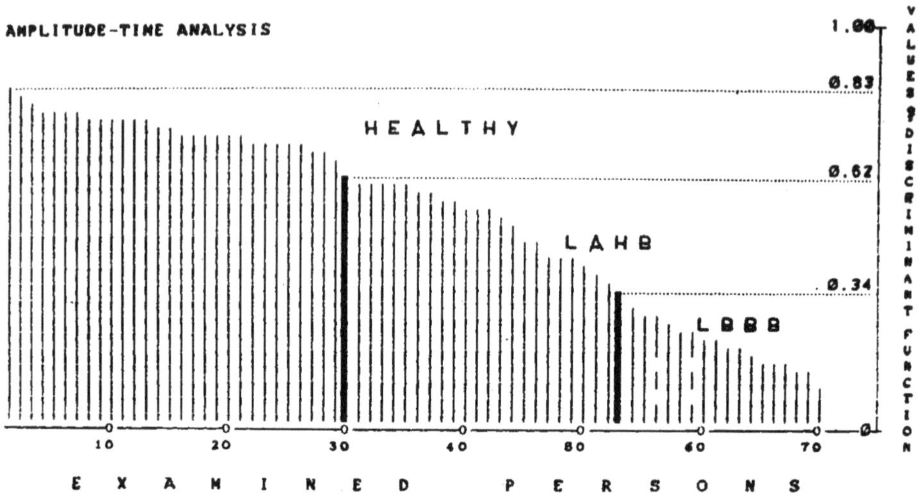

Figure 2. The distribution of persons examined according to values of the discriminant function.

values of the discriminant function and the intervals coressponding to the diagnostic groups. The height of each segment indicates the value of the discriminant function. With this method we were able to separate sharply the two groups: healthy and LAHB. Two patients with LAHB (dashed line) were included in the LBBB group.

4. Conclusions

Components A_{10} and A_{20} are most useful in differenciation the groups examined in visual assessment. The curve of the remaining components do not differ significantly in the two groups: LAHB and healthy. The similarities and differences in the course of all dipolar and quadrupolar components are the basis for defining measurable discriminant variables. To calculate those variables it is enough to examine only fragments of the multipolar curves. The variables represent mainly: surface, duration time and amplitude of QRS complex and ST segment.

5. Reference

1. B.Nowak, Dissertation, (1991), Medical Academy, Wrocław.

BSPD PROCESSING BY MAPPING SYSTEM CARDIAG 128.1

ANNA MALKOVA
Institute of Physiological Regulations,
Czechoslovak Academy of Sciences,
FN Bulovka, pav. 11, 180 85 Prague, CSFR

and

MILENA POLANKOVA, ZDENEK DRSKA, DAGMAR VALOVA
Institute of Physiological Regulations,
Czechoslovak Academy of Sciences,
FN Bulovka, pav. 11, 180 85 Prague, CSFR

ABSTRACT

A new equipment Cardiag 128.1 produced by ZPA Cakovice, Czechoslovakia enables simultaneous recording of standard 12-lead ECGs, VCGs using Frank lead system and matrix of 16x5 ECGs for body surface potential mapping.

Special electrodes set in the form of belts is applied on the sitting patient. Softwear includes analysis of ECGs and VCGs, mapping data are evaluated in the form of isopotential maps, integral maps, isopotential maps of asynchronous maxima or minima, isochronous maps and maps of divergence.

Cardiag is a new PC added ECG diagnostic system which enables simultaneous recording of standard 12-lead ECGs, VCGs using Frank lead system and matrix of 80 ECGs for body surface potential mapping.

Cardiag is composed of an input system, digitalization subsystem, numeric processing subsystem and on line personal computer (Fig. 1.).

The set of electrodes consists of six elastic belts attachable around the patient thorax on which special leads in their holders are fixed. The belt being locked electrodes are in contact with the patient body surface using only water as a contact medium.

The belt above is situated on the level of jugulum, the second one on the level of the second intercostal space and the others are every two intercostal spaces below. The first column is situated in the right mid axillary line, the fifth one on the sternum, the ninth one in the left mid axillary line and the thirteenth column is on the spinal column (Fig. 2.).

Three types of electrodes can be used, electrodes with springs or with cables enable to smooth the disproportionality of patient chest surface. Signal recording is made on the sitting patient.

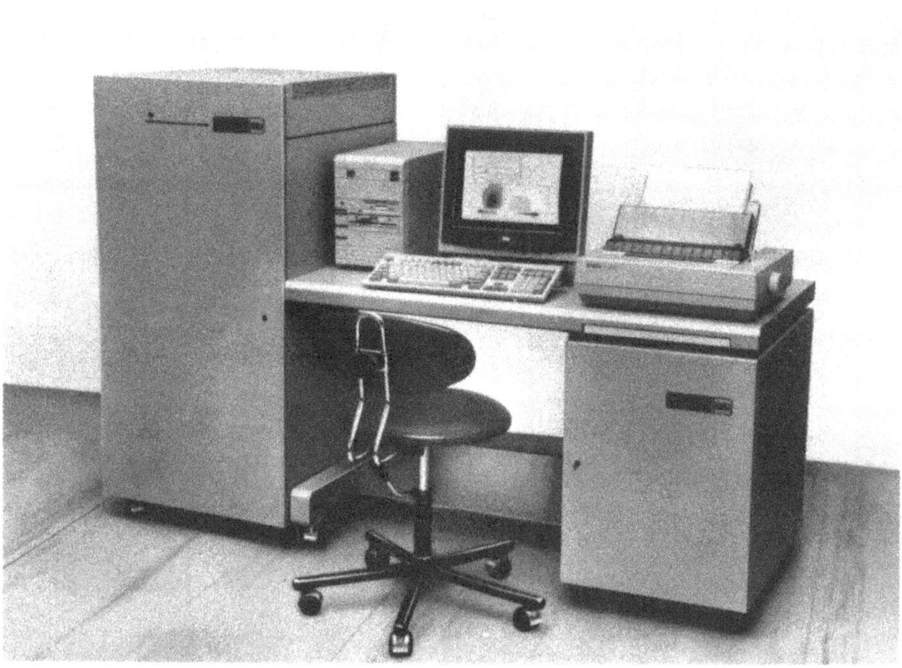

Fig. 1. Cardiag 128.1 is a PC added ECG diagnostic system.

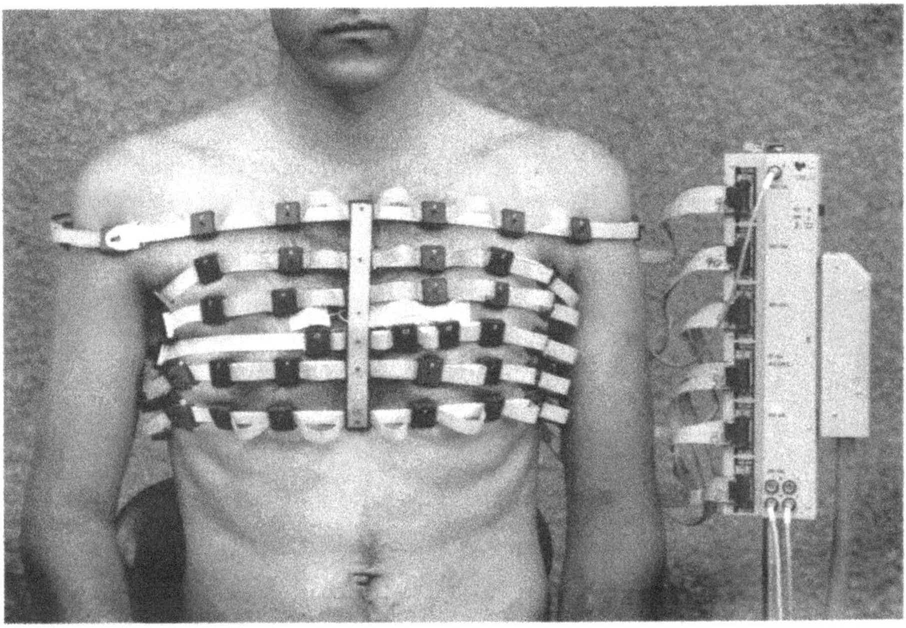

Fig. 2. The scheme of electrodes positions on the chest surface. For further information see text.

Cardiag provides automatic amplitude evaluation of ECG peaks and waves and evaluation of intervals duration. VCG signal can be represented in the form of time curves or loops in frontal, left sagital and transversal planes. Various calculated parameters as size of maximum vectors, maximum space vector angles, average circumference vector velocity etc. can be studied (1).

Matrix of 80 ECGs can be visualized as isopotential maps in selected intervals during atrial depolarization and ventricular depolarization or repolarization (Fig.3.). Special colour table can be used. Negative potentials are in various shades of blue colour, positive potentials are in the scale from yellow to black colour.

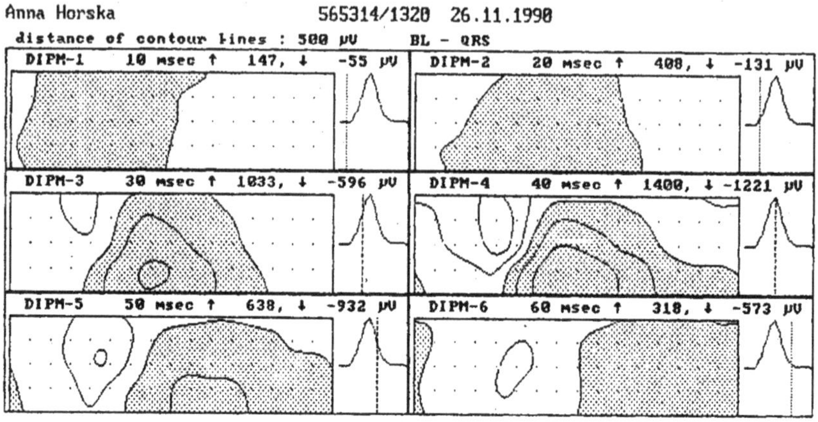

Fig. 3. The set of isopotential maps in 10 ms interval from the onset of QRS in healthy subject. Area of positive potentials is dotted. Interval between isolines is 500 uV. Maximum and minimum potential values are found out.

Maps of negative divergence enable detailed study of potential changes (1).

Integral maps can be visualized from QRS, STT and QT intervals.

Isochronous map of Q wave, integral map of Q wave and map of asynchronous potential minimum of Q wave enable to specify the localization and size of changes in body surface potential distribution (BSPD) of heart electrical field due to myocardial infarction.

In the near future softwear will be completed by programs for quantitative evaluation of maps (departure maps or maps of abnormal depolarization area). Probabilistic expert system for VCG, eventually for BSPD mapping classification of IHD patients, is being developed.

Reference:

1. Stojan, M.: Základy analýzy elektrického srdečního pole pro klinické účely. Praha 1991, printed

THE INITIAL PATIENT SELECTION FOR BODY SURFACE POTENTIAL MAPPING USING THE "MARVEL" SYSTEM

Leslaw Rusiecki, Krystyna Laszki-Szczachor, Dariusz Kalka

Department of Pathophysiology
Medical Academy of Wroclaw
Poland

The main purpose of the examination was a description of the state of electrical activity of heart in health people to make the supervisory group of normal electrocardiograms. In the next step the selected people were examinated in Fukuda Heart Potential Mapping System HPM-7100 to build standards for this group.

The "MARVEL" (Microcomputer Analysing Recorder of Various Electrocardiographic Leads) System was originally developed to run on personal computers and especially to diagnose blocks, axis deviations, ventricular hypertrophies and myocardial infarctions. In the begining of examination all parameters of recording and patient identification data are set manually. Eight bipolar standard leads are measured: two limb (II&III) and six precordial. The ECG signal picked up from the body surface is going by two preamplifiers to the 8-channel amplifier. The output signal is digitized by AD converter with an eleven-bit accuracy and the sampling rate of 500 samples per second for each channel. The data is stored on the hard disc in the wanted format and ready to be processed. Next 8 digital signals are transformed into 12 standard leads using simple mathematical operations. It is possibile to show some of signals (recorded or transformed) on the screen. Using three chosen leads, the function of "spatial acceleration" is built to locating QRS complexes. Recognition of onsets and ends of each of ECG waveforms is made. About 400 parameters are calculated to be useful for logical tree and decision tables for diagnosis.

The diagnostic criteria are based on some rules of Bonner Program. Tests applied to intervals and wave widths are adapted to the way of the pattern recognition and measurement determines such intervales. In the beginning all of preconditions are check to skip or to do each of tests. It is useful to make sure as to a possibility of existing of two different diseases. All results of diagnostic interpretation are stored in the memory to verify once again. The last step is printing of diagnosis with full, partial or condensed (Fig.1) morphological information [1].

In the system more than 70 cases were examinated: about 40 classified as heart disease (confirmed by cardiologists) and 30 normal electrocardiograms. To confirm the initial selection of the second group (normal) the USG examination was made. After that patients were sent to BPM System to make final examinations (Fig.2).

The Heart Potential Mapping for health people in Wroclaw shows an existing 3 types of HPM norms depending of patient constitution and heart position [2].

The "MARVEL" System and user's software were made originally applying both theoretical methods for digital processing of ECG signals and practical knowledge. The system is useful to make initial classification of electrocardiograms before body potential mapping of electrical heart activity and enable to increase effectiveness in routine medical practice.

R e f e r e n c e s:

1. J.Jagielski and K.Laszki-Szczachor and Leslaw Rusiecki, Automatic analysis and diagnostic interpretation of 12 electrocardiographic standard leads, Biosystems,vol.1, ed. J.Jagielski and W.Zmyslowski (Communication Publishers, Warsaw, 1991) p.291-302.
2. D.Kalka, Heart potential maps in electrocardiographic diagnostics. Analysis of HPM in health people (Doctor's dissertation, Medical Academy of Wroclaw, 1992)

Microcomputer Analysing Recorder of
Various Electrocardiographic Leads
"M A R V E L"

Forename:	Krystyna	Ident.No.:	238
Surname:	Krupinska	Age:	24
Adress:	Wroclaw	Reg.date :	03-10-1991
Street:	Borowska 207/6	Time:	10:03:24

Wave	P	P1	Q	R	S	R1	S1	T
Amp. [mV] I	0.24	0.00	-0.30	0.54	-0.44	0.00	0.00	0.16
Amp. [mV] II	0.30	0.00	-0.48	1.38	-0.24	0.00	0.00	0.77
Amp. [mV] III	0.18	0.00	-0.34	1.08	-0.26	0.00	0.00	0.56
Amp. [mV] aVR	-0.26	0.00	-0.79	0.45	-0.47	0.00	0.00	-0.18
Amp. [mV] aVL	-0.24	0.00	-0.20	0.47	-0.42	0.00	0.00	0.12
Amp. [mV] aVF	0.18	0.00	-0.16	1.38	-0.36	0.00	0.00	0.62
Amp. [mV] V1	-0.16	0.00	-0.14	0.78	-1.34	0.00	0.00	-0.31
Amp. [mV] V2	0.18	0.00	0.00	0.82	-1.39	0.00	0.00	0.29
Amp. [mV] V3	0.00	0.00	-0.18	0.86	-1.42	0.00	0.00	0.29
Amp. [mV] V4	0.18	0.00	-0.09	0.83	-1.53	0.00	0.00	-0.32
Amp. [mV] V5	0.16	0.00	0.00	0.79	-1.44	0.00	0.00	-0.32
Amp. [mV] V6	0.16	0.00	-0.09	0.76	-1.32	0.00	0.00	0.28
Intervals [sec]	PQ 0.114	ST 0.034	QT 0.330	PR 0.146	QRS duration: 0.094 sec			

Axis: P= 58°, QRS= 89°, T= 73°, grad.= 68°

Normal sinus rhytm
Heart rate 73 beats per minute

Observe that some of parameters are equal to 0.0 and it doesn't mean it's true but means that diagnostic role of this parameters is insignificant !

NORMAL ELECTROCARDIOGRAM

Fig.1 The output report presented in a short form.

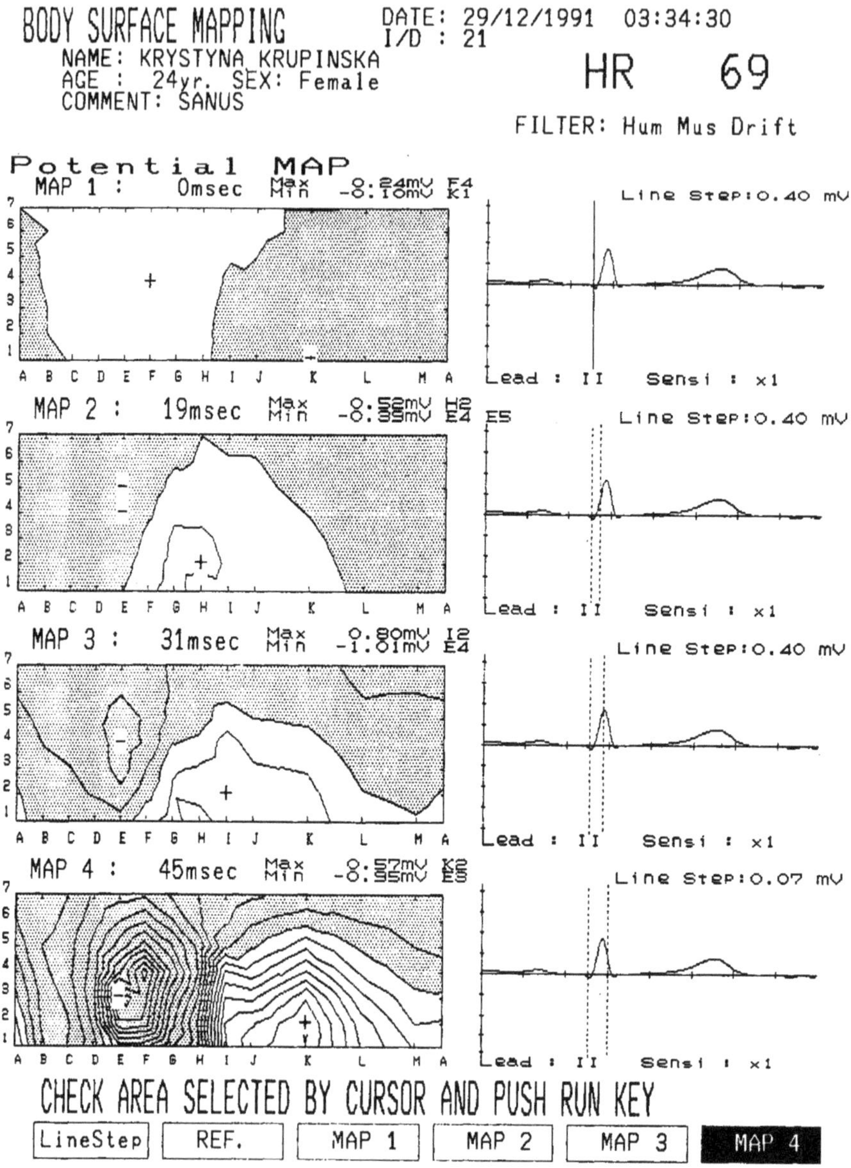

Fig.2 Isopotential maps at 4 stages made after selection in "MARVEL" System.

PART III
Clinical Diagnostics of Body Surface Mapping

BODY SURFACE ISOCHRONE MAPS IN YOUNG NORMAL SUBJECTS

KATARÍNA KOZLÍKOVÁ
Institute of Pathological Physiology, School of Medicine, Comenius University, Bratislava, Czechoslovakia

IVAN HULÍN
Institute of Pathological Physiology, School of Medicine, Comenius University, Bratislava, Czechoslovakia

PETER KNEPPO
Institute of Measurement Science, Slovak Academy of Sciences, Bratislava, Czechoslovakia

PETER POLAKOVIČ
Institute of Computing Technique, Comenius University, Bratislava, Czechoslovakia

ABSTRACT

A new method of displaying heart activation sequence on the body surface has been introduced. It is based on an inverse procedure to the potential mapping.
Electrocardiograms were recorded with the measuring and computing system CardioPC in 24 sites on the whole chest and then reconstructed to 150 point's maps. Body surface isochrone maps during the whole QRS complex were constructed in 89 normal young subjects of both sexes aged 9 to 19 years for the threshold potential of 0.1 mV.
The isochrone maps showed very high similarity in all observed subjects. The activation appeared in the sternal area first of all. The mean time of the earliest appearance was 7 ms after the QRS onset as established from the RMS signal. The activation spread from the sternal area downwards and leftwards to the back where it changed its direction upwards. It usually ended around the right shoulder at the latest mean time of 61 ms after the QRS onset. The mean duration was 55 ms.
An illustration of isochrone maps in myocardial infarction is given to show the obviousness of this kind of maps.

1. Introduction

Body surface mapping of the electrical heart field enables us to obtain the most total information about the electrical conditions of the heart that is nowadays available by noninvasive techniques. However, it is associated with large amount of data that have to be processed and interpreted. Therefore, there have been made some attempts to reduce the number of data using integral maps and several kinds of isochrone maps, e.g. maps displaying the activation time using R wave peaks[1], the duration of R waves[2] or the minimum of the first derivative during the QRS complex[3].

Another type of isochrone maps was briefly introduced in 1984[4]. It is called **isochrone maps with threshold potential** and it allows to display the heart activation sequence on the body surface in a simple but very clear way. A more detailed study has now been made in young normal subjects.

2. Materials and methods

The method of **body surface isochrone maps with threshold potential** is based in principle on an inverse procedure to body surface potential mapping[5]. Firstly, a potential value is chosen that is called the **threshold potential**, either positive or negative. The next step is to search for **the first time instant** in which the electrocardiographic curve **reaches or exceedes** this chosen potential. The **time instant distributions** over the whole chest are then displayed in the isochrone maps.

The described method has been used to study 89 young subjects who were regarded to be normal according to their medical history, physical examination and standard ECG. Their age distribution is listed in Table 1.

Table 1: Studied subjects

Group	Number	Age [y]
Men	23	18 - 19
Boys older	11	13 - 14
younger	6	9 - 10
Women	31	18 - 19
Girls older	14	13 - 14
younger	4	9 - 10

The electrocardiograms were recorded with the measuring and computing system CardioPC[6] according to Barr's system of electrodes[7,8]. The isochrone maps with threshold potential **U = 0.1 mV** were constructed during the **QRS complex**.

3. Results

When comparing the isochrone maps qualitatively very high similarity in all subjects has been observed (Figure 1). The activation always appeared in the sternal area. At first, it extended nearly symmetrically through the anterior chest. After this, the activation spread downwards and leftwards to the back where it changed its direction upwards. It usually ended around the right shoulder.

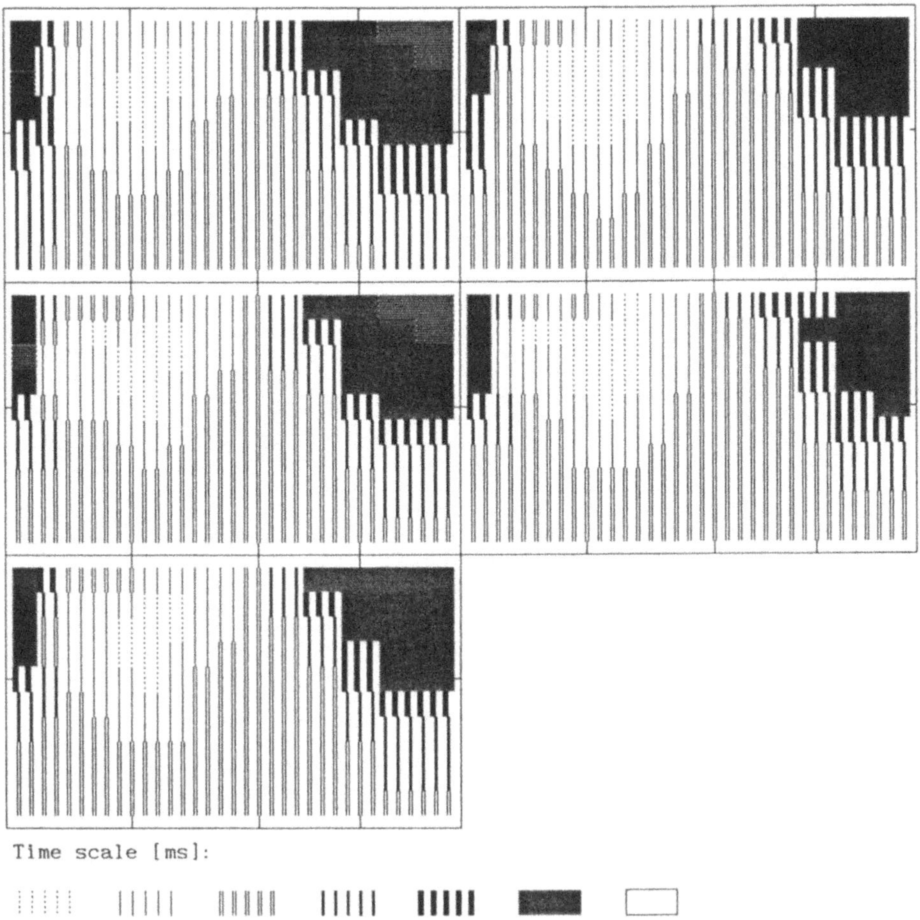

Figure 1: Mean body surface isochrone map with threshold potential U = 0.1 mV in all studied groups.
The map represents the chest from yugulum to umbilicus cut at the right midaxillary line. Short vertical lines display the positions of the sternum, left midaxillary line and spine, respectively. Short horizontal lines mark the 4th intercostal space. From the left to the right, the groups are men, boys, then women ang girls and the last map displays the mean of all studied subjects.

Potentials U ≥ 0.1 mV covered the left anterior chest and the lower left back during the QRS complex in more than 90 % of studied subjects and almost the whole chest in more than 50 % of cases (Figure 2).

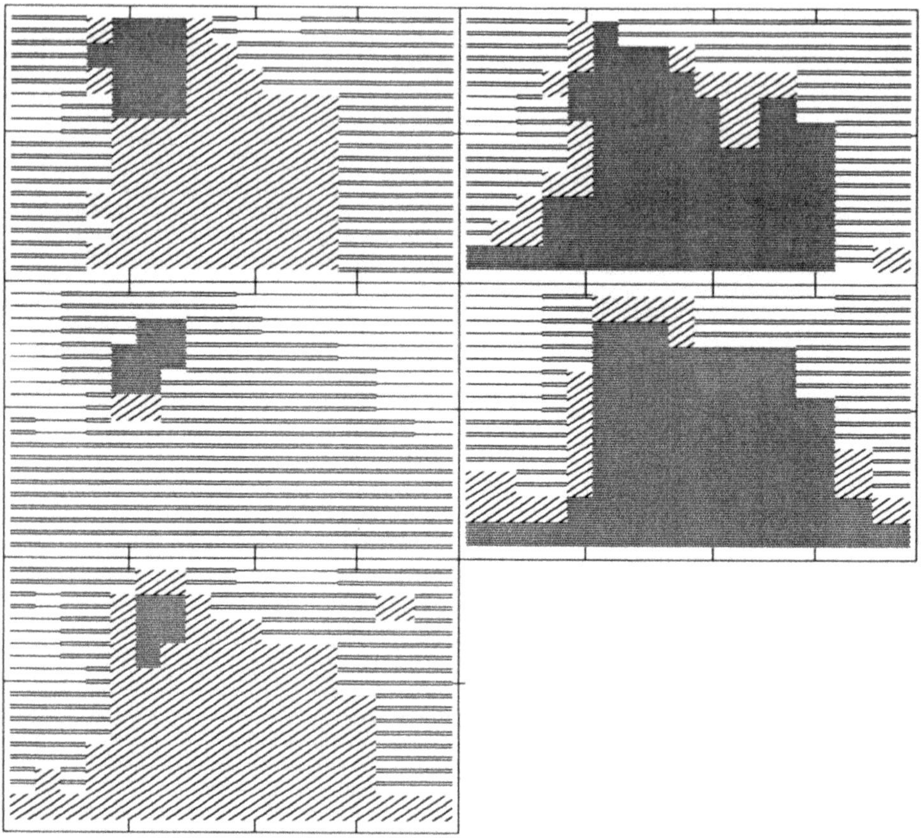

Frequency of appearance [%]:

0 1-10 11-50 51-90 91-99 100

Figure 2: Appearance of potential U ≥ 0.1 mV in body surface isochrone maps of all studied groups during QRS complex
The description of the maps is the same as in previous figure.

The beginning of the activation in the isochrone map is defined as the very first time instant in which the measured potential exceeded the threshold potential regardles of the measurement point. Alike, the end of the activation is the last time instant. The duration of the activation is the difference between them. These characteristics are listed in Table 2.

Table 2: Mean values and standard deviations of beginnings, ends and durations of activation in isochrone maps with U ≥ 100 μV of normal subjects

Group	Beg [ms]	End [ms]	Dur [ms]
M	7.5 ± 2.0	64.5 ± 6.2	58.0 ± 5.3
W	7.0 ± 2.5	59.6 ± 10.3	53.6 ± 8.9
B	6.1 ± 2.1	59.1 ± 6.5	54.1 ± 4.9
G	6.7 ± 1.8	58.2 ± 5.7	52.5 ± 4.4
All	6.9 ± 8.1	60.8 ± 7.5	54.9 ± 6.3

The activation in myocardial patients started in more different areas of the chest and its spread differed very much from normal subjects as illustrated in Figure 3.

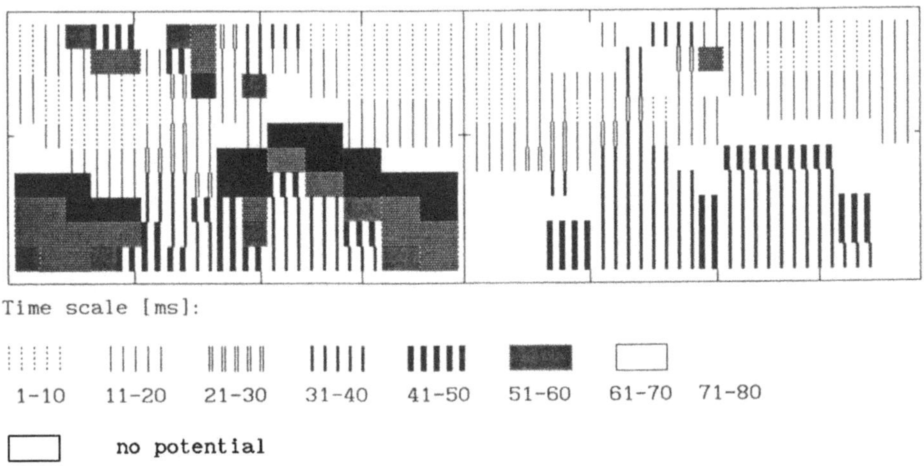

Figure 3: Mean body surface isochrone map with threshold potential U = 0.1 mV in two cases of myocardial infarction
The left panel displays an isochrone map of a 65 years old man with a 6 years old myocardial infarction and the right panel displays an isochrone map of a 63 years old man with a myocardial infarction 2 months old.

4. Discussion and conclusions

These isochrone maps were designed to display the heart activation sequence. We could confirm that this representation of the electrical heart activity doesn't depend on the used lead system as similar results were obtained earlier[9].

The isochrone maps with threshold potential have some advantages. They are simple to construct as they use the same algorithm for positive and negative potentials and for any wave of the electrocardiogram. The algorithm may be also repeated for the same wave.

These maps allow the choice of any level of potential so they can be used even for low level activities that are usually covered by higher potentials. They give us time information and, at the same time, spatial information about the propagation of the electrical heart field. They enable data reduction although the appropriate threshold potential will depend on the application.

The isochrone maps also allow studies of heart activation when using the projection of parts of the heart on the body surface[9,10]. The heart activation has been observed to begin in the septal area, to spread through the apex to the ventricles and to end in the base of the left ventricular wall. These observations are in good agreement with published data[11].

5. Acknowledgments

This research has been supported by the grant No 05/22 offered by the Ministery of Education of Slovak Republik.

6. References

1. Hayashi et al., *Jap. Circulat. J.* **45** (1981) 1182
2. Okajima, *Jap. Circulat. J.* **45** (1981) 347
3. Yamaki et al., *Circulation* **79** (1989) 312
4. Kozlíková et al., in *Sbornik abstrakt, 8. kongres ceskoslovenske patologicke a klinicke fyziologie* (Brno 1984)
5. Kozlíková and Hulín, *Bratisl. lek. Listy* **87** (1987) 194
6. Tyšler et al., *Biosignal'88* (Brno 1988)
7. Barr et al., *IEEE Trans. Biomed. Eng.* **18** (1971) 125
8. Miller et al., *Circulation* **62** (1980) 632
9. Kozlíková and Hulín, *Biosignal'88* (Brno 1988)
10. Selvester and Gillespie, *Adv. Cardiol.* **10** (1974) 120
11. Durrer et al., *Circulation* **41** (1970) 899

ATRIAL MAPPING IN THE DIAGNOSIS OF SILENT HEART FAILURE IN PATIENTS WITH MYOCARDIAL INFARCTION

TASHPOLOT BALTABAEVICH BALTABAEV
JULIAN ARKADIEVICH TILIS
ZHANNA VICTOROVNA SAVCHENKO

Department of Emergency Cardiology,Kirghiz Institute of Cardiology, Bishkek, 720361, USSR

ABSTRACT

The method of atrial mapping allows to estimate the response of atria to short-term volume load(VL) during quick depressurization of the chamber with negative pressure applied to the lower part of the body and to diagnose latent disturbances of left ventricular contractile function in patients with acute myocardial infarction(AMI)

1. INTRODUCTION

Heart failure(HF) is the most frequent complication of AMI [3]. As silent HF has no clinical manifestations, both invasive and non-invasive methods [6] including exercise tests are used for its determination [4].The search of other means allowing reliable diagnosis of silent HF in AMI is justified.

The aim of study was to work out the diagnostic criteria of silent HF using atrial mapping during short-term VL on the heart.

2. PATIENTS

We studied 31 patients aged 56.1±2.5 years, with acute primary extensive MI without signs of HF on the first day of the disease. Fifteen apparently healthy subjects aged 40.0±2.5 years served as controls.

3. METHODS

As an exercise test we used a short-term VL achieved

by a quick depressurization of the chamber applied to the lower body(negative pressure of -40 mm Hg was maintained in the chamber during 10 minutes)[4].

Atrial map was plotted basing on ECGs recorded from 90 points on the chest surface[1]. Location of negative and positive potentials, sums of amplitudes of negative and positive P waves(A^+ and A^-), and sums of their duration (D^+ and D^-) were estimated. Atrial maps were estimated at rest, at the peak of VL and on the 5th minute of restitution. Simultaneously, LV end-systolic and end-diastolic dimensions, LV ejection fraction, and maximal left atrial dimensions were determined by EchoCG.

4. RESULTS

During the short-term VL in the control group increases in left heart dimensions and LV ejection fraction were insignificant. On atrial maps A^+ and D^+ increased by 10 % and 7.4 %, respectively, from the baseline values, and A^- and D^- did not change. These changes returned to normal values by the 5th minute of restitution. All the patients were divided into 2 subgroups by their responses to VL. In group 1 patients(n=10) changes similar to those in control group were revealed, and this was regarded as the absence of HF. In group 2 patients(n=21) during VL A^- incresed by 11.3 %, A^+ by 19.0 %, D^- by 13.5 %, D^+ by 18.9 %($p<0.05$). By the 5th minute of restitution negative P waves continued to increase (A^- by 25.5 % and D^- by 20.7 % in comparison with control values); A^+ was higher than the baseline level by 22.9 %, D^+ tended to decrease, but still its values exceeded basal values by 8.08 %. Revealed deviations were regarded as the manifestations of silent HF and this was also confirmed by EchoCG data : in response to VL dimensions of the left heart increased($p<0.05$), LV ejection fraction reduced by 30 %. All these changes were still present on the 5th minute of restitution.

5. DISCUSSION

In patients without signs of HF and in healthy subjects quick inclusion of some part of deposited blood into circulation is accompanied by A^+ and D^+ increases without significant A^- and D^- , and P-wave increases on atrial electrocardiograms. These changes in parameters result from a more pronounced load on right atrium and right ventricle. Due to the deposition of on additional volume of quick blood inflow to the lungs, left heart chambers receive a much lesser blood volume does not inducing their overload. According to the principles of heart heterometric autoregulation, short-term VL increases the baseline length of myocardial fibers, that is accompanied by the increased myocardial contractile function (LV ejection fraction increases).

In contrast to aforementioned, during VL in patients with silent HF the values of A and D , and both negative and positive P-waves increase, suggesting that increased venous return is accompanied by oveload of not only right heart,but of left one,too. LV ejection fraction decreases. During the first days of MI there occurs a decrease in right ventricular contractile function, representing a compensatory mechanism which prevents lung edema formation [2,5].

These data tally with ours: by the 5th minute of restitution period on the atrial ECTG A^+ and D^+ did not return to basal values, whereas A^- and D^- continued to grow, suggesting the deterioration of LV contractile function. Atrial ECTG data are in accordance with EchoCG data: at maximal VL left heart dimensions increased ($p<0.05$), LV ejection fraction decreased in comparison with basal values,and these changes persisted till the 5th minute of restitution.

6. CONCLUSION

6.1. On atrial maps in healthy subjects and AMI patients without sings of HF, during VL, A^+ and D^+ increased by 10% and 7.4%,respectively, from the basal values and no changes in A^- and D^- were revealed. These changes return to baseline values by the 5th minute.

6.2. On atrial maps of AMI patients with silent HF during maximal VL A^- increased by 11.3%,A^+ -by 19.0%, D^- -by 13.5%, D^+ -by 18.9%. By the 5th minute of restitution negative P-wave potentials continued to increase, suggesting the further hemodynamic overload of left atrium.

7. REFERENCES

1. R.Z. Amirov, Integral topograms of cardiac potentials (Moscow,1973)p.109.
2. V.S.Volkov, V.Z. Gabinsky,I.E. Oransky.Kardiologya, (USSR),6(1970)99.
3. A.P.Golikov,V.A.Ruabinin, Kardiologya,(USSR),9(1986)5.
4. M.M. Mirrakhimov, T.B. Baltabaev, T.A. Azhimamatov, Kardiologya,(USSR),9(1985)83.
5. A.V.Fandeev, G.M.Kapustin,Sovetskaya Meditzina,(USSR), 8(1983)17.
6. W.U. Bussmann, Acute and Chronic Heart Failure(Berlin, 1986)p.286.

IMPORTANCE OF QRS INTEGRAL MAPPING FOR THE EVALUATION OF THE MYOCARDIAL INFARCTION EXTENT AND LEFT VENTRICULAR FUNCTION

Slavomíra FILIPOVÁ, Jozef BARTÚNEK, Stanislav CAGÁŇ

Department of Internal Medicine IV, School of Medicine, Comenius University, Bratislava, Czechoslovakia

Electrocardiography of acute myocardial infarction (MI) is focused not only on diagnosing the acute coronary event presence, but also on the assessment of its localization and extent. The immediate and partly the long-term prognosis of acute MI patients depends on the dimension of ischemic lesion. The extensive MI accompanied with the serious regional wall motion disturbance leads to the significant fall of rogional ejection fraction and subsequently to the fall of global ejection fraction. It threatens the patient in acute MI stage with the acute cardiac failure, sudden cardiac death and in the next stage with the development of chronic cardiac failure. Under the impact of our experiences with surface ECG-mapping of acute MI, we begat to consider the question of the integral QRS and ST-T mapping parameters if they reflect the importance of MI not only as far as its extension is considered, but also in connection with the functional consequences on the myocardium.

We have examined 92 patients with completely documented acute MI (Q-wave and non-Q wave type according to 12 lead ECG). We have used the equipment Kardio-SMEP 01 with the limited 30-lead system for total surface ECG-mapping. Every patient has been analyzed according to: 1) isopoten-

tial QRS maps; 2) integral QRS and ST-T maps.
Except of the quantitative topographic description of surface distribution of cardioelectric field we have evaluated numerical values from all types of maps (maxima and minima of the maps and ratios between minimum and maximum).

Every patient was underwent 2-dimensional echocardiography on the informative evaluation of segmental wall motion (normal kinesia-N, hypokinesis- H, akinesis- A, dyskinesis- D). On the basis of the echocardiographic results we have divided the patients into 4 groups: 1) N: (normal kinetics in all segments); 2) H: hypokinesis at least one segment; 3) A: akinesis at least 1 segment; 4)D: dyskinesis at least one segment.

FIG. 1

M459- V. T./1923/ AC. ANTERIOR M.I. /dyskinesis /

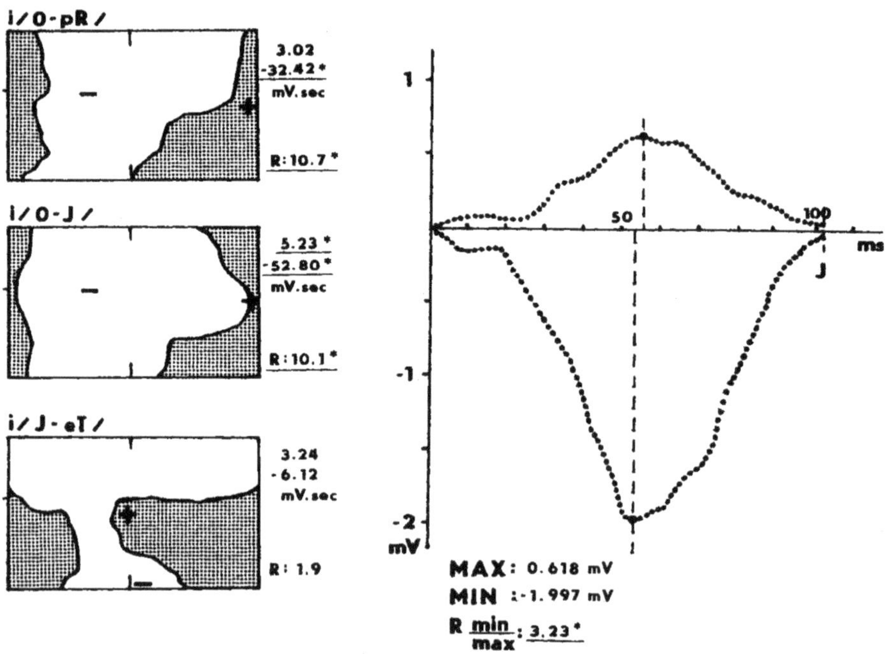

Results.

In the case of the extensive anterior Q-wave MI (Fig. 1) with apical dyskinesis is typical the large negative area on the anterior and left lateral thoracic wall on the integral QRS maps. There are striking high values of minima of integral QRS and ST-T maps and on the graph from the isopotential QRS maps.

The quantitative parameter of isopotential QRS maps, ratio min/max of total QRS complex, grows from the group N to the group D. None of the patients with the normal wall motion has this ratio higher than 2.5 and ratio 5.0 and higher we can find only in the dyskinetic group.

Under the impactof the results of integral QRS maps we can say that: 1) the ratio between min/max on the integral map (0-30 msec)QRS is higher than 3.0 only in patients with akinesis and dyskinesis; 2)the ratio min/max on the integral (0-peak R) map exceeds the value 3.0 only int the group D; 3) equally, ratio between min/max for total QRS (0 to J of QRS) map exceeds 5.0 only in the group D (Fig. 2); 4) the single values of minima and maxima for

Fig. 2

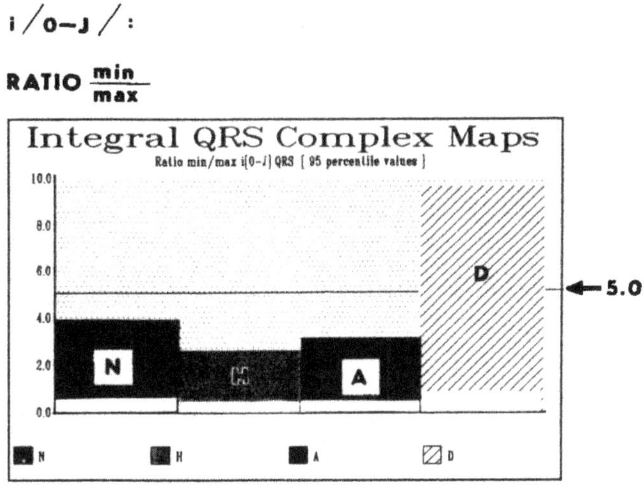

Fig. 3

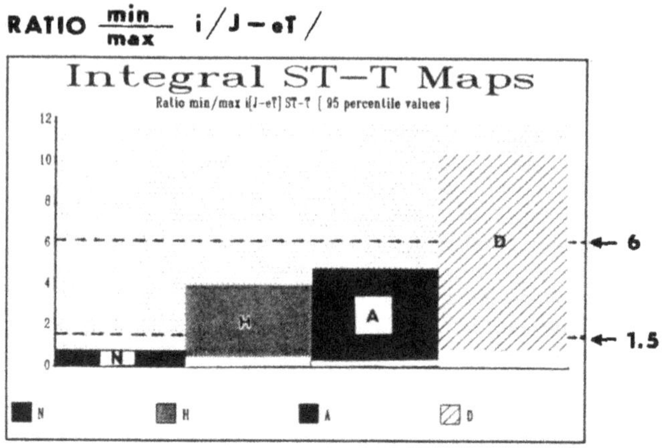

total QRS integral maps are very variable, but with the tendency for the fall of maximum and for the growing of minimal values in the direction from the group N to D. 5) The ratio between min/max of integral ST-T map (Fig.3) in patients N is below 1.5; values higher than 6 were calculated only in patients with dyskinesis.

Conclusions.

The quantitative evaluation of the integral QRS and ST-T maps has the definite limitation, caused by the great variability of cardioelectric field potentials. However, these limitations are valid more or less for all surface electrocardiographic methods (12-lead ECG, VCG, ...). Our results show that integral QRS and ST-T maps have the certain signs, behalf which we can evaluate the infarct area and the stage of the left ventricular functional damage, before the morphological, independent on the electrocardiographic examinations, procedures.

A QUANTITAIVE ANALYSIS OF INTEGRAL TOPOGRAMS IN THE PATIENTS WITH POSTERIOR LEFT VENTRICULAR MYOCARDIAL INFARCTION

R.Z. AMIROV

INSTITUTE OF PHYSICAL THERAPY, MOSCOW, USSR.

ABSTRACT

Overall ST elevation on the whole map is the most reliable index for quantification. Overall negative potential at the area of MI and overall potential at the site of transmural damage are also reliable and informative.

1. GENERAL ASPECTS

Many aspects of efficacy ofuse of cardiac surface potential mapping to reveal posterior myocardial infarction (MI) are still not completely understood, clinical trials are scanty and they do not cover all multiple problems.

At present, about ten modifications of a topographic study of electrical cardiac field (ECF) are offered. Instant and integral maps are most widely used. Maps of time and velocity of potential spreading, differential topograms, maps of areas of basic waves of a ventricular complex and othershave been also developed.

To estimate the obtained maps a variety of absolute and relative indices are used. Thus, ECF characteristics relative to amplitude values includes over 100 indices. Classification of this richest set must help a specialists to find out and use the most informative indices in his studies.

The aim of this studs is to promote an improved diagnosis of posterior MI and its complete qualitative and quantitative description. For it the following goals are to be solved: development of a classification of all indices of external ECF irrespective of a way and method of a topographic study, to find indices most reliably reflecting changes on topographic in posterior MI on the basis of a computer analysis.

2. MATERIAL AND METHODS

In 120 patients (114 men and 6 women) with confident posterior MI ECG was registered accroding to the accepted scheme (ECG-12), as well as from 90 points located over the whole chest surface, a system of Wilson's unipolar leads - integral topography (ITG-90). The obtained data and constructed topograms were treated according to the previously described method proposed by us (R.Z.Amirov,1965,1973).

A quantitative analysis of ITG-90 was done by means of Agat computer. Twenty-one amplitude indices were statistically treated.

RESULTS

Taking into account presence of various methods of mapping of superficial cardiac potentials we offer to distinguish the following classes:

1. Amplitude ECF charcteristics includes ECF indices proceeding from values of positive and negative ECG waves.

2.Time ECF parameters : proceeding from dipole circular movement, there is possibility to study time indices of QRS period by means of wave duration maps.

3. Velocity parameters of ECF: a study of velocity of electrical zone distribution on the chest surface.

4.Characteristics of ECF relative to ventricular wave area on ECG.

While studying numerous indices used during an analysis of maps we paid attention to various approaches to selection of that or this parameter out of the whole mass. A part of them is obtained during a study of individual ECG leads (mainly of maximal extremums) The following group of ECF parameters is a general sum of map indices. Other parameters may be united relative to the sign with which they caharcterize separate zones and areas of graphic ECF representation, which are obtained by means of different ariphmetic decisions. Therefore in each class we may distinguish the following groups:

1.Indices of individual leads.
2.Overall indices of maps.
3. Indices for certain zones and areas.
4. Estimated (calculated) indices.

For a quantitative analysis of ITG-90 we used indicesincluded into "Amplitude characteristics of ECF" class. The parameters shown in table I are most frequently used.

Classification of ECF parameters studied during a study of mapping of superficial cardiac potentials is simple and convenient. It may added by other indices without any change in the structure of this classification.This systematization has allowed to construct algorithm and a program for automatic ITG-90 estimation.

Realized statistical treatment of 21 parameters included into all classification groups of the "Ampltude ECF characteristics"class has proved, that a degree of information in each of them is quite different,

Results of the statistical analysis has confirmed, that all main indices of individual leads are low informative. They have either low criterium of reliablility of mean ariphmetic value (t   3), or a high degree of variability of these events, or high confidence interval at P=0.05. Thus, for example, an index of maximal depression of ST segment at P=0.05 has the following values:

$x = 0.138 \pm 0.078 \ (0.021 + 0.297)$
$t = 1.767$
$K_V = 304.78\%$

For this index an error in mean ariphmetic value is rather high, hence, this value is not reliable. It is confirmed by a high degree of dispersion of other values of a variation raw around this mean value. In the first group attention must be paid to an index of maximal elevation of ST segment above an isoelectrical line. Its values at P = 0.05 are as follows:

$x = 1.276 \pm 0.139 \ (0.992 \div 1.560)$
$t = 9.148$
$K_V = 58.86\%$

As for informativity of the examined indices maximal elevation of ST segment above an isoelectrical line ranks the fifth place. As for a reliability degree it ranks the first place in our studies. Mathematical description of this index at P=0.05 is as follows:

$x = 16.793 \pm 1.885 \ (12.948 \div 20.638)$
$t = 8.911$
$K_V = 60.45\%$

In the third group indices of certain zones and areas: two indices are most informative: overall negative potential from MI area and overall potential from the area of transmural damage. Their mean values are:

$X_1 = 48.618 \pm 4.649 \ (39.413 \div 57.823)$
$X_2 = 47.031 \pm 5.749 \ (35.303 \div 58.759)$

and their reliability criteria and variation coefficients are:

$t_1 = 10.457$ $\quad K_{VI} = 88.68\%$
$t_2 = 8.180$ $\quad K_{V2} = 65.83\%$

Relative indices of the fourth group are least informative.

Thus, the examination results allow us to arrive at the following conclusions:

1. A quantitative analysis of ITG provides a more complete description of posterior MI and hence this method per se helps for the diagnosis.
2. Classification of quantitative indices of ECF allows to approach more differentially to their selection during studies.
3. For quantitative characteristics of posterior MI the most reliable index is overall elevation of ST segment on the whole map, reliable and informativeindices are overall negative potential from MI area and overall potential from the area of transmural damage.

References

1. Amirov R.S. Integral topograms of cardiac potentials. (1973). Nauka, Moscow.
2. Amirov R.Z. Differential aliquot maps in the diagnosis of the left ventricular myocardial hypertrophy electrocardiology. (1988), Ed. H.Abel, Excerpta Medica, p. 347

INTEGRAL TOPOGRAMS IN PATIENTS WITH BRONCHIAL ASTHMA

R.AMIROV

and

Sh. ZAGIDULLIN, V.SHAKIROV, R. ZOULKARNEEV

Central Institute of Physical therapy, Moscow, USSR

ABSTRACT

Myocardial disorders, hypertrophy in particular, seen in various areas deteriorate a clinical course and prognosis in bronchial asthma (BA). An effort has been made to determine specific features of electrical cardiac area relief in patients with BA.

1. MATERIAL AND METHODS

Ninety-nine patients with BA of an infectious allergic form have been examined at the end of in-hospital treatment because of an aggravated status. Myocardial hypertrophy was diagnosed by means of electrocardiography. Widimsky's criteria (1973) were used for a diagnosis of the right ventricular hypertrophy (RVH) and Sokolow's and Lion's ones (1949) modified by Sh. Yanushkevitchius and Z. Shilinskite (1973) were used for a diagnosis of the left ventricular hypertrophy (LVH). The patients with BA were divided into four groups: without hypertrophy (WH) (52 patients) with RVH (21 patients), with LVH (21 patients and with biventricular hypertrophy (5 patients).

A control group (CG) consisted of 21 practically healthy persons.

Registration of standard 12-lead ECG was done in all patients. Electrical cardiac area relief was examined with the help of integral topography offered by R.Amirov (1969). Ninety-evenly distributed unipolar leads (5 lines, 18 raws) were registered from the chest surface. Q, R,S,T wave amplitude and ST segment deviation were measured with 0.5mm accuracy. The obtained data were computer treated by the authors. The results were presented as integral body surface maps (IBSM) of potential distribution of electropositivity (EP) and electronegativity (EN) during depolarization and of ST deviation and T wave during repolarization.

2. RESULTS AND DISCUSSION

IBSM seen in the control group was characterized with dipole potential distribution. EP (R wave) maximums were located inferiorly and to the left of EN (S wave) maximums. In most patients overlapping zones were found. Overlapping zones (OZ) were located on the anterior chest surface superiorly and to the left of V_1-V_2 leads. QRS in OZ were found on the left chest surface between a median clavicular and posterior axial line. Zero zones (ZZ) of EP were registered mainly in the left upper part and ZZ in EP on the right lower anterior chest surface.

ST elevation was registered in 38% of CG mainly by 2-3 intercostal space higher than V_3-V_6 lead area and no more than in 5 leads. ST depression was found in 14% of the cases in single leads, 1-2 intercostal spaces higher than V_2-V_4. Registration area +T was 1.4 times as much prevailing over -T area. Bell-like +T was distributed mainly in the left anterior lateral area.

In all groups of patients with BA common differences from CG were more significant in WH group. IBSM showed decreased local and total EP and EN potentials evidently caused by reduced pulmonary electroconductivity seen in bronchial obstruction, emphysema and pneumosclerosis (K. Ikeda et al.,1984,1985). It was noted, that at the phase of reduced aggravation, at the reduced bronchial obstruction the amplitude indices became normalized in all groups.

Displacement of maximal potential registration zones downwardly can be explained by cardiac displacement as a result of compressing action of emphysematous lungs.

It is evident, that a certain role is played by diffuse distrophic changes in the myocardium as a result of chronic hypoxaemia and excessive adrenergenic effect (Thomas,1972).

Higher frequency of total amplitude and ST deviation area caused by ST depression is of particular interest as well as an overall decrease of amplitude indices. Of course, myocardial hypertrophy, LVH in particular influence ST deviation. However, they were found in the patients with BA but without signs of myocardial hypertrophy.

It is known, that overall ST deviation and its area reflect a hemodynamic load level and associated subendocardial perfusion (Amirov R., 1975, L.Polonetsky et al., 1985, S.Yasui et al.,1985, N.Marchionni et al., 1986). At the stage of lowered aggravation and at tendency to amplitude increase on IBSM a reduced frequency, overall amplitude and ST deviation area were noted. They mas be used as an index of improved subendocardial perfusion.

In addition, Objective IBSM features were revealed in the patients with BA of RVH,LVH and R-LVH.

EP (R wave) and EN (S wave) maximums are approximating at the expense of displacement of R-maximum to the right and S maximum to the left and dawnwardly, a decrease in ZZ and displacement of EP ZZ to the anterior chest surface and EN ZZ to the anterior median chest surface were typical for the patients with RVH. OZ RR' had a larger area, seen more frequently and located much lower than in CG including V_1-V_3 lead area. OZ QRS area was extended and displaced to the left between anterior and posterior axilary line. Divergence in ST elevation and depression zones at the expense of +ST zone displacement to the left and -ST zones to the right was found.

IBSM in the patients with LVH have the following specific features: EP (R wave) maximum in amplitude surpasses a CG index and is located inV_1-V_2 area,its amplitude is less than in CG. Tendency to divergence in EP (R wave) and EN (S wave) maximums is mild. It proves a complex character of cardiac anatomic position and rotation shifts in the patients with BA and prevalence of clock-wise rotation along a longitudinal axis (N.Mukharlyamov,1973; K.Ikeda et al.,1985). Prevalnce of EP sum over EN was 1.25, ZZ areas in comparison with CG were enlarged by 7-9 leads. Moreover, location was reverse: ZZ in EP part of the left chest area. OZ RR' were registered over a less area, inferiorly and to the right of V_1, OZ QRS appeared more rarely, than in CG and RVH with less area and located to the right of R maximum. A tendency to to obtaining T+ and to -T, shift of +T maximum to the right was traced.

On IBSM of five patients with biventricular hypertrophy there were no specific differences. Different combinations of RVH and LVH most frequently of overall and local amplitude differences were increased at less area of ZZ, enlarged OZ RR' and QRS and at significantly displaced ST segment were noted

SUMMARY

Inferior maximum location on IBSM, lowered amplitude indices and a tendency toward normalization at the stage of aggravation decline were typical for all patients with BA. In addition frequency of overall amplitude and ST deviation were mainly seen because of depression and tendency towrd reduced aggravation was noted.

Relationship between overall ST deviation indices and other IBSM may characterize a degree of pathological load on the cardiopulmonary sytem i n the patients with BA. Typical LVH and RVH signs on IBSM were found. Disordered relationship betwen IBSM and lung function requires to reestimate myocardial hypertrophy criteria in the patients with BA.

REFERENCES

1. Amirov R.Z. Instant and total relief of electrical cardiac field in QRS.Kardiologia (Russ.)(1969)9,156.
2.Amirov R.Z., Minaeva I.N. A relief of electrical cardiac field according to integral topographic data in healthy persons and in that ones with hypertrophy. Kardiologia (Russ.) (1973),6,59-63.
3. Ikeda K., Kubota J., Watanabe V. et al. Electrocardiographic study of chronic emphysema by means of body surface mapping. Jap.Heart J. (1984), 25,5,689-700.
4. Ikeda K., Kubota J., Yasui S. Effects of lung volume on body surface electrocardiogram. Isointegral analysis of body surface maps in patients with chronic pulmonary emphysema. Jap. Circulat.J. (1985), 49,3,284-291.
5.Marchionni N., Moschi I., Lambardi A., Tozzi P.,Salani et al. Prediction of left ventricular function in acute anterior myocardialinfarction by serum creatine activity and precordial ECG Mapping. Clin. Cardiol.(1986),9,5,187-190

Thomas A.I.Chronic pulmonary heart diseases. Brit.Heart J. (1972) 34,7, 653-657.

7. Yasui S., Kubota I., Ohyama T. et al. Diagnosis of coronary artery diseases by body surface mapping. Body surface distribution of exercise-indices, ST changes in patients with myocardial infarction. Jap. Circulat.J. (1985),49,7,727-732.

DIFFERENTIAL ELECTROCARDIOGRAPHIC DIAGNOSIS OF DILATED CARDIOMYOPATHY AND ISCHAEMIC HEART DISEASE (PRECORDIAL MAPPING DATA)

G. V. RYABYKINA, M. M. SALTYKOVA, A. V. SOBOLEV
All-Union cardiology research center of the USSR
Academy of Medical Science, Moscow, USSR.

Computer analysis of the ECG wave areas in 35 precordial leads was performed in 60 cases of DCMP, 34 of them had ECG-pictures liked OMI (slow Rv1-v3, destroyed "R-line" in v1-v6, pathological Q). The group of 23 cases CAD with OMI and dilatation of heart cavities was used as control.

The sum ΣaS+aR of areas S-wave in left low region and R-wave in right high region was chosen as most informative parameter. Appearance of relation ΣaS+aR > 0.55mv*c is an indication of OMI absence. Using this rule the absence of OMI was defined in 82% cases of DCMP and 80% cases CAD.

The uncertainty of etiology and pathogenesis of dilated cardiomiopathy (DCMP), the severity of the disease and the variety of clinical manifestations are reasons for a high interest to this type of pathology and search for new diagnostic parameters of instrumental methods of investigation [1].

Echocardiography and scintigraphy of the myocardium take a special place among the methods of functional differential diagnosis of DCMP and CAD. However, data obtained by there methods not always enable the final diagnosis to be made. In this connection the electrocardiographic method of diagnosing DCMP has not last its value though the use of a 12-lead ECG in this type of pathology involves certain difficulties related to polymorphism of ECG changes in DCMP and focal scars of the myocardium [3].

The aim of this study was to work out an algorithm of differential diagnosis of DCMP on the data of 35-lead precordial mapping [5].

Material and methods

60 DCMP patients were examined. DCMP was diagnosed on the basis of complex clinical and instrumental examination including coronaroangiography (CAG), left ventriculography (VG) and myocardial biopsy. The results of the examination excluded such diseases as CAD, myocarditis, congenital and acquired heart defects, arterial hypertension and other

pathologies. In 9 dead the diagnosis were confirmed by autopsy.

The comparison group consisted of 60 IHD patients with myocardial infarction in the past.

All patients of this group during the present investigation in different leads of ECG-12 manifested disruption of "line R" or pathological Q or QS. Old myocardial infarction (o.m.i.) of inferior localization were observed in 13 patients. 27 patients manifested anteroseptal o.m.i. and 20 anterolateral o.m.i. 23 patients of this group with dilated of heart cavities with left ventricular end-diastolic dimension exceeding 5.9 cm comprised a subgroup which will be marked with index "d".

The analysis of cartograms was made by a computer. Areas "a" of waves Q, R, S, T, of the whole QRS complex and segment ST [4] and length L of QRS complex were calculated.

Results

Table 1 shows data on ECG-12 changes in the DCMP and CAD groups. As is seen from the table scar-like ECG changes manifested in 34 cases. In 24 cases there were signs of o.m.i. changes of anteroseptal localization, 8 cases manifested signs of anterolateral localization and 2 cases there were o.m.i. changes of inferior localization. In 24 cases the absence of o.m.i. was confirmed by Echo-CG, CAG and VG , 4 cases of which were confirmed by autopsy. The group of 34 DCMP patients with scar-like ECG changes hereinafter will be marked with index "s".

Tab. 1. The old myocardial infarction (o.m.i.) electrocardiographic features in patients with dilated cardiomyopathy (DCMP) and coronary artery disease (CAD).

	Groups of patients		
Criteria for o.m.i.	DCMP n=60	CAD n=60	CADd n=23
Q, QS and/or r<2mm v1-v3	40%	45%	21.5%
Rv4 > Rv3 < Rv2 and/or Q	13.3%	33.3%	43.5%
Q,QS II,III,avF	3.3%	21.7%	35%
Without Q and/or QS	43.3%	0%	0%

Table 2 shows the results of classifying the ECG material according to voltage criteria of Sokolov-Lyon hypertrophy. Among 23 patients suffering from IHD complicated by insufficient blood circulation accompanied by dilatation of heart chambers, positive criteria of Sokolov-Lyon were determined in 20% and among 34 DCMP patients with pseudoinfarction. ECG changes in 53% of cases. Criterion Sv1+Rv5>35mm, for instance, was observed in 13% and 26% of cases respectively. Mean value of sum Sv1+Rv5 for the IHD group was 21.6mm with dispersion equal to 9.1 and for the DCMPs group 25.4mm with dispersion 11.2. According to Fisher's criterion [2] there mean values have no confidence differences.

Tab. 2. Criteria of Sokolov-Lyon for the diagnosis myocardial hypertrophy.

ECG criteria of hypertrophy	DCMP n=60	DCMPs n=34	CAD n=60	CADd n=23
LVH	20%	14.7%	11.7%	17.4%
RVH	31.7%	23.5%	6.7%	4.2%
BVH	11.7%	14.7%	1.7%	0%

Fig.1 shows two examples of ECG-12 registered on a DCMP patient (A) and a IHD patient (B). In both cases there are signs of o.m.i. changes of anteroseptal localization without signs of hypertrophy.

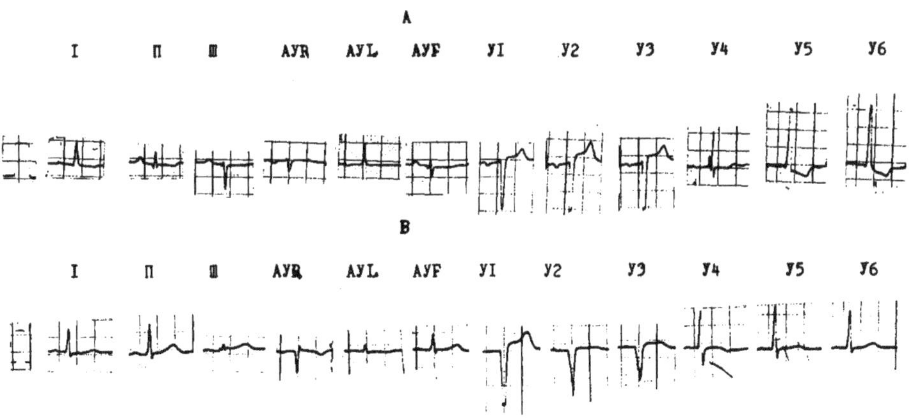

Fig. 1.

To show graphically a more informative diagnostic criterion automated search for parameters with the use of methods of dispersion analysis was carried out. Of the most significance for distinguishing DCMP and CAD groups were parameters $\sum aS_{1-3}^{V-VI}$ and $\sum aST_{-6-7}^{II-VI}$ (ST depression area). Histograms of distribution of these parameters are given in Fig. 2, 3. As is seen from the histograms, DCMP is characterized by a far more significant diminishing segment ST in left leads of the cartogram and by deeper S in lower right leads as compared to CAD.

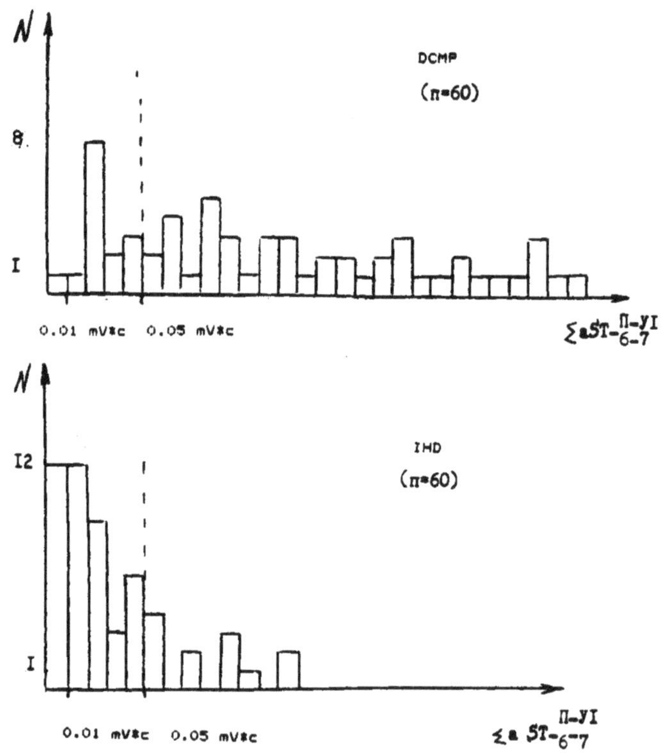

Fig. 2. Distribution histograms of parameter aST_{6-7}^{II-VI} in groups DCMP and CAD. Abscissa - parameter values $\sum aST_{-6-7}^{II-VI}$ ordinate - number of observations.

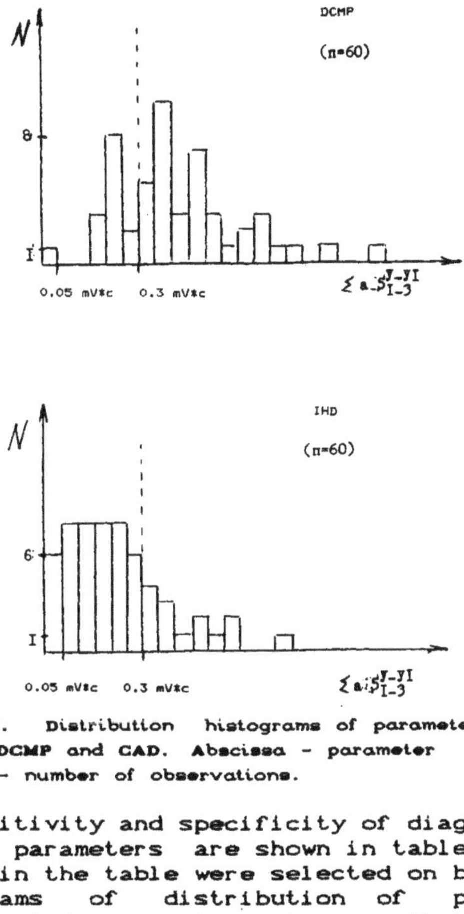

Fig. 3. Distribution histograms of parameter aS in groups DCMP and CAD. Abscissa - parameter values aS, ordinate - number of observations.

Sensitivity and specificity of diagnosis by each of the chosen parameters are shown in table 3. The constants given in the table were selected on basis of the type of histograms of distribution of parameters on the investigated groups in such a way that a maximum of cases showed be diagnosed correctly. It us necessary to note that parameters characterizing the area of segment ST do not give additional information as compares to aS. Waves R in left upper leads(parameter ΣaR_{6-7}^{II-IV}) an DCMP group cartograms are on the average higher than in CAD group. The authors investigated parameter $\Sigma aR_{6-7}^{II-IV} + \Sigma aS_{1-3}^{V-VI}$ which have given maximal information. This parameter makes it possible to come to a correct conclusion in 70% of DCMP and 80% of CAD cases. For DCMPs and CADd groups a correct conclusion can be made in 82% and 80% of the cases respective.

Tab. 3. ECG-35 indices used to distinguish DCMP and CAD

ECG-35 indices (mV*c)		DCMP n=60	DCMPs n=34	CAD n=60	CADd n=23
$\sum aS^{\overline{V}-\overline{VI}}_{1-3}$	> 0.3	77%	77%	23%	33%
$\sum aST^{\overline{II}-\overline{VI}}_{6-7}$	> 0.05	70%	70%	30%	30%
$\sum aR^{\overline{II}-\overline{IV}}_{6-7}$	> 0.15	66%	52%	33%	24%
$\sum aR^{\overline{II}-\overline{IV}}_{6-7} + \sum aS^{\overline{V}-\overline{VI}}_{1-3}$	> 0.55	70%	82%	20%	20%

Roman indices mean intercostal space, arabic indices - vertical lead columns.

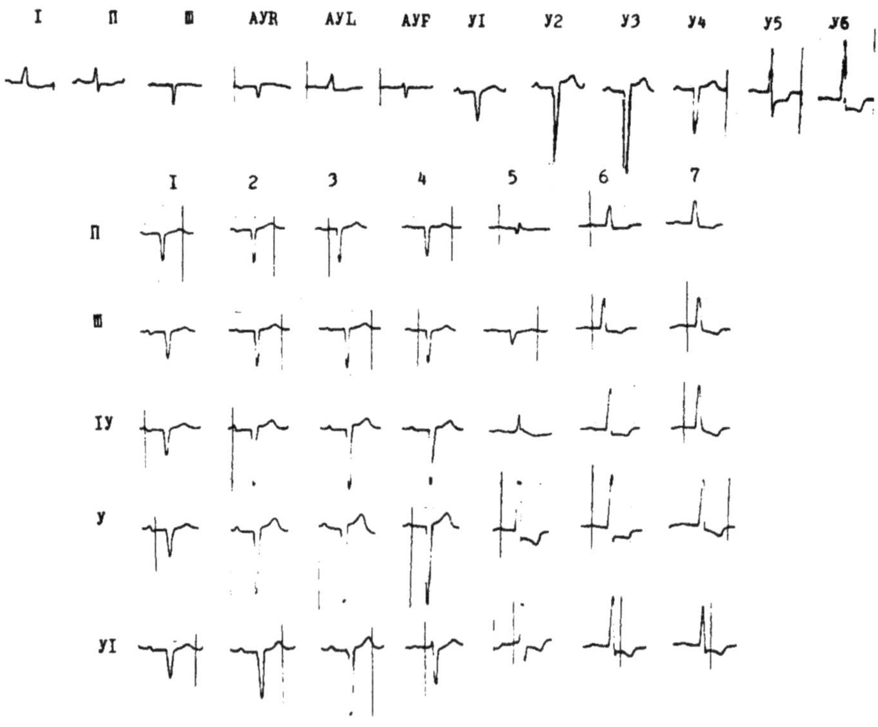

Fig 4. The ECG-12 and 35 in patient with DCMP.

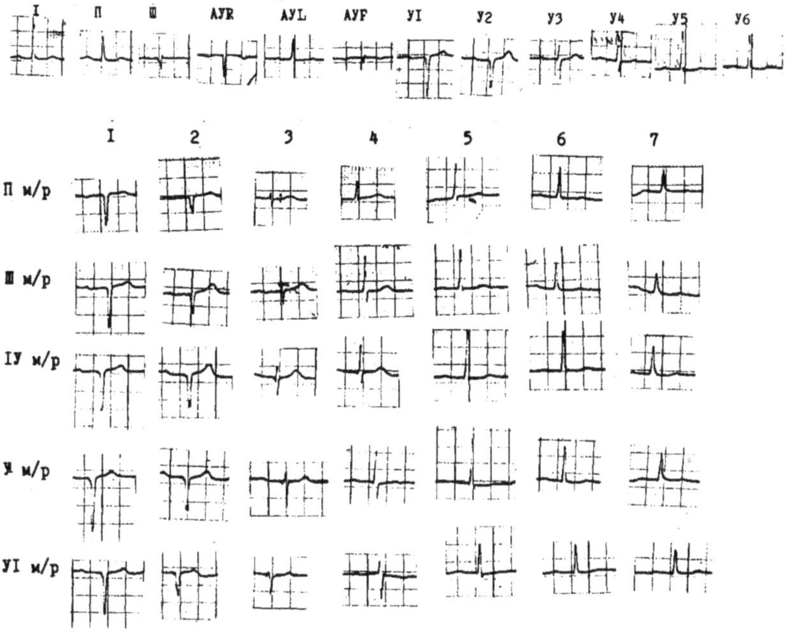

Fig 5. The ECG-12 and 35 precordial leads in patient with CAD and hypertensive cardiovascular disease.

Fig. 4 and 5 show examples of ECG-35 of DCMP and CAD patients with o.m.i. in the anterior and anteroseptal wall correctly identified with the help of the mathematical apparatus applied.

Discussion

The result of the investigation show that signs Q, QS and "disruptions of line R" in dilated heart cavities are not sufficiently informative. In the case of IHD with o.m.i. changes and ventricular dilatation ECG in 20% of cases show voltage signs of hypertrophy. Mean value of QRS complex voltage indices give no ECG confidence differences in IHD and DCMP patients with scar-like type of ECG curve due to which this sign proves to be insufficiently reliable for differential diagnosis.

On the contrary, precordial mapping used for these purposed is sufficiently effective. Parameter $\sum aR^{II-IV}_{6-7} + \sum aS^{V-VI}_{1-3}$

obtained from the summing up R wave areas in leads 6, 7, 13, 14, 20, 21 and the summing up S wave areas in leads 22, 23, 24, 29, 30 and 31 makes it possible to identify cases of DCMP and IHD in 82% of DCMP cases with infarct-like ECG changes.

It should be noted that the ST segment depression indicator proves to be a more characteristic sign of DCMP than IHD. Depression of the ST segment goes along with growing voltage in the ventricular complex. This indicator evidently is not a specific sign of IHD.

Conclusions

ECG in DCMP in comparison with CAD is characterized by deeper waves S in right lower leads of cartogram and more depressed segment ST in left columns of ECG-35 leads.

The algorithm proposed makes it possible to differentiate infarct-like ECG in DCMP from ECG in CAD with o.m.i. sensitivity 70-82% and specificity 80%.

References

1. Goodwin J.F., Oakley C.M., *Br. Heart. J.*,1972, v.34, p.545.

2. Kramer G. *Mathematical methods of statistic* (Moscow, Nauka, 1975) p. 631 (Russian)

3. Mucharliamov N.M., Popovitch M.I., Zatushevski I.F. *Dilatational cardiomyopathy* (Kishinev, Shtiintza, 1983) p. 157 (Russian).

4. Saltikova M.M., Ryabykina G.V., Sobolev A.V., *Cardiology*, 1990, N 7, p. 52-57 (Russian).

5. Maroko P., Libby J., Covell J. e.a., *Am. J. Cardiol.*, 1972, v. 29, N 2, p. 223 - 230.

PART IV
Clinical Diagnostics of Electro- and Vectorcardiography

VECTORCARDIOGRAPHIC DIFFERENTIATION BETWEEN RIGHT VENTRICULAR DILATATION AND HYPERTROPHY

IVAN RUTTKAY-NEDECKÝ, VAVRINEC SZATHMÁRY, RÓBERT OSVALD
Institute of Normal and Pathologic Physiology, Slovak Academy of Sciences, Sienkiewiczova 1, Bratislava, Czech and Slovak Federative Republic

and

EVA VANŽUROVÁ, KATARÍNA KANÁLIKOVÁ, ĽUDMILA STANOVÁ, MARTA VALENTÍKOVÁ
Institute for Cardiovascular Diseases, Partizánska 2, Bratislava, Czech and Slovak Federative Republic

ABSTRACT

The relation between vectorcardiographic parameters and hemodynamic variables was investigated in 55 cases of secundum type atrial septal defect (right ventricular volume overload) and in 67 patients with congenital pulmonic stenosis (right ventricular pressure overload). Vectorcardiographic signs of right ventricular hypertrophy were related to increased pulmonary to systemic blood flow ratio and to echocardiographic measure of right ventricular dilatation in the volume overloaded group, and to elevated right ventricular pressure in the pressure overloaded group. Computer simulation of pure ventricular wall dilatation or hypertrophy resulted only in an increase of the to the right amplitude of the simulated horizontal plane VCG loop accompanied by a decrease of the magnitude of to the left and posteriorly oriented vectors. It did not elicit anterior displacement and clockwise rotation of the loop. These latter changes appeared only when dilatation and hypertrophy were combined in computer simulation experiments.

1. Introduction

The vectorcardiogram representing right ventricular enlargement shows a much greater variation in its configuration and orientation than it does in left ventricular hypertrophy.[1] However, it has not yet been satisfactorily clarified to what extent and how do the shape and the parameters of the VCG loop depend on hemodynamic alterations caused by the underlying heart disease. Confusing results have been obtained especially when the relation of right ventricular pressure to vectorcardiographic parameters was compared between patients with pulmonic stenosis and patients with atrial septum defect.[2]

This study was undertaken to examine the pertinent points of difference in the vectorcardiogram of pediatric age group patients with pressure versus volume overload causing right ventricular enlargement.

Patients with secundum type atrial septal defect served as a natural model of primarily right ventricular dilatation, patients with pulmonic stenosis as that of primarily right ventricular hypertrophy.

Computer simulation of the effects of right ventricular hypertrophy and/or dilatation on the shape of the vectorcardiogram was utilized to analyze the role played by separate as well as combined changes of diastolic chamber volume and ventricular wall thickness in more detail.

2. Material and Methods

The study groups consisted of 55 patients with ostium secundum type atrial septal defect (ASD) and of 67 patients with pulmonic stenosis (PS). All of them were studied by the Pediatric Cardiology Service of the Cardiosurgical Department, Institute for Cardiovascular Diseases in Bratislava. They had cardiac catheterization and echocardiography (M-mode, 2-D, Doppler). Their age distributions and right ventricular peak systolic pressures are presented in Table 1.

Table 1.

		ASD	PS
N:		55	67
Age(years):	Mean	9.9	10.6
	SD	4.9	4.3
	Median	9	10
Right ventr. systolic pressure mmHg	Mean	34.4	47.6 $p<0.001$
	SD	7.4	27.7
	Median	33	40

For vectorcardiographic studies, the McFee-Parungao axial lead system[3] was used. Left sagittal and horizontal plane loops were photographed from the screen of a Hewlett-Packard 1520 A Vectorcardiograph system and optically enlarged (1 mV corresponded to 42 mm). The vectorcardiographic variables under study were: planar projections and spatial magnitude of instantaneous vectors at 10 ms intervals of QRS, as well as maximum amplitudes and sense of rotation of the horizontal loop.

Students t-test and correlation analysis were used for statistical evaluation. The $P < 0.05$ level of significance was adopted.

Our computer model[4] was constructed for simulation of ventricular excitation wavefronts: the left ventricular wall was bounded by 2 coaxial half-spheroids and the right ventricular wall by 2 coaxial quarter-spheroids. In the "normal" case, the ratio of left to right ventricular wall thickness was 2.28. More than 160.000 equally spaced elements of an imaginary three-dimensional integer field corresponded to points in a three-dimensional cartesian network and filled the space of ventricular walls.

The simulation program for myocardial activation sequence was a simplified modification of Huygens's geometrical method of wavefront construction. The excitation sequence started from carefully defined points on the left and right endocardial surfaces, corresponding to the experimentally determined areas of initial activation.[5]

3. Results

3.1. Loop Configuration

It is known, that the configuration of the VCG loop in the horizontal plane gives an additional parameter to use in conjunction with the right maximum spatial vector in assessing severity of obstruction in patients with pulmonic stenosis.[6]

Grouping the VCGs according to the evolving pattern of the horizontal plane loop (type C to A), as observed with increasing severity of right ventricular hypertrophy, the expected relation to increasing values of right ventricular systolic pressure (RVsP) was observed in PS patients (Fig.1).

In ASD patients significant elevation of the RVsP was found only in cases with clockwise rotation of the horizontal VCG loop (type A).[7] However, the loop configuration did reflect the severity of hemodynamic alterations in the ASD group if it was related to the pulmonary to systemic blood flow ratio instead of to RVsP (Fig.2).

This discrepancy should not be unexpected. While in PS with pressure overload the RVsP is a fair indicator of the degree of right ventricular wall hypetrophy, this is not the case in volume overloaded ASD patients with normal, or only moderately elevated resistance in the lesser circulation. Hemodynamic and echocardiographic indicators of right ventricular dilatation are here the appropriate non-electrocardiologic measure of the degree of right ventricular hypertrophy.

RVsP did not exceed the value of 50 mmHg in our ASD group. Dividing the PS patients into two subgroups according to lower or higher than 50 mmHg values of RVsP, it could be demonstrated (Fig.3), that distinct configurational changes of the group mean horizontal loop appeared only in the subgroup of PS patients with higher RVsP, but even in those, they did not attain the loop deformation observed in the ASD group. Our reference mean VCG loop was constructed from data obtained in an earlier study of 145 healthy persons.[8] PS patients with lower than 50 mmHg RVsP differed from the normal pattern only by a significant increase of instantaneous vector magnitudes.

3.2. Spatial Vector Magnitude

The time course of spatial instantaneous QRS vector magnitudes was compared to normal values published by Liebman et al.[9] for the age group of 2 to 19 years.

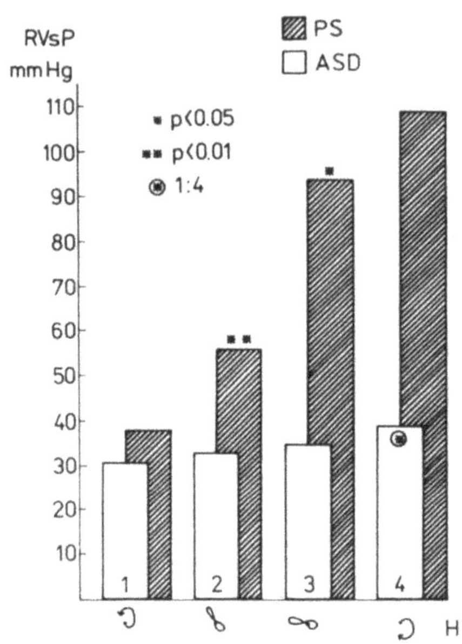

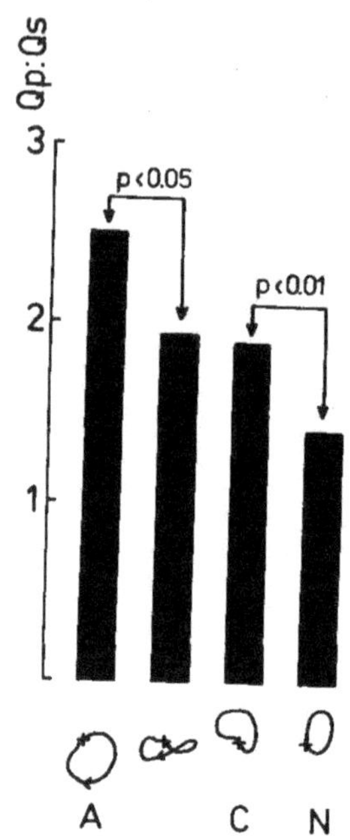

Fig.1. Group means of right ventricular systolic pressure (ordinate) in patients with different patterns of horizontal VCG loop. 1:counterclockwise, 2:figure of eight posterior, 3:figure of eight anterior, 4:clockwise anterior. Empty columns atrial septal defect, hatched columns:pulmonic stenosis.

Fig.2. Group means of pulmonic to systemic blood flow ratio (ordinate) in patients with atrial septal defect grouped according to horizontal VCG loop configuration (type A to C).

The group means were significantly greater at all measured instants of QRS in the ASD and PS patients as compared to normal values, with the exception of the 40 ms QRS vector where the difference between the norm and the ASD group did not reach significance (Fig.4). The values of the PS group were significantly higher than the values of the ASD group at 30,40,50 and 70 ms of QRS. There was no significant difference between sample means of spatial vector magnitudes of PS patients with lower or higher RVsP than 50 mmHg.

The correlation between QRS instantaneous spatial vector magnitude and RVsP or right ventricular gradient attained positive significance only at 50 and 60 ms of QRS (Fig.5)

It should be noted, that most of the scatter of points occurs at pressures below 50 mm Hg and significant values of the coefficient of correlation can be attained only if the sample contains a sufficient number of patients with higher than 50 mm Hg values of RVsP. In this study, the coefficient of correlation between maximum

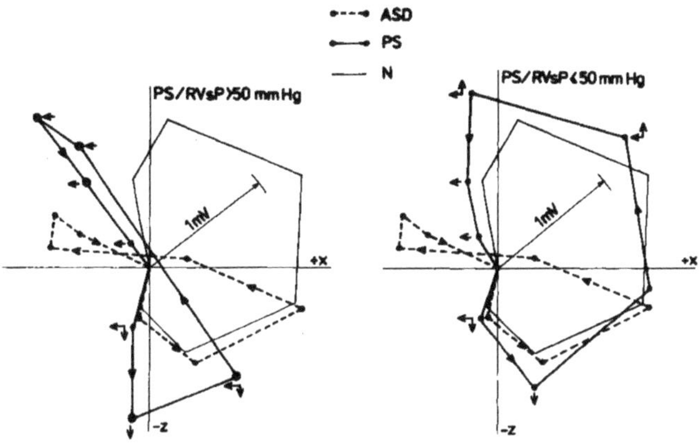

Fig.3. Horizontal plane loops constructed from medians of x,y,z amplitudes at 10 ms intervals of QRS. Broken line: atrial septal defect, thin line: reference sample, thick line: pulmonic stenosis. On the left panel patients with higher, on the right panel with lower than 50 mm Hg right ventricular systolic pressure. Significant displacement of the PS loops with respect to norm is indicated by arrows.

right amplitude of the horizontal plane loop and RVsP was only 0.125 in PS patients with less than 60 mm Hg RVsP, but 0.890 in those with higher RVsP values.

3.3 Computer Simulation Studies

Factors which may play a role in VCG configurational changes were analyzed by computer simulation experiments.[10,11] Simulation of eccentric right ventricular hypertrophy, by gradually increasing the model right ventricular wall thickness up to 100% increase, resulted in a gradual decrease of the magnitude of horizontal plane QRS vectors oriented to the left and posteriorly, along with an increase of the right posterior amplitude of the loop. The sense of rotation remained counterclockwise.

Increase of the short axis of the right ventricle, without changing the wall thickness, simulating ventricular dilatation, led to the same pattern of changes as above, only they were of lesser extent. Again, no change of the sense of rotation occurred.

Combination of the increase of right ventricular wall thickness by 100%, along with increase of the right ventricular short axis by 20% (hypertrophy and dilatation) resulted in a figure of eight configuration of the horizontal plane loop.

Similar changes as due to hypertrophy or dilatation of the right ventricle have been demonstrated to occur also by gradually delaying the beginning of right ventricular activation. Therefore, we combined all the three factors, i.e. delay of right ventricular activation by 5 time steps, increase of the short axis and of ventricular wall thickness by 100%. This simulation resulted in a full blown pattern of type A right ventricular hypertrophy, with a clockwise rotated and to the right and anteriorly displaced horizontal plane loop as well an increased to the right amplitude.

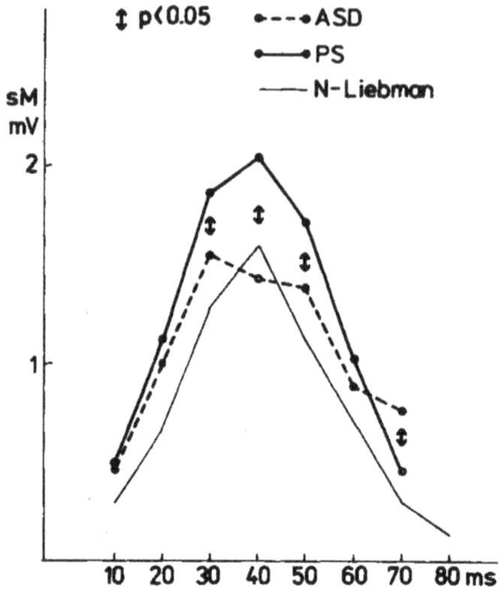

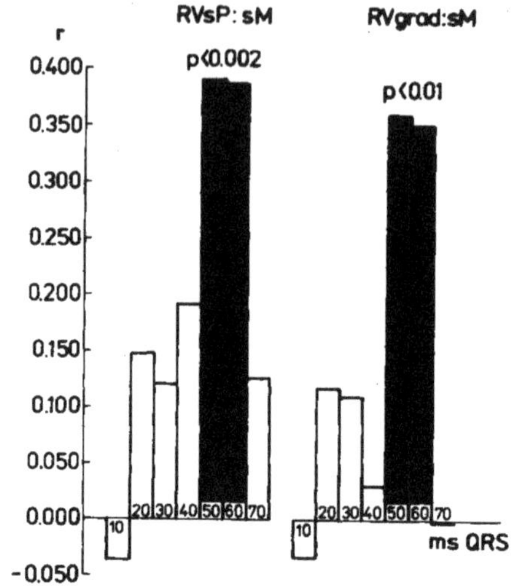

Fig.4. Mean spatial vector magnitudes at 10 ms intervals of QRS. Broken line: atrial septum defect, heavy full line: pulmonic stenosis, thin line: normal values published by Liebman et al. Arrows indicate moments of significant difference between PS and ASD. The difference between ASD and norm is significant at all instants with the exception of the 40th ms.

Fig.5. Values of correlation coefficients (r) between spatial vector magnitude and right ventricular systolic pressure (left panel), as well as right ventricular systolic gradient (right panel) for 10 ms intervals of QRS. Significant values of r are indicated by black columns.

4. Discussion

Since the right ventricular wall responds differently to different types of hemodynamic overload, primarily by dilatation to volume overload and primarily by hypertrophy to pressure overload, the independent hemodynamic variables to be related to vectorcardiographic parameters in order to evaluate their ability to reflect ventricular enlargement (hypertrophy, dilatation, or both) are also different: pulmonary to systemic blood flow ratio, or echocardiographic right ventricular to left ventricular dimension ratio in volume overloaded patients and right ventricular systolic pressure in pressure overloaded patients.

Increase of right ventricular wall thickness increases the right posterior maximum amplitude of the horizontal plane loop and decreases the magnitude of to the left and posteriorly oriented vectors more than diastolic dilatation of right ventricular chamber. However, the effects of simulated pure hypertrophy and pure dilatation of the right ventricle on the VCG loop are qualitatively the same. The deformation of the loop in this case results evidently from electromotive distributions in which the orientation and size of the unopposed activation fronts plays the major role, structural or anatomical changes of the left ventricular wall are not required for the explanation of observed displacements. An additional factor as demonstrated in an earlier study may be rotation of the heart around its long axis which occurs in right ventricular dilatation.

The figure of eight and clockwise rotation of the horizontal loop are the consequence of a combined increase of wall thickness and diastolic chamber volume. The role played by delay of right ventricular activation is as yet only hypothetical.

Ventricular enlargement, as observed in cardiac pathology, is practically always a combination of dilatation and hypertrophy, but one of these components may prevail.

Evaluation of the results of this study shows that in patients with primarily right ventricular dilatation (ASD) a figure of eight or clockwise rotating anterior horizontal plane loop speaks for additional ventricular wall hypertrophy, but not necessarily for elevated pressures in the lesser circulation. In patients with primarily pressure overload (PS) the increase of the to the right amplitude of the loop is related to increasing ventricular systolic pressure, white a clockwise rotated anteriorly displaced horizontal plane loop indicates very probably also additional dilatation of the ventricle.

5. References

1. T.C.Chou, R.A.Helm and S.Kaplan, *Clinical Vectorcardiography* (Grune and Stratton, New-York, 1947).
2. A.Calhoun Witham, in *Advances in Electrocardiography*, ed.R.G.Schant and J.W.Hurst (Grune and Stratton, New-York, 1972).
3. R.McFee and A.Parungao, *Amer.Heart J.* **62** (1961) 93.
4. I.Ruttkay-Nedecký, A.Drkošová and V.Szathmáry, in *Advances in Electrocardiology*, ed. P.d'Alché (Centre de Publications de l'Université de Caen, Caen, 1985).
5. D.Durrer, R.van Dam, G.E.Freud, M.J.Janse, F.Z.Meijler and R.C.Arzbaecher, *Circulation*, **41** (1984), 401.
6. R.Curtis Ellison and N.J.Restieaux, *Vectorcardiography in Congenital Heart Disease* (Saunders, Philadelphia, 1972).
7. I.Ruttkay-Nedecký, E.Vanžurová, M.Čulen and K.Kanáliková, *Electrocardiology 1988*, ed.H.Abel (Elsevier Sci.Pub., Amsterdam, 1989).
8. I.Ruttkay-Nedecký and P.Ruttkay-Nedecký, *Bratisl.lek. Listy*, **77** (1982) 403.
9. J.Liebman, Th.D.Downs and A.Priede, in *Vectorcardiography 2*, ed.I.Hoffman, R.I.Hamby and E.Glassman (North-Holland Publ.Co., Amsterdam, 1971).
10. V.Szathmáry and I.Ruttkay-Nedecký, in *Simulation of Systems in Biology and Medicine* (Proceedings of 7th Prague Symposium, Prague, 1990).
11. V.Szathmáry, I.Ruttkay-Nedecký, Th.Eifrig and Š.Šajban, in *Electrocardiology 1988*, ed.H.Abel (Elsevier Sci.Publ., Amsterdam, 1989).

NEW ECG/VCG-PARAMETERS SHOW EARLY REGRESSION OF LEFT VENTRICULAR HYPERTROPHY

HAIN, P.

KLINIK LINDENHOF, ZUGSBRADL KG, BAD NAUHEIM

FRG

Since 1987 we are writing VCG-loops always at the same procedure, ECG is done, using conventional leads (limb- and chest leads). SCHILLER, Switzerland, equipment is used, but our version utilizes lead I and aVF for the frontal and V2 and V6 for the horizontal plane. Providing VCG-loops and echocardiograms of all patients over years, we gradually came to know, that same particular configurations of loops are representing left ventricular hypertrophy (LVH), when conventional ECG criterions were inconspicuous.
In some patients we were able to document worsening of LVH while they did not take their drugs suffering from hypertension (Fig. 1) and so got an idea, what was to expect regarding improvement:

- the angle representing left axis deviation (LAD) is growing less
- superior forces are drawing back to inferior
- terminal right forces in the horizontal plane are shifting to the left
- posterior forces are growing less, while the anterior are increasing.

Fig.1

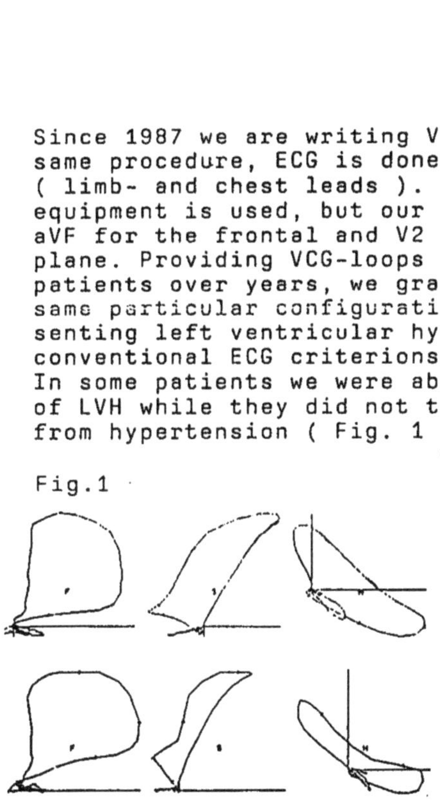

Loops of a 66 years old man with long lasting hypertension and polyglobulism. Loops above show mild LVH, beneath, two years later, a severe worsening is seen after a periode without therapy

A score was established with a range up to 80 points and was correlated with diastolic septal thickness 54 patients (learning group):

Fig.2

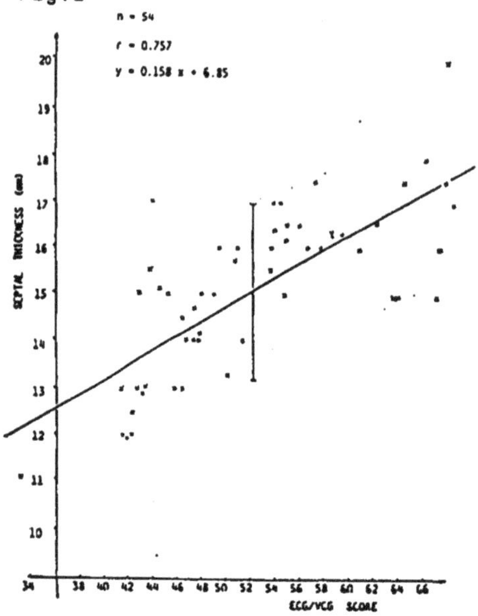

Correlation of LVH, measured by septal thickness, with score received by VCG-loops

1. sum of sinus of the frontal angle of LAD, which is devided to portions of 90 degrees, multiplied by 10; up to 20 points.
2. 1/5 of percentage of right maximal vector compared with maximal left; up to 20 points.
3. 1/5 of percentage of maximal superior vector compared with the sum of superior and inferior; up to 20 points.
4. 1/5 of percentage of maximal posterior vector compared with the sum posterior and anterior; up to 20 points.

Using that score (Fig.2) coefficient of correlation between thickness of septum and VCG-score turned out of be far higher than expected (r = 0,76). Score values over 60 however are often adjoined by obviously too small septal measurements. That may be due to mighty obesity, sturdy thoraxes or other difficulties concerning echocardiography. We then found out, which time it takes to realize regression of LVH by VCG-loops.
48 patients with LVH based on only recently detected hypertension were treated with an comination of Nifedipine and Metropolol for 4 up to 6 weeks ($\bar{x}$ = 4.4) and movement of loops were compared with 15 patients under long lasting different therapies.
All but three patients of the 48 showed certain movements concerning good improvement, while only two of the comparing group were improving, one showed even worsening while we detected a leak problem after aortic valve replacement.

Fig.3

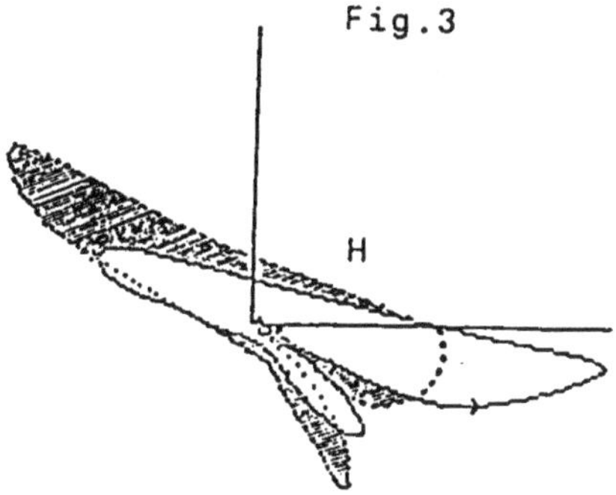

46 years old Italian with so far untreated hypertension. Hatched loops before, white one,5 weeks after onset of therapy with Nifedipine and Meropolol. There is a markable shift from right posterior to left anterior.

In the following you see a typical example of improvement after therapy (Fig.3). While the above mentioned score turned out to be too sluggish for routine, improvement could easily be detected at the first glance especially when a steady movement was seen during all examinations over the whole time. Loss of weight did not play that role we had thought. Althought reduction of weight was one what was better in the comparing group (4.3$\pm$ 3.6 kg) than in the testing group (3.7 $\pm$ 3.5 kg) there was a far better improvement in the latter, what was astonishing for us, as we had thought the body weight to be an important parameter for LVH.
49 % of patients showed remarkable movements of loops only in the frontal plane with loss of superior and gain of inferior extension. Only 14 % of loops were moved in horizontal loops alone with loss of right posterior and gain of left anterior extension.
In 36 % there were both, frontal and horizontal movement. By the way, a tendency of narrowing of the T angle in the horizontal plane was seen, but the difference of the testing group (-14 $\pm$ 32 degrees) and the comparing group (0.5 $\pm$ 17 degrees) was too small to be significant. Unfortunately septal thickness did not change at all showing an increased value of 14 $\pm$ 1,4 mm before and after regression. That may be due to a better visibility of septal structure after weight loss, hiding a real decrease.
Regression of LVH occurs far quicker than expected and may be made visible in VCG loops within few weeks after onset of therapy, motivating both, patient and physician. Hence changes of VCG-loops during regression of LVH reveal new parameters for its detection.

ECHO- AND ELECTROPHYSIOLOGIC CORRELATIONS IN RIGHT AND LEFT VENTRICULAR APICAL HYPERTROPHY OF UNKNOWN ORIGIN

MIRSAID M. MIRRAKHIMOV
RAISA I.RUDENKO
ZUKHRA U. KABAEVA

Kirghiz Institute of Cardiology, Bishkek, 720361, USSR

ABSTRACT

A set of noninvasive clinical and instrumental criteria of right and left ventricular apical hypertrophy of unknown origin was determined in 41 patients (mean age 35±4.6 years).

The diagnosis of right ventricular hypertrophic cardiomyopathy (RVHC) was based: on the increase in RV apical thickness to ⩾ 1.5 cm in local RVHC and to ⩾ 2 cm in extensive RVHC, decreases in RV anterior-posterior dimensions, disturbances in RV diastolic performance by 2D and pulse Doppler ECHO; on the presence of abnormal q waves (> 1.3 R, ⩾ 0.04 sec), and negative T waves of different magnitude in standart leads - mainly in extensive RVHC; on the changes in the direction of initial vectors to the left and downwards on VCG; and on either increase or sharp decrease in R-wave voltage in lower and mid-chest areas on ECG maps.

Left ventricular hypertrophic cardiomyopathy (LVHC) was diaghosed on the basis of increase in LV apical thickness to ⩾ 1.5 cm, in the ratio between LV apical thickness and posterior-basal segment to ⩾ 1.7 cm, disturbances of LV diastolic performance by 2D and pulse Doppler ECHO, presence of negative T waves of different magnitude in the following ECG leads; I-III, aVR, aVF, aVL, V1-V6, and sings of LV hypertrophy on VCG; on the increases in R-wave voltage in the 5th-6th intercostal spaces, and in electrical activity of LV free wall on ECG maps.

1. MATERIALS AND METHODS

Using a complex clinico-functional study, acquired and congenital heart diseases were excluded in 32 patients (mean age 32±3 years) with right ventricular (gr.1) and in 9 patients (mean age 36±4 years) with left ventricular (gr.2) apical hypertrophy. The diagnosis of apical hypertrophic cardiomyopathy was based on 2D and pulse Doppler ECHO data recorded from standard views[1,2,3]. The groups were studied using 12-lead ECG, VCG according to MacFee-Parungao, ECG mapping (90 leads). Ten healthy subjects served as controls.

2. RESULTS AND DISCUSSION

Group 1 patiens were divided into 2 subgroups: (a) - with local apical hypertrophic cardiomyopathy (n=18, mean age 29±2.8 years) and (b) extensive apical hypertrophic cardiomyopathy (n=14, mean age 34±3.6 years).

Subgroup (a) subjects had right ventricular (RV) apical hypertrophy ⩾ 1.5 cm (mean value 1.68±0.04 cm) by ECHO, IVS apical segment thickness 1.42±0.02 cm (versus 0.89±0.2 cm in controls, $p < 0.05$), hypokinesia of the latter segment (0.51±0.03 cm versus 0.78±0.06 cm in controls, $p < 0.05$), the increase in the apical to basal IVS thickness ratio to ⩾ 1.4 (IVS regional hypertrophy ratio), the decrease in anterior/posterior RV dimensions at the analysed IVS level (0.51±0.03 cm versus 0.91±0.07 cm in controls, $p < 0.05$). Right ventricular anterior wall thickness did not exceed the normal range (0.33±0.02 cm), mean pulmonary artery pressure was also normal (13.9±1.19 mm Hg).

Gr.2 (b) subjects had RV apical hypertrophy ⩾ 2 cm (mean value 2.6±0.08 cm) and hypertrophy of the adjacent 2/3 of IVS (2.44±0.22 cm, $p < 0.05$), the increase in the IVS regional hypertrophy ratio (1.94±0.12), hypokinesia of the above mentioned IVS segments (0.54±0.02) cm versus 0.78±0.06 cm in controls, $p < 0.05$),the reduction of RV cavity dimensions (anterior - posterior dimension at the middle level of IVS segment was 0.89±0.15 cm versus 1.48±0.13 cm in healthy subjects, ($p <0.05$), moderate thickening of RV anterior wall (0.42±0.04 cm versus 0.31±0.02 cm in controls, $p < 0.05$). Mean pulmonary artery pressure was normal (13.4±0.08 mm Hg). There was an increase in the right atrial systolic and diastolic sectional plane area in both subgroups - in (a) the values were 17.6±0.8 and 11.7±0.6 cm, and in (b) - 16.3±1.7 and 10.3±0.8 cm versus 11.8±0.5 and 6.7±0.17 cm in controls, respectively; the disturbance of RV diastolic performance - decceleration time in (a) was 167±4.2, in (b) - 158±9.3 msec versus 133±8 msec in controls, $p < 0.05$).

Clinical symptoms included cardiac pains (n=15), exertional dyspnea (n=11) (n=11), palpitations (n=12). Eleven of 18 subgroup (a) patients had no complaints. Physical examination revealed pulsation along the left sternal edge (n=14), systolic murmur at the apex of the heart (n=9) and along left sternal edge (n=13).ECG demonstrates signs of RV hypertrophy in 16 patients. Abnormal q waves (> 1/3 R, $\geq$ 0.04 sec) and T-wave inversion of various grades were present in 11 and 10 subgroup (b) patients, respectively, and in 2 and 3 patients in subgroup (a), respectively. VCG study showed changes in the direction of initial vectors (downwards and to the left) in 17 patients, signs of RV hypertrophy - in 19. ECG-mapping revealed 2 types of changes of dipolar activity of the heart.Type 1 was characterized by an increased voltage of R-wave in lower and middle sternal planes (n=17); type 2 - by the decrease of R-wave voltage down to zero values in the same area (n=15). Five-year follow-up revealed the decrease in RV dimensions in both subgroups - RV anterior-posterior dimension achieved 1.57±0.18 cm in (a) and 1.34±0.16 cm in (b) versus basal values 1.25±0.12 and 0.89±0.15 cm, respectively, ($p<0.05$). In left ventricular (LV) hypertrophic cardiomyopathy ECHO study demonstrates the increase in the thickness of LV apex (1.8±0.04 cm), of IVS apical segments (1.36±0.02 cm, $p<0.05$), its hypokinesia, the increase in IVS regional hypertrophy ratio (1.54±0.05, $p<0.05$). The ratio of LV apical to posterior basal segment thickness achieved 1.9±0.04. There were disturbances of LV diastolic performance: decceleration time turned to be increased (153±19 msec versus 118±13 msec in controls). Six of 9 gr. 2 subjects had no complaints. ECG study revealed T-wave inversion of different grades in standard and chest leads; VCG study revealed signs of LV hypertrophy in 8 subjects studied. ECG-mapping demonstrated increases of R-wave voltage in the 5th-6th intercostal space and electrical activity of LV free wall.

Thus, noninvasive diagnosis of right and left ventricular apical hypertrophy is based on the combined use of 2D, pulse Doppler, ECHO,ECG, VCG, and ECG-mapping data.

3. REFERENCES

1. H. Feigenbaum, in Echocardiography(Philadelphia, 1976)
2. G. Keren, B.Balshassen, J.Cherez et al.Circulation D71(1985)45
3. J.G. Webb, Z.Sasson etal., Am.J.Cardiol. D15(1990)83

ORTHOGONAL ECG-3 IN DIFFERENTIAL DIAGNOSIS OF IHD AND CCMP

F.U.GADZHAEVA, Z.Z.DOROFEEVA, T.A.SACHNOVA,
A.V.SOBOLEV, I.A.DAVIDOVA

All-Union cardiology research center of the USSR Academy of Medical Science, Moscow, USSR.

The new approach to differentiation of IHD from congestive CMP, the analysis of certain diagnostic criteria based on use of ECG-3 (lead system by McFee - Parungao), may be evaluated as very useful for clinical practice. If routine ECG reveals QRS complexes of low amplitude such criteria are as follows: $Sx > 4mm$, $Sz > 12mm$, $Rx + Sz > 27mm$, $\Sigma Rxyz + \Sigma Sxyz > 45mm$, $\Sigma Rxyz \; \Sigma Sxyz < 1,5mm$.

New approaches to the differential diagnosis of the different forms of so called cardiomyopathies, including congestive cardiomyopathy (CCMP) are intensively studied in the last years. CCMP is one of widespread and severe forms of heart disease [2-8]. It may manifests as a chronic, subacute or acute pathological process and its clinical symptoms and signs are often evaluated as myocarditis, ischemic or rheumatic heart disease in the stage of decompensation. Life time diagnosis of CCMP is very difficult because it is based on the comparison of the clinical data with the results obtained by means of instrumental investigations. Such comparison due to the practical necessity requires the correct use of the invasive methods (cardiocatheterisation, myocardial biopsy, ventriculography and selective coronarygraphy) as well as series of noninvasive methods. Not uncommonly observed uniformity of ECG-12 changes in CCMP and ischemic heart disease (IHD) (low voltage of QRS complex, T wave inversion, arrhythmias, disorders in atrioventricular and intraventricular conduction and other) caused us to search some electrocardiographic quantitative signs which may be diagnostically significant either for chronic IHD or for CCMP.

Material and methods

217 persons including 83 apparently healthy persons, 60 patients with chronic IHD (without episodes of myocardial infarction) and 74 patients with CCMP were investigated by means of ECG-3 (Mc Fee - Parungao system) as compared with ECG-12. Results of quantitative characteristics analysis of heart electrical field according to ECG-3 axial system with modification polarity of the lead Z are presentated in this report. This data were obtained in such patients (including 24 - with CCMP and 30 patients with IHD) which ECG-12 have not appearance the sign of 1) myocardial hypertrophy, 2) intraventricular conduction disturbances and 3) focal myocardial affection.

In other words, those part of our material, in which the common ECG investigation could not reveal significant deformation of QRS complexes or voltage signs of myocardial hypertrophy (according to the criteria of Sokolov - Lyon), is presented below. Such ECG were designed as not enough informative from the point of view, of their diagnostic significance in patients with ischemic heart disease and congestive CMP. In all the cases of our material, including 54 patients with enough informative ECG-12, clinical diagnosis was verified with data of coronarygraphy, and Echo.

Diagnosis was verified in 14 cases by means of postmortal investigation. The quantitative analysis of R and S waves in leads X, Y, Z, (ECG-3) was performed. Calculation of corresponding summary and relative data was based on the principles of grouping according to leads used in our previous work [1].

Results

Two types of QRS complex configuration in leads X, Y, Z were revealed. Type 1 may be characterized as having only R wave or prevalent R wave (qR) in leads X and Y; it was conditionally designed as "R-type". The specific feature of type 2 is appearance of S wave only in leads X and Y; thus configuration of ventricular complex may be described as qRS ("S-type"). In the same time in the healthy persons "S-type" is systematically registered in lead Z (prevalently in the ventricular complex forms rS, rs, RS ECG of rate of "S-type" in the leads X and Y) but not in Z \ was different in groups of apparently healthy persons, patients with ischemic heart disease and with congestive CMP and consisted correspondingly 41 case or 49,9% (near half a case in the lead X), 26 per cent and 75% (in both last groups prevalently in the lead Y). Thus, a significant prevalence of "S-type" in patients with congestive CMP in comparison with a control group and its relatively low rate in patients with IHD according to the data of ECG-3 was established.

Quantitative data obtained by means of ECG-3 in three studied groups are represented in the table.

ECG-3 Param. (mm)	Control: All Group N =83		Control: S-type N=41 for X, N=31 for Y		IHD: All Group N =30		IHD: S- type N =6 for X, N =8 for Y		CCMP: All Group N =24		CCMP: S-Type N=15 for X, N=18 for Y	
	M	σ	M	σ	M	σ	M	σ	M	σ	M	σ
Rx	13,3	4,2	12,9	4,2	13,2	4,0	10,2	3,7	12,7	6,4	10,3	5
Sx	1,1	1,8	2,3	1,9	0,5	1,1	2,9	1,1	4,2*	3,8	5,4**	2
R/Sx	-	-	8,1	4,6	-	-	4,2*	1,8	-	-	3,0*	3
Ry	9,1	4,2	7,5	4,2	6,4*	3,6	3,8	2,5	4,8*	3,8	4,2	4
Sy	0,9	2,1	2,5	2,9	0,8	1,7	2,9	2,0	3,4*	3,2	4,2*	3
R/Sy	-	-	5,4	4,5	-	-	2,3*	1,8	-	-	2,9	6
Rz	4,8	2,3	-	-	5,2	2,9	-	-	4,3	4,1	-	-
Sz	8,1	4,0	-	-	9,4	5,1	-	-	16,6**	6,0	-	-
R/Sz	0,7	0,5	-	-	0,9	1,5	-	-	0,3*	0,3	-	-
ΣRxyz	27,4	6,3	-	-	24,8	6,3	-	-	21,8*	10,9	-	-
ΣSxyz	10,2	5,3	-	-	10,7	5,5	-	-	25,0**	6,9	-	-
ΣRxyz + ΣSxyz	37,3	7,7	-	-	35,5	6,2	-	-	45,5**	10,5	-	-
ΣRxyz / ΣSxyz	4,0	2,6	-	-	3,7	5,0	-	-	1,1**	0,8	-	-
Rx+Sz	21,3	5,5	-	-	22,6	6,2	-	-	30,0**	8,3	-	-
Rz+Sx	5,9	2,9	-	-	5,7	2,9	-	-	7,6	5,5	-	-

* - significant difference from control P < 0,01

** - significant difference between two groups of pathology (IHD and CCMP) in addition to significant difference between the both groups and control (P < 0,01).

Since "S-type" in the lead Z could be detected in all studied groups, relations R/Sz were calculated as averages for all investigated contingent in the limits of every group. Relations R/Sx,y were calculated according to the number of cases of "S-type" detection.

As it may be seen from the data presented in the table, the most ECG-3 features in the patients with IHD and congestive CMP have obviously different direction, although the routine ECG is unable to reveal any signs of left or right ventricular hypertrophy. Diffuse myocardial affections, consequent decrease of myocardial contractility and enlargement of both ventricles in congestive CMP in concidence with increased common electric potential lead to appearance of the signs of both left and right ventricular dilatation on ECG-3 curve ($Sz > 12mm$, $Rx + Sz > 27mm$ and $Sx > 4mm$, and $\Sigma Rxyz / \Sigma Sxyz < 1,5$), although the pattern of routine ECG remains near to be normal.

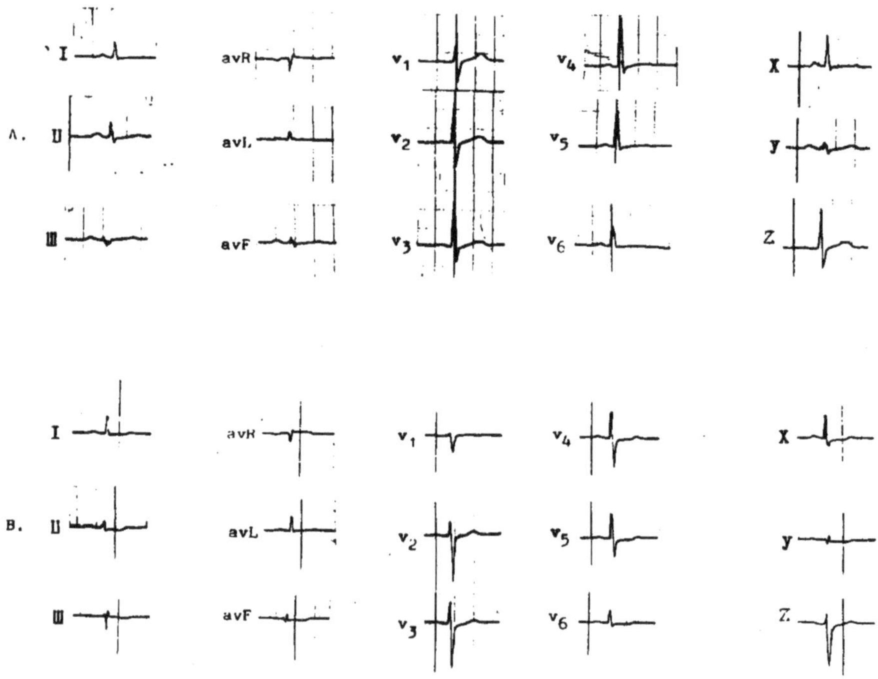

Fig. 1. A - ECG-12 and ECG-3 of patient with IHD, B - ECG-12 and ECG-3 of patient with IHD and hypertension. Tlere are no signes of myocardial hypertrophy on the ECG-12 and ECG-3 in both cases.

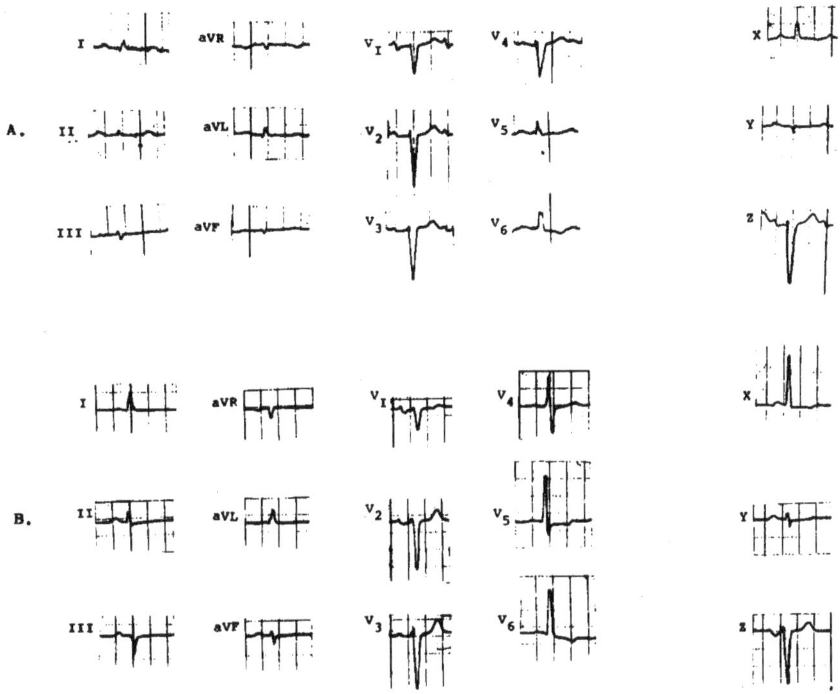

Fig. 2. A, B - ECG-12 and ECG-3 of patients with CCMP. There are no signes of myocardial hypertrophy on the ECG-12 in both cases. There are signes of left ventricular hypertrophy on the ECG-3 in both cases (Sz >12 mm, Rx +Sz >27 mm).

References.

1. Gadzhaeva F.U., *Ter. archives*, 1978, N 4, p. 82
2. Goodwin J.F., *Brit. Heart J.*, 1982, N 48, p. 1
3. Maron B.J., Wolfson J.K., Ciro et al., *Am. J. Cardiol*, 1983, N 51, p. 189
4. Motomura M., Kawaguchy Y., Fukunara T. et al., *JPN. Circulat. J.*, 1985, N 49, p. 292
5. Mucharliamov N.M., Popovich M.I., Zatushevsky I.F., *Congestive cardiomyopathy*. Kishinev, Shtiintza, 1986.
6. Ryabykina G. V., Lobova N.M., Dauletbaeva C.M., *Ter. Aarchives*, 1983, N 3, p. 128
7. Sumarokov A.V., *Ter. Archives*, 1985, N 4, p. 153
8. Yonesaka S., Becker A.E., *Brit. Heart J.*, 1987, N 58, p. 156

ANALYSIS OF DECARTO PARAMETERS FOR PREDICTION OF THE ECHOCARDIOGRAPHIC LEFT VENTRICULAR MASS AND LEFT VENTRICULAR MASS INDEX.

G.A.MUROMTSEVA, S.P.POTAPKIN, V.M.SHAMARIN

USSR Research Centre for Preventive Medicine,USSR Ministry of Health,Petroverigsky Str.,10,Moscow 101953,USSR

V.G.TRUNOV

Institute for Problems of Information Transmission,Acad.Sci.USSR,Ermolovoy St.,19,Moscow 101447,USSR

ABSTRACT

Multiple stepwise regression methods were used to identify an optimal subset of DECARTO (dipolar electrocardiotopography) parameters derived from orthogonal Frank ECG measurements, for prediction of the echocardiographic left ventricular mass (LVM) and LVM Index using data of 148 subjects of both sexes. We investigated 52 parameters including some demographic, anthropometric and DECARTO parameters as well as 3 parameters of scalar ECG in common and sex patient groups. As a result the following parameters were rather chosen: sum of Rx and Rz amplitudes, time of recording of maximal excitation area in the "Excitation arrival" map, additional excitation area at 10 ms, excitation area in the left upper anterior octant and systolic blood pressure. The correlations between echocardiographic and investigated electrocardiographic estimates of LVM and LVM Index were r=0.69 and 0.58 respectively. Selected parameters produced a moderate informativity (sensitivity 66.7 per cent, specificity 91.9 per cent for LVM and 26.6 and 92.7 per cents respectively for LVM Index). The informativity of selected parameters in the female group is higher than the informativity in the male group for LVM prediction as well as for LVM Index prediction. DECARTO parameters of investigated models are more informative for LVM detection as compared with informativity for LVM Index detection.

1. Introduction

Dipolar electrocardiotopography (DECARTO) is a new noninvasive technique for the representation of electrical processes, taking place in the heart during one cardiac circle. The diagnostic abilities of DECARTO parameters for left ventricular mass (LVM) and LVM Index prediction are studied in this report.

The aim of this investigation was determination of optimal subsets of DECARTO parameters for LVM and LVM Index prediction by means of multiple stepwise regression procedure. As well as the diagnostic informativity of DECARTO method and correlative relationships between decartographically and echocardiographically estimated LVM and LVM Index were examined.

2. Materials and Methods

The groups of investigated patients are listed in table 1. In all subjects 3 orthogonal Frank ECG and M-mode and two-dimensional echocardiograms were recorded. Frank ECG were used for construction of the decartograms by means of the method discussed in detail elsewhere[1]. LVM was verified by means of echocardiography. For LVM Index detection (LVM Index = LVM/Body Surface Area) body surface area calculated with formula by Dubois[2] was used.

We investigated 52 parameters including 41 DECARTO parameters, 8 demographic and anthropometric and 3 scalar ECG parameters. DECARTO parameters used: maximal vector magnitude, in mV; instantaneous vector magnitudes (IVM), in mV; area of decartogram, where excitation duration exceeds 40 ms (S), in relative units; integral index of prolonged excitation (II), in relative units * ms; depolarization duration (DD), in ms; time of recording the maximal excitation area in the "Excitation Arrival" map (TMEA), in ms; area of decartogram excited during every 10 ms (ADE), in relative units; additional excitation area at every 10 ms (AEA), in relative units; ADE:AEA at every 10 ms of cardiac circle; S in the octants. Demographic and anthropometric parameters used: sex, age, height, weight, chest circumference at levels of the 4th

Table 1.

Patient groups investigated in the study

	Groups for LVM prediction: common	male	female	Groups for LVM Index prediction: common	male	female
Healthy subjects	37	20	17	55	30	25
	echocardiographical LVM <= 180 g			echocardiographical LVM Index <= 91 g/m^2		
Subjects with LVH	66	47	19	79	51	28
	echocardiographical LVM > 180 g			echocardiographical LVM Index > 91 g/m^2		
Threshold state *	45	22	23			
Total	148	89	59	134**	81	53

LVH is the left ventricular hypertrophy; * - patients with threshold state have increased intraventricular septum and/or left ventricular wall thickness, or enlargement of the cavity, without any increase in LVM. ** - 14 patients excluded from examination as a result of uncorrected verification.

and 5th intercostal spaces (CC-4 and CC-5), systolic (SBP) and diastolic blood pressure (DBP). 3 scalar ECG parameters used: sum of Rx and Rz amplitudes (Rx+Rz), in mV; Rx amplitude, in mV; Rz duration, in ms.

3. Results

The optimal subsets of investigated parameters for prediction of the echocardiographic LVM and LVM Index on a continuous scale are demonstrated in table 2.

Table 2

Models for the LVM and LVM Index prediction in studied groups

Parameters	Coefficients in groups: common	male	female
	For LVM prediction:		
Intercept	-65.4	-98.7	-17.8
Weight	1.3		1.3
CC-4		2.0	
SBP	0.3		0.3
II		0.3	
Rx+Rz	19.4	15.0	22.3
Rz duration		-1366.4	
TMEA	1.0	2.1	
IVM at 60 ms		-0.2	
ADE at 10 ms	-28.5	2.7	
AEA at 10 ms	30.4		
S in left upper anterior octant		-6.8	
R^2	0.47	0.48	0.53
	For LVM Index prediction:		
Intercept	11.55	124.1	36.7
Height		-0.6	
SBP	0.2		0.2
DBP		0.3	
Rx+Rz	10.7	6.6	12.6
DD		-0.4	
TMEA	0.5	1.1	
IVM at 10 ms	-2.2		
ADE at 10 ms		1.2	
AEA at 10 ms	2.6		
R^2	0.34	0.36	0.40

We identified by a stepwise regression procedure that in common group the models consist of 6 and 5 parameters respectively for LVM and LVM Index prediction, in male group - of 8 and 6 parameters and in female group - of 3 and 2 parameters respectively. The following parameters take an important part: the sum of Rx and Rz amplitudes in all studied groups, the additional excitation area at 10 ms in common group and temporary parameters in the male group. Chest circumference at level of the 4th intercostal space or height was chosen by the step-up procedure according to the models for men and weight and blood pressure for women.

Multiple correlations in the female groups are always slightly higher than correlations in the male groups. The R^2 values indicate that 48 per cent of the echocardiographic LVM variation in men and 53 per cent in women as well as 36 per cent of the LVM Index in men and 40 per cent in women could be accounted for by the DECARTO models. These results do not agree with results by Wolf et al.[3], predicting LVM Index by means of 12 lead ECG. Correlation relationships between LVM estimated by the regression models and LVM estimated by echocardiograms show that the models slightly underestimate large LVM as well as large LVM Index values in studied groups.

Sensitivity of the model for detection of LVM in the common group was 2.5 times higher than for detection LVM Index (sensitivity 66.7 per cent, specificity 91.9 per cent for LVM and 26.6 and 92.7 per cents respectively for LVM Index). The informativity in the female group (sensitivity 84.2 per cent, specificity 94.1 per cent) is higher than the informativity in the male group (72.3 and 95 percents respectively) for LVM prediction as well as for LVM Index prediction (28.6 and 96.0 per cents for women, 15.7 and 96.7 per cents for men, respectively).

It is concluded that the DECARTO parameters describe the real LVM more accurately than LVM Index, i.e. LVM normalized with respect to the body surface area. Thus, DECARTO parameters of investigated models are more informative for LVM detection as compared with informativity for LVM Index detection.

4. References

1. L.I.Titomir and I.Ruttkay-Nedecký, *Intern.J.Bio-Med.Comput.* **20** (1987) 275.
2. D.Dubois and E.F.Dubois, *Arch.Intern.Med.* **17** (1916) 863.
3. H.K.Wolf, G.W.Burggraf et al., *J.Electrocardiology* **24** (1991) 121.

DIAGNOSTIC VALUE OF RIGHT THORACIC ECG-LEADS IN PULMONARY HYPERTENSION IN CHRONIC OBSTRUCTIVE LUNG DISEASE

ABDERRAHMAN MACHRAOUI, M.D., ANDREAS HELFEN, M.D., STEFAN VON DRYANDER, M. D., JÜRGEN BARMEYER, M.D.

Department of Cardiology and Angiology, University Medical School Bergmannsheil Bochum, Gilsingstr. 14, D-4630 Bochum, Germany

and

DIETER SCHÖTT, M.D., WOLFGANG.T. ULMER, M.D.

Department of Pulmology, University Medical School Bergmannsheil Bochum, Gilsingstr. 14, D-4630 Bochum, Germany

ABSTRACT

By considering the right thoracic ECG leads (Vr) we tried to develop a sensitive and specific criterion for the diagnosis of pulmonary hypertension in chronic obstructive lung disease (COLD).

We examined 75 patients by bodyplethysmography, right heart catheterization and blood gas analysis. We developed a modified Sokolow-Lyon-Index (SIm) as a sum of R amplitude in Vr3 and S amplitude in V6 and a combination of SIm with PaO_2 (SIm-PaO_2) following the formula SIm + 0.02 (100 - PaO_2). We found a good linear correlation between the mean pulmonary artery pressure (PAPm) and SIm (r = 0.80) or SIm-PaO_2 (r = 0.84). For recognition of pulmonary hypertension (PAPm > 20 mmHg) the criterion SIm $\geq$ 0.3 mV (positive SIm) showed a specifity of 84% and a sensitivity of 64%. It was found in 48% of the patients. PAPm was higher in patients with a positive SIm than in patients without this criterion (33 ± 13.9 mmHg and 20 ± 8.1 mmHg, respectively; p < 0.0001). Using the criterion SIm-PaO_2 $\geq$ 0.7 mV the sensitivity increased to 81.5%.

Conclusion: Frequency, sensitivity and specifity of the two new criteria facilitate the diagnosis of pulmonary hypertension and suggest the application of lead Vr3 in patients with COLD in clinical routine use.

Introduction

There are many electrocardiographic criteria of pulmonary hypertension and cor pulmonale. These criteria are generally highly specific but not sensitive. Therefore many patients with pulmonary hypertension remain undetected. The aim of this study was to develop a specific as well as a sensitive ECG parameter for non invasive prediction of pulmonary hypertension under special consideration of the right thoracic leads.

Patients and methods

Seventy-five patients in a stable cardio-pulmonary state were included in this study, 62 male and 13 female, mean age 62.7 ± 9.5 years. All presented with chronic obstructive lung disease known since 12.1 ± 9.7 years. The underlying disease had been confirmed clinically and by bodyplethysmography. Laboratory and lung function data showed a high air way resistance with a mean value of 6.8 ± 3.3 cm H_2O/l/s and a high intrathoracic gas volume of 149.1% of the expected value. The severity of hypoxemia was variable but generally moderate with a PaO_2 of 65.3 ± 11.6 mmHg on average. All patients applied aerosols with ipratropiumbromid, fenoterol and glucocorticoids. Ninety-one percent additionally received aminophylline and 87.0% oral glucocorticoids. Diuretics and glycosids were prescribed in 50.0% and 34.8% respectively.

Exclusion criteria of the study were diseases of the left heart, patterns of myocardial infarction in the ECG, regional or diffuse contractility disorders, dilated left ventricle at echocardiography or raised pulmonary capillary pressure at rest as well as congenital heart diseases

The four right thoracic ECG leads Vr3-Vr6 were recorded in addition to the common 12 leads I-III. aVR, aVL, aVF and V1-V6. A modified Sokolow-Lyon-Index (SIm) as a sum of amplitudes of R in lead Vr3 and of S in lead V6 (n = 75) and the combination of SIm with PaO_2 (SIm-PaO_2, n = 44) according to the formula SIm + 0.02 (100 - PaO_2) were established. PaO_2 was expressed in percent of the sex and age corrected reference value according to Ulmer et al[1]. Immediately after the ECG recording a right heart catheterization by Swan-Ganz technique was performed.

Results

The mean values of hemodynamic data demonstrated a constellation of precapillary pulmonary hypertension with high PAPm and pulmonary artery resistance (Rp) and low pulmonary capillary mean pressure (PCPm) (26.4 ± 12.9 mmHg, 396.0 ± 294.0 dyn·s·/cm^5 and 8.7 ± 4.2 mmHg, respectively). Patients with pulmonary hypertension were better discriminated from those with normal pulmonary artery pressure applying the right thoracic lead Vr3 than using the common ECG leads alone. PAPm was higher in patients with positive SIm (SIm ≥ 0.3 mV) than in patients without this criterion (33 ± 13.9 and 20.2 ± 8.1 mmHg, respectively; table 1).

The best correlations were found between PAPm and the ECG parameters involving right thoracic leads, SIm and SIm-PaO_2 (r: 0.80 and 0.84, respectively; table 2, figure 1).

TABLE 1. ECG criteria and pulmonary artery mean pressure (mean value and standard deviation)

ECG parameter	n	PAPm (mmHg)	p<
R/S(V1) < 1	64	23.9±10.2	
R/S(V1) ≥ 1	11	40.5±17.9	.0006
R/S(V6) > 1	69	24.4±11.1	
R/S(V6) ≤ 1	6	42.6±15.8	.0025
R(Vr3)+S(V6) < 0.3	39	20.2±8.1	
R(Vr3)+S(V6) ≥ 0.3	36	33.0±13.9	.0001

R: R amplitude. S: S amplitude. n: Number of patients.

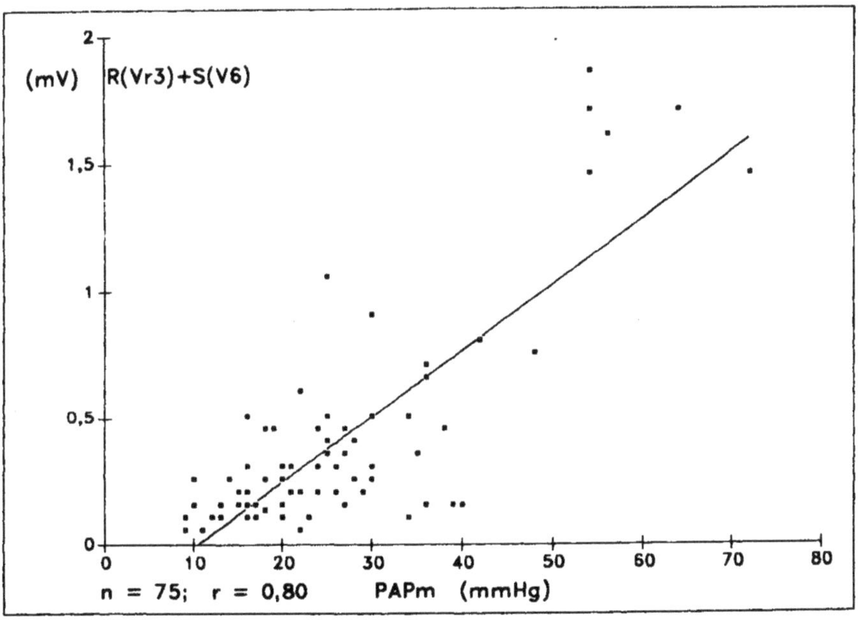

FIGURE 1: Correlation between pulmonary artery mean pressure (PAPm) and the modified Sokolow-Lyon-Index, R(Vr3)+S(V6). Linear equation: $y = -0.27 + 0.026\ x$. n= number of patients. r: correlation coefficient.

TABLE 2: Correlation between ECG parameters and pulmonary artery mean pressure

ECG parameter	n	r
R(V1)	75	0.52
R(V1) + S(V6)	75	0.69
R(Vr3)	75	0.73
R(Vr3)+ S(V6)	75	0.80
R(Vr3)+ S(V6)	44	0.75
SIm-PaO_2	44	0.84

R: R amplitude (mV). S: S amplitude (mV). SIm-PaO_2: R(Vr3)+ S(V6) + 0.02 (100 - PaO_2).
n: Number of patients. r: Correlation coefficient.

Finally the new criteria SIm $\geq$ 0.3 mV and SIm-PaO_2 $\geq$ 0.7 proved to be more sensitive (64.0 and 81.5%, respectively) than others like P pulmonale, R/S(V1), R/S(V6) or R(V1)+S(V6) with a sensitivity of 16-28% only.

Discussion

Chronic obstructive lung disease, emphysema, right heart hypertrophy and dilation lead to topographical changes resulting in orientation of the main electrical vector more to lead Vr3 than to V1[2]. The better correlation between pulmonary artery mean pressure and the modified Sokolow-Lyon-Index R(Vr3)+S(V6) in comparison with the Sokolow-Lyon-Index R(V1)+S(V6) can be explained by these topographical changes.

Right ventricular hypertrophy was reported to be detected earlier from right thoracic ECG leads than from common ECG leads[3,4]. So far however ECG criteria using right thoracic leads were not referred to invasively measured pulmonary artery pressures. We found the highest sensitivity in predicting pulmonary hypertension by the new criterion R(Vr3)+S(V6) $\geq$ 0.3 mV.

Hypoxemia is one of the pathophysiological mecanisms resulting in pulmonary hypertension[5,6]. According to findings of Gassner et al[7] PaO_2 showed a negative correlation with pulmonary artery pressure in the present study (r = 0.54). A combination of PaO_2 with ECG patterns of pulmonary hypertension seemed to be usefull therefore. The developed criterion R(Vr3)+S(V6) + 0.02 (100 - PaO_2) $\geq$ 0.7 raised the sensitivity from 64 to 82.3% without loss of specifity.

Conclusion: Frequency, sensitivity and specifity of the two new criteria facilitate the diagnosis of a pulmonary hypertension and suggest the application of lead Vr3 in patients with COLD in clinical routine use.

References

1. W. T. Ulmer, G. Reichel and D. Nolte, *Die Lungenfunktion. Physiologie, Pathophysiologie und Methodik* (Thieme, Stuttgart 1986).
2. F. D. Holford, *The electrocardiogram in lung disease*, ed. A. P. Fishman (McGraw-Hill Books Co., New York, 1980) p. 139.
3. F. Camerini, J. F. Goodwin and M. Zoob, *Brit. Heart J.* **18** (1956) 13.
4. H. Warembourg, A. Schouller, P. Pauchant, G. Nadiras, G. Duloux, P.E. Masure and G. Fossati, *Arch. Mal. Coeur* **58** (1965) 344.
5. U. S. von Euler and G. Liljestrand, *Acta. Physiol. Scand.* **12** (1946) 301.
6. A. P. Fishman, *Amer. Rev. resp. Dis.* **114** (1976) 775.
7. A. Gassner, H. Tizek, L. Fridrich and M. Pichler, *Schweiz. med. Wschr.* **115** (1985) 266.

EXTRACTING INFORMATION ABOUT THE LOCATION OF CARDIAC ACTIVATION PROCESSES FROM NELSON LEADS. RESULTS FROM NORMAL MAN.

TH. EIFRIG and S.SIKORRA
Institute of Pathological Physiology of the University, Liebigstr.27, D-7010 Leipzig, Germany

ABSTRACT

A type of NELSON lead system with 20 electrodes is used to determine besides the vectorcardiogram the locuscardiogram in men, too. The latter can be obtained straightforward using the same electrodes as for the estimation of the vectorcardiogram. The result has a simple geometrical meaning. Therefore, it can be interpreted in relation to cardiac topography.

The experimental data from normal men show a locuscardiogram, characterized by typical dipole locations inside the heart at the begin and the end of the QRS complex, but dominance of non-dipolarities in the middle of the QRS complex.

1. Introduction

In electrocardiological research for clinical purposes the electrical source of the heart is in general assumed to be a time dependent dipole. The characterization of such a kind of source is quite simple: it is completely defined by two vectors $\vec{D}$ and $\vec{R}$, where $\vec{D}$ is the cardiac dipole moment, which describes magnitude and direction of the source, and $\vec{R}$ is the vector pointing at the electrical center, which desribes the location of the dipole inside the body (Fig.1).

During the cardiac activation process both vectors change their magnitude and direction. Their pathes are called the vectorcardiogram, and the locuscardiogram of the heart, respectively. The commonly used corrected ECG lead systems provide information about the cardiac activation process in form of a vectorcardiogram only. Usually any information about the location of the dipole is missing, although just that kind of information could be essential for diagnostic predictions, because of its strong relation to the cardiac topography.

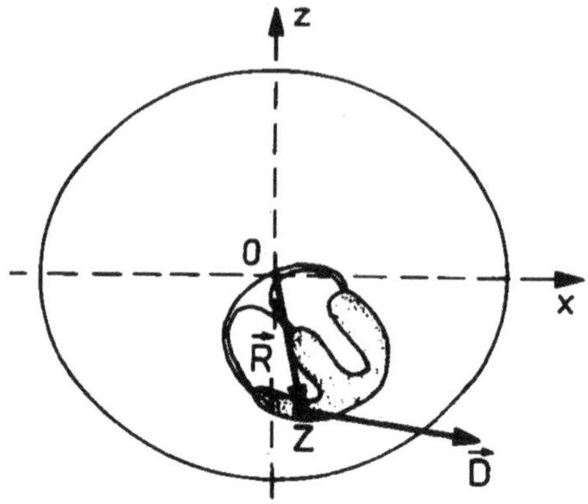

Fig.1 Horizontal cross section of the chest, with origin 0 of the chest related coordinate system and cardiac electrical center Z.

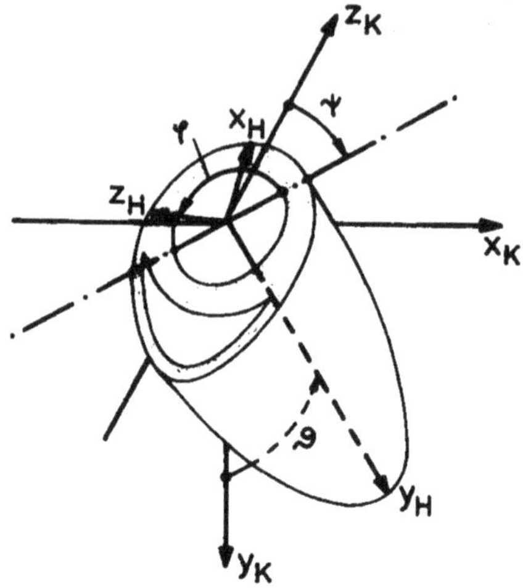

Fig.2 Position of the heart in the chest, with axes of chest related coordinate system (index k) and heart related coordinate system (index h).

2. Methods

In the last years we developed a lead system, which allows to determine both, the dipole moment and the cardiac electric center in an inexpensive manner. It is a modified NELSON[1] lead system with 20 lead points, located on the body surface in 5 equidistant planes . The system is described elsewhere[2,3]. It enables the determination of the 3 orthogonal components of the dipole moment, and additionally the determination of the cardiac quadrupolar moments, too.

From all these measured electrical moments we can calculate the electrical center of the heart[4]. The corresponding mathematical algorithm is a simple minimizing procedure for the squared sum of the quadrupolar moments, yielding an unique solution for the electrical center.

The obtained data are represented firstly using the common vectorcardiographic coordinate system, refering to the orientation of the chest, with origin at the 5th ICS, and axes in left, inferior, and posterior directions (see Fig.1). Additionally we take into account the tilted and twisted position of the heart within the chest (Fig.2), and we transform the results from the chest coordinate system into the cardiac coordinate system by rotation around standard angles.

3. Results and Discussion

Our investigation includes the electrocardiographic measurements on 12 healthy untrained young men (mean age of 23 years). The vectorcardiogram of all the probands shows the typical leftward directed vector loop in the usual chest related representation. Refering to the heart, however, the vector loop is frontally directed (Fig.3). We remember, that no information about the location of the activation processes is included in the vectorcardiograms.

In Fig.4 the locuscardiogram (i.e. the path of the cardiac electrical center during QRS) is represented in both coordinate systems. Unlike the cardiac dipole moment the electrical center has a simple geometrical meaning. Therefore, we will try to interprete the results in relation to cardiac topography. To do this, we use the cardiac coordinate system. Inscribing the locuscardiogram into a standard shape of a normal human heart (shown on the top of Fig.4), we can follow up the path of the electrical center from the begin of ventricular activation to the end of the

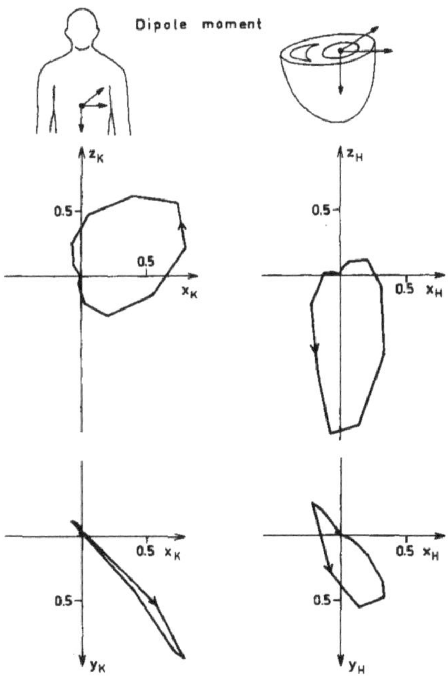

Fig.3 Vectorcardiogram of normal man in the chest related coordinate system (left), and in the cardiac coordinate system (right).

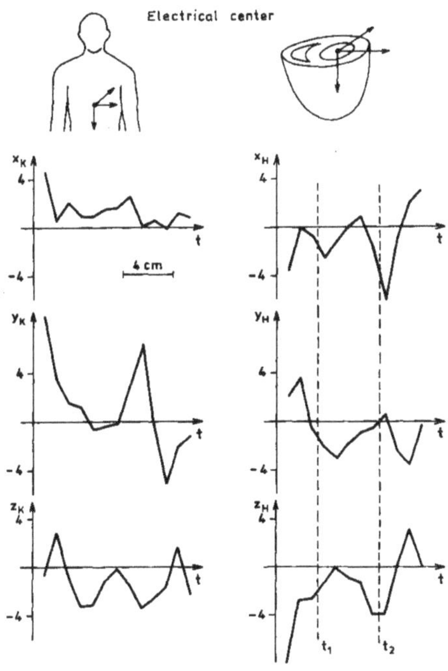

Fig.4 Locuscardiogram of normal man in the chest related coordinate system (left), and in the cardiac coordinate system (right).

QRS complex. At early QRS times $t < t1$ we find the resulting activation region in the outer wall of the right ventricle (obviously at this time the activation fronts in the left ventricle cancel each other in normal men!). At late QRS times $t>t2$ the electrical center moves along the ventricular basis from right to left, corresponding to the latest activated parts of the heart.

Using this information we can inscribe the cardiac dipole moment in the corresponding cardiac regions, which shows into the direction of propagation of the instantaneous activation front. So we find propagation in basal direction in the right ventricular wall at the begin of QRS, and propagation to the left in the basal regions at the end of QRS.

At middle QRS times $t1 < t < t2$ the calculated electrical center moves irregularly inside a central region of the heart. However, at these times the minimizing procedure for the determination of the electrical center gives poor results. That means, the character of the cardiac source is actually quadrupolar at this time, presumably because of contributions of large activation fronts from distinct parts of the heart. In such a case the calculated location of the resultant dipole is without any practical meaning.

Summarizing, we obtain two kinds of information from the locuscardiogram: first we get a measure for the degree of nondipolarity of the cardiac source from the result of the minimizing procedure; then, if we found that the source is actually dipolar, we can relate the time dependent activation process to the chest topography.

If we are able to use additional informations from other noninvasive diagnostic methods, e.g. echocardiography, regarding the actual cardiac position and dimensions, then we can relate the activation process directly to the cardiac topography.

4. References

1. C.V. Nelson, P.R. Gastonguay, A.F. Wilkinson and P.C. Voukydis, in *Vectorcardiography 2*, eds. I.Hoffman, R.I. Hamby and E. Glassman (North Holland, Amsterdam, 1971) 85-97.
2. Th.Eifrig, A. Joel and H.Schwartze, *Ergebn. Exp. Med.* **46** (1985) 274-284.
3. Th. Eifrig, *Zur Theorie des kardioelektrischen Feldes in der postnatalen Wachstumsperiode* (Thesis, University of Leipzig, 1989) pp. 67-84.
4. D.B. Geselowitz, in *The theoretical basis of electrocardiology*, eds. C.V. Nelson and D.B. Geselowitz (Clarendon Press, Oxford, 1976) 202-212.

MEASUREMENT OF CARDIAC DIPOLE MOMENT IN CHILDREN. REFLECTION OF CARDIAC GROWTH.

R. KLUGE, H. SCHWARTZE, and TH. EIFRIG
Institute of Pathological Physiology of the University,
Liebigstr.27, D-O-7010 Leipzig, Germany

ABSTRACT

A modified NELSON lead system is used for estimating the dipole moment in a total of 100 healthy children between two weeks and 59 months of age. A continuous enlargement of the size of the vector loops is observed, predominantly in the left lower posterior direction with growing age. First results from children with aortic or pulmonic stenosis indicate the suitability of this method for accurate diagnoses of left or right heart hypertrophies in children.

1. Introduction

The electrical dipole moment of the ventricles corresponds to the sum of the synchronously generated electromotive forces. Its magnitudes and directions are determined mainly by the mass distribution of the myocardium. The cardiac growth during infancy and childhood is associated with an increasing dipole moment and also with a change of its direction, caused by the developing dominance of the left ventricle.Characteristical alterations of the cardiac dipole moment are conditioned by pathological heart growth too, which is caused by pressure- or volume overload of the various parts of the heart.

The voltages, measured from the body surface, however, don`t increase according to the growing heart mass, because they are highly influenced by the synchronously changing body dimensions. Thus, newborns with a heart mass of about only 18g [1] generally show larger body surface potentials then scool children . An exact reflection of cardiac growth can only be obtained by calculating the electrical dipole moment of the heart from measured body surface potentials. The procedure will be successfull by applying the orthogonal ECG-lead system developed by NELSON[2], modified by EIFRIG et al.[3], taking into account the thorax dimensions of the individual child.

2. Method

18 electrodes arranged in three rows to six electrodes around the thorax are connected to a resistor network which carries out numerical integrations for estimating the x and the z vectors[3]. Two electrodes are placed in the neck and beside the Spina iliaca ant. sup., respectively, for the y vector. A potentiometer is used to adjust for thorax eccentricity estimated from left-right and anterior-posterior thorax dimensions.

The measured voltages are multiplied by the mean electrical tissue conductivity and by geometrical factors. These factors represent the thorax crossectional area and the thorax surrounding, respectively, being estimated from the measured thorax dimensions. A computer programm delivers on-line the course of the dipole moment components during the QRS-time, the constructed vector loops in the three plane projections and the maximal spatial dipole moment. The needed time for measuring the thoracic dimensions, the exact placing of the 20 electrodes, the registration of the ECG, the isolation of one QRS-complex on the computer screen and the print-out of the automatically estimated results takes about 15 minutes. The influence of physiological heart growth on the dipole moment has been studied in 100 healthy children. In addition, results of 2 clinical cases with left- or right ventricular hypertrophy are presented.

3. Results

Physiological heart growth

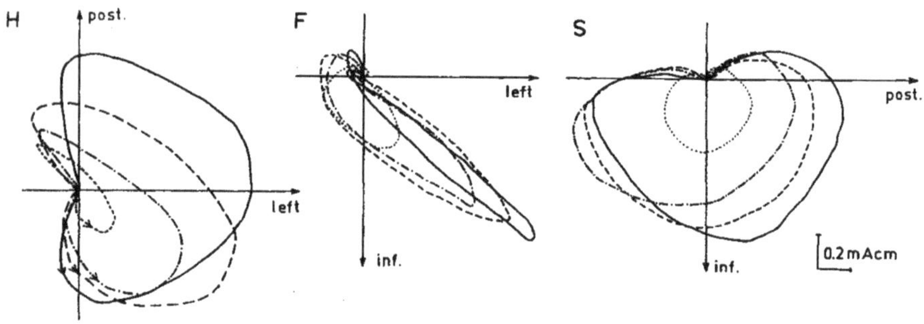

Fig.1: Increase of vector loops with growing age. Horizontal, frontal, and sagittal projections of calculated mean spatial vector loops of healthy children 0 - 2 months (···),6 - 9 months (-·-), 12 - 18 months(---), and 36 - 60 months (——) of age. n = 25 per age group.

Mean spatial vector loops calculated for the four age groups show a remarkable and continuous increase with growing age. The dipole moment expands mainly to the left, to the inferior, and to the posterior, resulting in a changed form of the loop (fig.1).

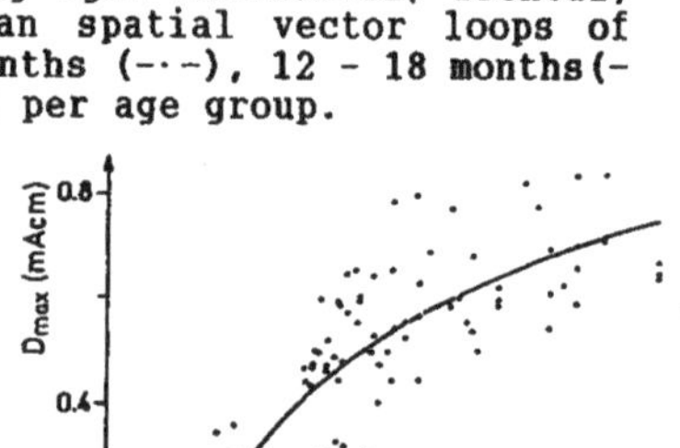

Fig.2: Dmax in dependence on the body mass in 100 healthy children. r=0.85.

The magnitude of the maximum dipole moment (Dmax) rises in close connection with the body mass (fig.2) from about 0.2 mAcm in 3 kg weighing infants to nearly 0.8 mAcm in 20 kg weighing children. This dependence follows the adaptation to a logarithmical function to a satisfying degree.

Left and right ventricular hypertrophy

The QRS-vector loops of a patient suffering from severe supravalvular aortic stenosis are presented in fig.3 in comparison to the normal values of his age group. The remarkable increase of size of the dipole moment directed to the left, to the posterior and to the inferior is obvious, the magnitude of the maximum spatial dipole moment exceeds the normal value.

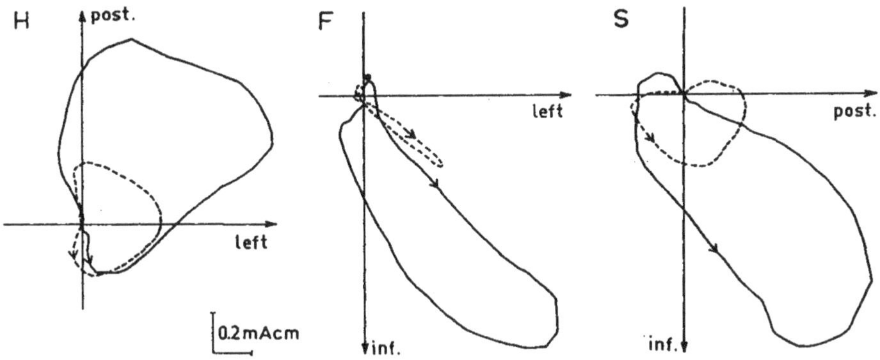

Fig.3: The spatial vector loop of a boy - 4 years 10 months old - suffering from subvalvular aortic stenosis (peak systolic gradient 78 mm Hg). Horizontal, frontal, and sagittal projections in comparison to the normal values.

Fig.4 represents the course of the QRS-vector loops of a 3 years old girl suffering from a valvular pulmonic stenosis in comparison to the normal mean loop of her age group. This girl was investigated twofold - shortly before and 3 month after ballonvalvuloplasty. The echocardiographical estimated peak pressure gradient before the therapy amounted to 95 mmHg, after the ballonvalvuloplasty remained a systolic gradient of about 25 mmHg.

This severe right heart hypertrophy can be recognized by the change of the rotation direction of the horizontally projected vector loop. In contrast to the norm, it rotates clockwise. In addition, the enlargement of those loop parts directed to the right becomes evident. Only three months after the pressure disloading of the right ventricle the finding evidently shows the tendency to normalize - the horizontal projection now shows a figure-of-eight configuration, and the loop parts directed to the right are much smaller.

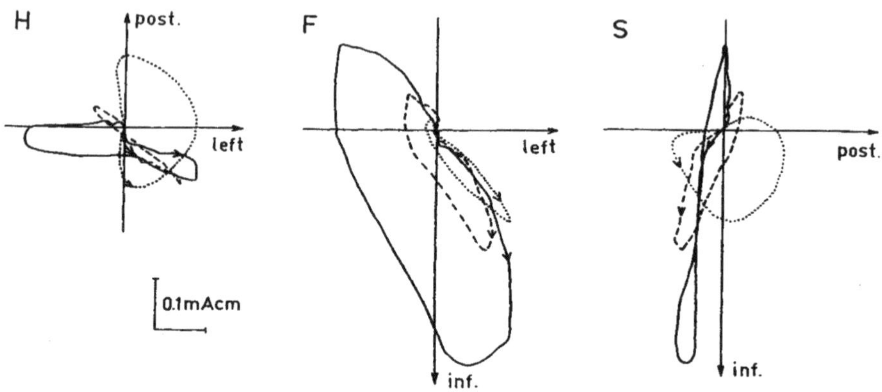

Fig.4: Horizontal, frontal, and sagittal projections of spatial vector loops in a patient suffering from pulmonic stenosis before (—) and after ballonvalvuloplasty (--) in comparison to the normal mean loop(··).

4. Discussion

The measurement of the dipole moment vector loops in healthy infants and children shows characteristical changes of form and magnitude according to increasing age. Similar form changes can also be detected by other vectorcardiographical methods like the FRANK-ECG, however, the magnitude growth can only be ascertained by determining the dipole moment. The pathological ECG-findings, demonstrated in the above two examples allow to expect that, the presented method will enable us to quantify the degree of the chamber hypertrophy. If the cardiac dipole moment reflects the development of the heart mass, it should also be possible to find the relation between the dipole moment and the degree of an unknown ventricular mass of a particular patient. A decisive improvement is to be expected especially by the evaluation of the severity of right heart hypertrophies as well as by the differentiation between hypertrophies and BBB.

5. References

1. D.G. Scholz, D.W. Kitzman, P.T. Hagen, D.M. Ilstrup, and W.D. Edwards, *Mayo Clin. Proc.* **63** (1988) 126-136.
2. C.V. Nelson, P.R. Gastonguay, A.F. Wilkinson, P.C. Voukydis, in *Vectorcardiography 2*, eds. I. Hoffman, R.I. Hamby and E. Glassman (North Holland, Amsterdam, 1971)85 - 97
3. Th. Eifrig, A. Joel und H. Schwartze, *Ergebn. Exp. Med.* **46** (1985) 274-284.

CORRELATIONS BETWEEN UNEXPECTED VCG CHANGES AND THE L.V. DIASTOLIC FUNCTION IN TYPE I DIABETES MELLITUS PTS.

Gotti G.,Barducci E.,Borgioni L.,Cattarini G.,Magris R.,Mastrobuoni G.,Moratti P.,Zilio G. and Palmieri M.

CCU and Cardiologycal Service - General Hospital MONFALCONE (Italy)

Palmieri Mauro MD
v. S. Marco 54
34074 MONFALCONE (Italy)

With the purpose to recognize the early markers of diabetic cardiomyopathy (DC),50 normotensive IDDM pts (21 m, 29 f) aged 20 - 75, free of cardiac symptoms were studied without knowledge of their clinical and metabolic data. The Frank-VCG QRS loops were examined for bites, ischemia or LVH (see FIG. A); then a 2D-ECHO was performed, the mitral flow investigated and the Doppler derived E/A wave velocity ratio obtained (see FIGG. B and C).

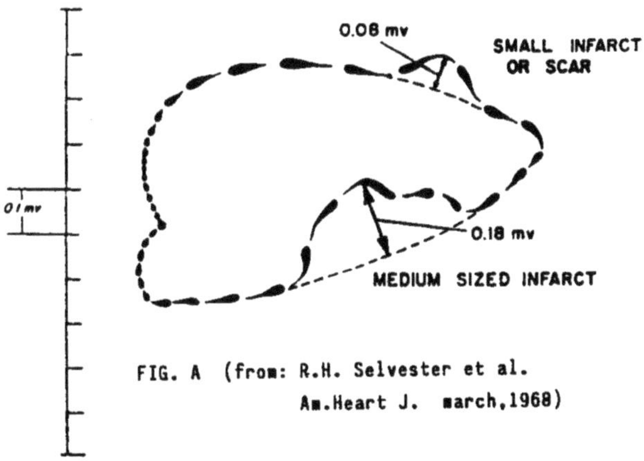

FIG. A (from: R.H. Selvester et al. Am.Heart J. march,1968)

2D-ECHO: were assessed LV hypertrophy or dilatation and LV wall motion abnormalities (LVWMA).

2D-DOPPLER: the mitral flow was investigated and mostly the E/A waves ratio considering the early (E) and late (A) filling rates as indirect markers of the LV compliance.

STANDARDIZATION PROCEDURE: to avoid false positive findings, only the inversion of the normal E>A ratio in A>E ratio was considered pathologyc.

The LV E.F. and the Fractional Shortening were considered for the systolic phase.

Lastly, the Glicosylated Hemoglobin (HB_{A1c}) and ratio of the age of onset of DM and the actual age of pts (DA/PA) were given by the diabetic out-patients clinic.

A group of 20 normal subjects matched for age and sex served as controls. According to the VCG findings, two groups were recognized: GROUP I, with normal VCG: 30 pts (60%), mean age 39.03 (20-74); 6 (20%) with $A > E$ ratio; mean DA/PA = 0.43; mean HB_{A1c} = 7.38 . GROUP II, with VCG abnormalities: 20 pts (40%), mean age 55.45 (31-75). At the VCG: bites in 9 (45%), necrosis in 2 (10%), ischemia in 4 (20%), LVH in 7(35%), IVC defects in 6(30%).

The 2D-ECHO was abnormal in all (100%) cases: $A > E$ ratio in 17 (85%), LVH in 11 (55%), a calcific mitral annulus in 51 (25%).

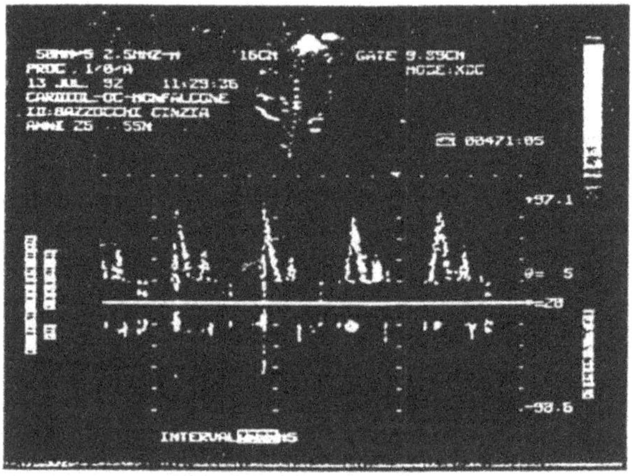

FIG. B - Normal Pattern ($E > A$)

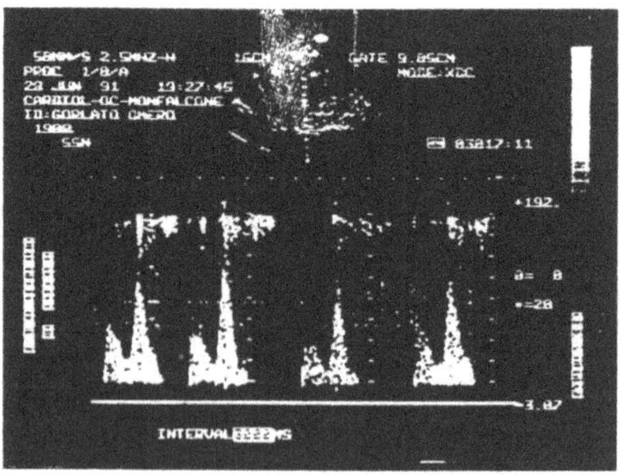

FIG.C - Pathological Pattern ($A > E$)

In these: mean DA/PA=0.52 and the mean HB_{A1c}=7.81.Clinical findings differentiated the II from I Group as follows: no complications in 3(25%) vs 14(46.6%); retinopathy in 12 (60%) vs 10(33.3%) and microaneurisms in 2(10%) vs 2(6.6%); neuropathy in 8 (40%) vs 6 (20%); nephropathy in 7 (35%) vs 3(10%); arteriopathy in 9(45%) vs 4 (13.3%).

VCG - 2D ECHO FINDINGS AND DM NON - CARDIAC COMPLICATIONS WITH RESPECT TO AGE OF PATIENTS

	AGE (yrs)	2 D - E C H O		V C G		CLINICAL FINDINGS	
		normal	abnormal	normal	abnormal	normal	abnormal
I GROUP 30 PTS	<50 23 pts (76.7%)	20 (86.9%)	3 (13.1%)	23	/	12 (52.2%)	11 (47.8%)
	>50 7 pts (23.3%)	4 (55%)	3 (45%)	7	/	2 (28.9%)	5 (71.1%)
		24 (80%)	6 (20%)	30	/	14 (46.7%)	16 (53.3%)
II GROUP 20 PTS	<50 6 pts (30%)	2 (33.4%)	4 (66.6%)	/	6	1 (16.6%)	5 (83.4%)
	>50 14 pts (70%)	2 (14.3%)	12 (85.7%)	/	14	2 (14.3%)	12 (85.7%)
		4 (20%)	16 (80%)	/	20	3 (15%)	18 (85%)

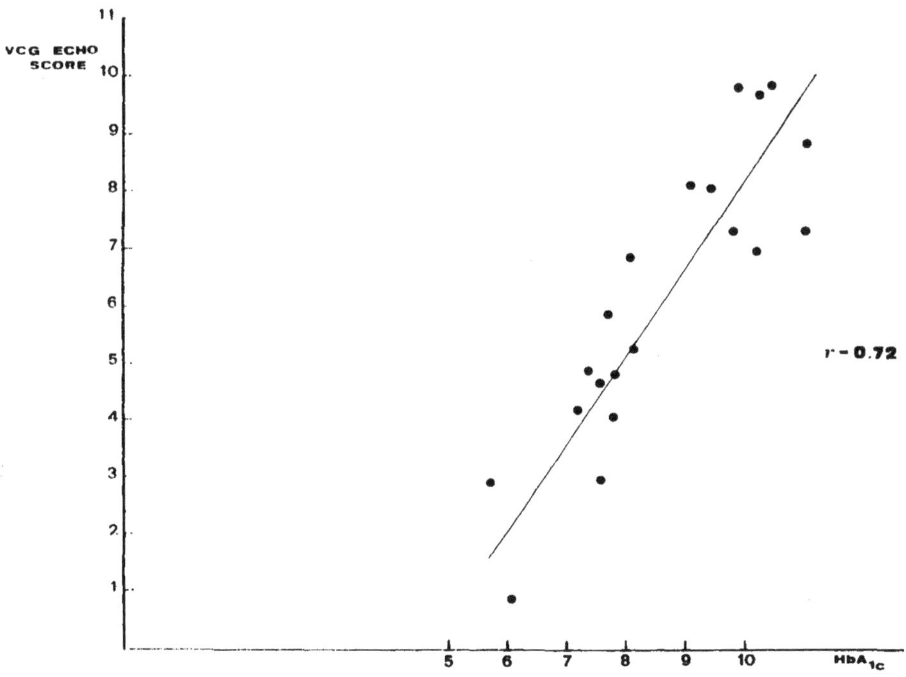

CORRELATION BETWEEN DM NON-CARDIAC COMPLICATIONS AND HbA_{1c}

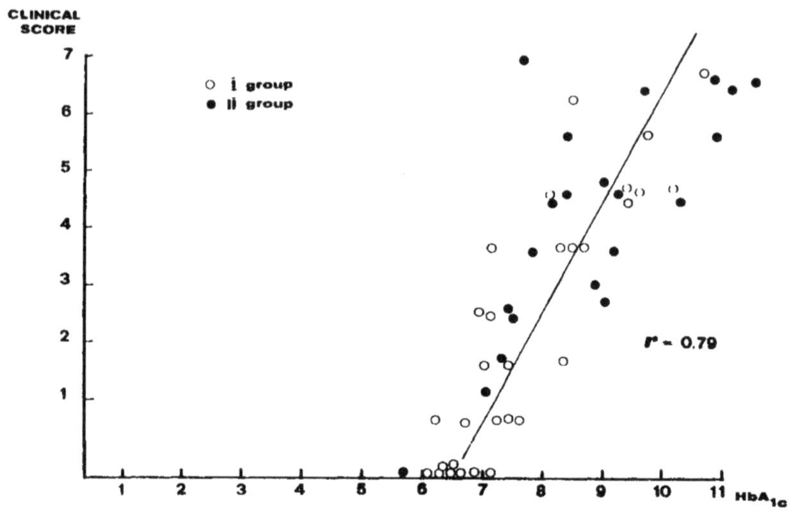

O V E R A L L:

50 PTS WITH IDDM
- ABNORMAL VCG: 20 (40%)
- ABNORMAL 2D-ECHO: 26 (52%)

20 NORMAL SBTS
- ABNORMAL VCG: 2 (10%)
- ABNORMAL 2D-ECHO: 2 (10%)

CONCLUSIONS

1) VCG changes (mostly bites) and 2D-ECHO abnormalities (mostly A > E ratio) have been shown in our IDDM pts asymptomatic for cardiac symptoms in a percentage much higher than in 20 sex age-matched controls (40% and 52% respectively v.s. 10% and 10%). So, especially when other DM non-cardiac complications are present, such findings deserve a peculiar interest as possible markers of pre-clinical DCM.

2) A correlation has also been found between VCG-2D ECHO abnormalities and HB_{A1c} as well as between clinical non-cardiac complications and HB_{A1c}, while only the age of pts beyond 50 years seems to be a marker of severity for the prognosis of the illness.

TRIAXICARDIOMETRIC AND IZOTOPE DIAGNOSTIC METHOD TO CLASSIFY THE DIFFERENT TYPES OF LEFT BUNDLE BRANCH BLOCKS.

L. REGÖS, I. BALOGH, Z. ANTALÓCZY, K. SZABÓ

Postgraduate Medical School, Budapest - 1389 P.O.B.: 112
Hungary

ABSTRACT

In left bundle branch blocks cases 3 subgroups were differentiated by the frontal plain ECG leads. Studiing the Conventional ECG leads, triaxicardiograms data of 42 patients suffering from LBBB.

1./ LBBB with an extreme left axis deviation, left anterior hemiblock type.

2./ LBBB with middle axis electrical position.

3./ LBBB with extreme right exis deviation, is in accordance with the left posterior hemiblock type.

In the LAH type group there were 19 patients, in the second group 20 patients and in LPH type, there were only 3 patients.

The patients whose anamnestic data contains myocardial infarction, were not taken into account in the following examination. Afterwards we used the radionuclid ventriculography multigated acquisition (MUGA) and on the basis of this examination, helped by phase analysis, the sequence of the left vantricular activation was definable. It was proved that the left ventricular depolarisation which was established earlier, coincided with the ECG morphology.

Introduction

More than eighty years ago Eppinger and Rothberger were the first to describe the nature of intraventricular conduction defects, simulated by an experimental setting (6). On humans, in nineteen-twenty, Fahr made the original observations and published his paper dealing with intraventicular conduction abnormalities (7). Ten years later, Barker, Macleod and Alexander finally clarified the ECG morphology of these conduction defects (3). In spite of this, the sequence of intraventricular conduction and its relation to the conventional 12 lead ECG is still a matter of interest; mostly because of its high incidence (from

0.4 to 1.1% according to Katz-Pick and Edmands) and also of the front linkage to organic heart diseases (5,8,14).

As a synthesis of the experimental and human observations, different subtypes of the left bundle branch block (LBBB) have been described by Myerburg (1973), Rosenbaum (1969) and Dhiuga (1977). (4,11,14) Our work-group has also actively contributed to this work (Antaloczy 1973 and 1974) by a triaxicardiometric classification of the left bundle branch blocks. (1,2)

According to the information accumulated in the literature two main types of LBBBs can be distinguished, taking into account the main QRS axis deviation in the frontal plane, as LBBB with normal axis and those with left axis deviation, morphologically similar to the left anterior hemiblock (LAH), but QRS widens more than 0.12 sec. The present clinical observations also comprise a third group in which the QRS pattern is very similar to the left posterior hemiblock (LPH), but also widens according to the aforementioned measure.

Patients and Methods

Since the electrocardiological and polarcardiographic (triaxicardiometric) body surface patterns of left ventricular (LV) activation in LBBB were previously described and the data available were compared with another selective method of LV activation or ventricular contraction sequences, the ECG gated myocardial technetium scintigraphy, the so-called phase display method (9). Similarly comparative methods using ECG, VCG and body surface mapping measurements, already proved earlier to be valuable by our working-group, in the localization of premature ventricular contraction on WPW patients (10,12) with different bypass tracts (Mester and Preda et al). In another study we also investigated the electro-cardiological similarities of different forms of intra-ventricular conduction defects and ECG patterns related to subtypes of ventricular preexcitation (Regös) (13).

In the present series the study population consisted of 42 subjects. By all of the them traditional 12-lead ECG, the 3 paravertebral leads and the orthogonal Frank leads were registered. The triaxicardiograms were derived by an analogic computer, using the Frank system (1,2).

Based on the measurements three subgroups have been distinguised:

1./ LBBB with normal axis in the frontal plane; 20 patients.

2./ LBBB with left axis deviation in the frontal plane, LAH type 19 patients.

3./ LBBB with extreme right axis deviation in the frontal plane, LPH type, 3 patients (Figure 1.).

Patients who suffered chronic myocardial infraction visualized by 201-thallium scintigraphy were excluded prior to the study, from further evaluation. Patients belonging to group, suffered from dilated cardiomypathy and because of their limited number, are not to be discussed in the present study.

Using the multigated (MUGA) acquisition radionuclid ventriculography (phase analysis) the most valuable scintigraphy photos were taken from the left anterior oblique 45° angle (LAO-45) projections (10). Since the left and right ventricular shapes could be clearly separated, and the activation delay and changes in the left ventricular contraction sequences could be well defined from this view. The spread of left ventricular contarction reflecting the depolarization sequences in this projection could be properly traced (Figure 2.). Two main identification points were used,

a./ Entry point of left ventricular contraction (the beginning of LV activation) from the right ventricular projection;

b./ Site of left ventricular shape activated the last (the end of LV activation).

Discussion

As it is known in LBBB, in the horizontal plane the left ventricular depolarisation vectors, are directed from the anterior side to the posterior . Regarding our first and second groups the inportant changes in the run off of the left ventricular activation were found to be along the Y axis, that is, to say alterations occurred primarily from the horizontal plane. If the changes in depolarization sequences point from the horizontal plane superiorly, the ECG leads reveals an LAH type of left bundle branch block. Contrarily if the vectors point inferiorly from the horizontal plane, it coincides in the frontal plane with a normal LBBB axis.

By taking into consideration these interrelations it can be established that in LPH type LBBB cases, the activation sequence, in anterior phase display projections, should be directed from left to right.

Evaluating the different examinations it seemed to be easy to determine the momentaneous-vectors on ECG and triaxicardiometric tracings. This cannot be carried out on the basis of phase display pictures, where the spread of activation (contraction) can be determined at distant points, but the detection of the exact pathway of LV activation would require a more sophisticated software. Furthermore studies using such a computer program and surface mapping registration of left ventricular activation are one of the possible ways of continuing the present study. The general problems are, by using the above method that we are unable to show and demonstrate, the transmyocardial activation.

References

1.) Z. Antalóczy, M. Strommer, L. Regös, B. Tomor: Quantitative vector analysis of bundle branch block by the triaxicardiometer analog computer. II. International Symposium on Electrocardiology. New trends in Electrocardiology. (Yerevan, 1973.)

2.) Z. Antalóczy, M. Strommer, L. Regös, B. Tomor: A szárblockok quantitativ vektoranalízise analóg computerrel, triaxicardiometerrel. M. Belorv. Arch. **27** (1974) 76.

3.) P.S. Barker, A.G. Macleod, J. Alexander: The excitatory process in the exposed human heart. Am. Heart J. **5** (1930) 720 .

4.) R. Dhiuga, J. Cummings, P. Deedwania, F. Amat-y-Leon, K.M. Rosen: The clinical significance of left axis deviation in patients with left bundle branch block. Clin. Res. **25** (1977) 217A.

5.) R.E. Edmans: An epidemiological assessment of bundle branch block. Circ. **34** (1966) 1081 .

6.) H. Eppinger, C.J. Rothberger: Folgen der Durchschneidung der Tawaraschenkel. Z. Klin. Med. **70** (1910) 1.

7.) G. Fahr: Analysis of the spread of the excitation wave. Arch. Int. Med. **5** (1920) 146.

8.) L.N. Katz, A. Pick: Clinical Electrocardiography. Lea and Febinger, Philadelphia (1956) Part I.

9.) J. Mester, E. Máté, L. Regös, Gy. Marosi, Z. Antalóczy, L. Csernai: Aussagekraft des Phasendisplayverfahrens zum Nachweis des WPW-Syndroms. Nuc. Compact. **16** (1985) 13.

10.) Mester J., Préda I., Kozmann Gy., Máté E., Regös L., Marosi Gy., Antalóczy Z., Cernay L.: Localization of accessory conduction pathways in Wolff-Parkinson-White syndrome through phase display and body surface mapping; A comparative study. Nuclear Med. Communication **7** (1986) 497.

11.) R.J. Myerburg, K. Nellson, H. Gelband: Physiology of canine intraventricular conduction and endocardial excitation. Circ. Res. **30** (1972) 217.
12.) I. Préda, J. Mester, Z. Antalóczy, Gy. Kozmann, L. Csernay: A testfelületi potenciális térképezés (surface mapping) értéke a kamrai preexcitatio helyének meghatározásában WPW syndromában. Cardiol. Hung. **19** (1990) 243, 1.
13.) L. Regös: A kamrai preexcitatio átfogó elektrokardiológiai rendszerezése. Ph. D. Thesis (Budapest 1983).
14.) M.B. Rosenbaum: Types of left bundle branch block and their clinical significance. J. Electrocardiography **2** (1969) 197.

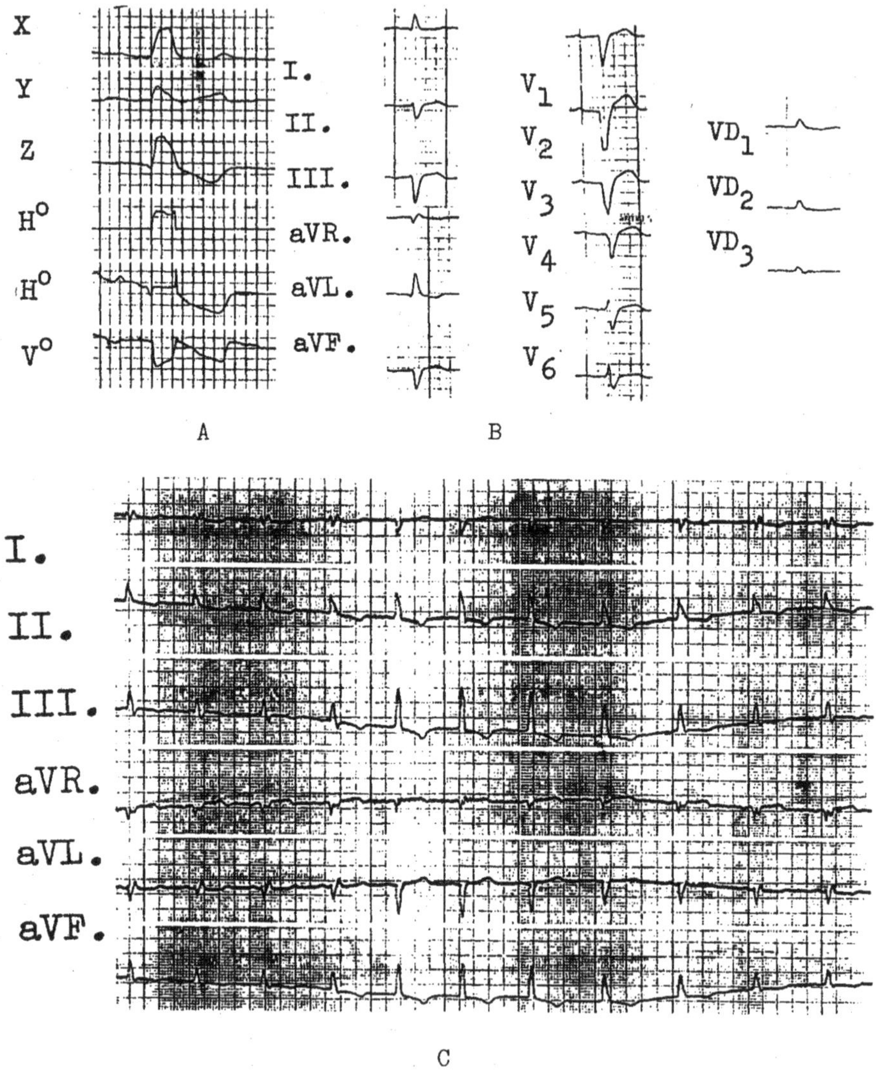

Figure 1.: A.: Frank leads and the triaxicardiograms in a case LBBB with normal axis in the frontal plane. B.: Conventional 12 leads and the 3 paravertebral leads in a case LAH type LBBB. C.: Intermittent LBBB type LPH.

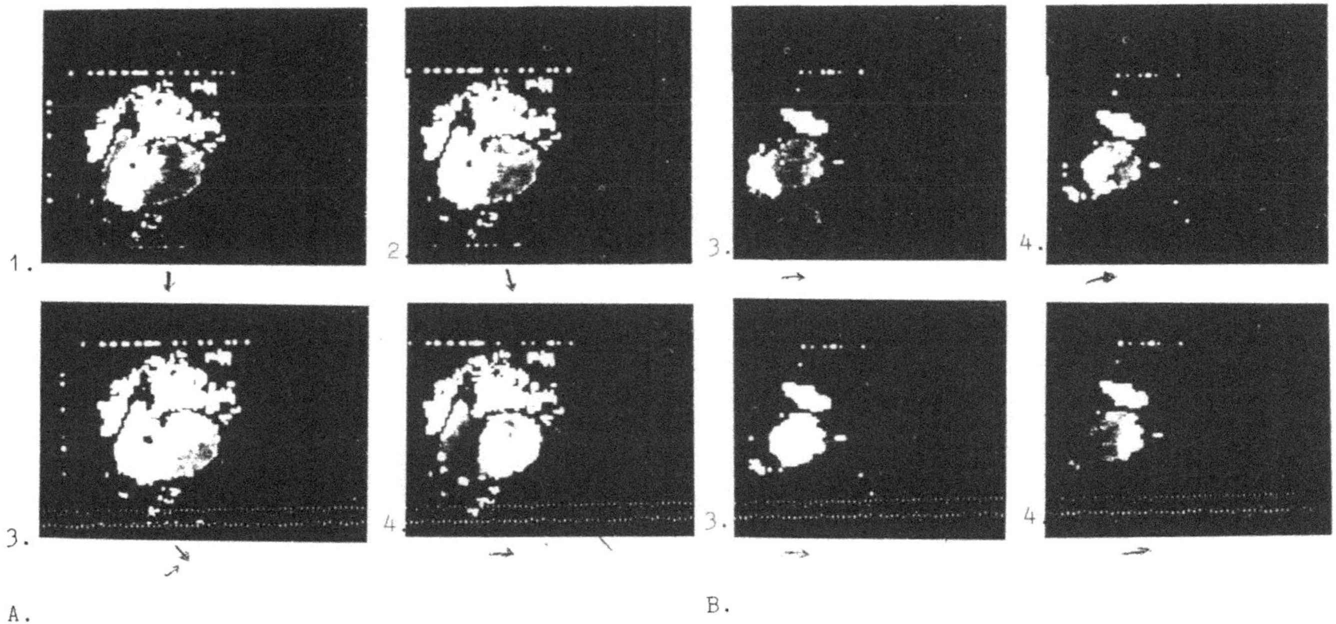

Figure 2.: Multigated acquisition radionuclid ventriculography. The pictures shows the activarion sequences of left ventricle in LAO-45.
A.: The narrows shows the LV activation sequance in a case of LBBB , with middle axis deviation.
B.: The narrows shows the activation sequance of LV, in a case of LAH type LBBB.

THE DISCREPANCIES BETWEEN ELECTRICAL AND MECHANICAL CONTRACTION TIMES IN HUMAN HEART

YASURO SUGISHITA
Cardiovascular Division, Department of Internal Medicine,
Institute of Clinical Medicine, The University of Tsukuba,
Tsukuba 305, Japan

and

TOHRU KURIHARA, IWAO YAMAGUCHI, HIROSHI MAEDA,
TOSHIYUKI ISHIMITSU, MASAE ENDO and TAKASHI MIYAUCHI
Cardiovascular Division, Department of Internal Medicine,
Institute of Clinical Medicine, The University of Tsukuba,
Tsukuba 305, Japan

ABSTRACT

It is generally believed that electrical contraction time is correlated with mechanical contraction time. However, in the kangaroo heart, there is a discrepancy between these two contraction times, and this is supposed to be a factor to induce sudden cardiac death of the animal. In this study, to evaluate the relationship between electrical and mechanical contraction times in the human heart, we measured QT interval (QT) and ejection time (ET) before and after hemodialysis (HD) in 21 patients with chronic renal failure (Group I), and before and after disopyramisde (D) 100 mg i.v.in 6 patients with arrhythmia (Group II). In Group I, although the no change of QT was not significant (an increase in 6 patients and change in 15 patients), all 21 patients showed a significant shortening of ET (0.30±0.03 sec → 0.26±0.04 sec, mean±SD, P<0.01). In Group II, QT prolonged significantly by D i.v. (0.38±0.03 sec → 0.43±0.04 sec, mean±SD, p<0.01), but ET was unchanged. In conclusion, electrical and mechanical contraction times do not change necessarily correspondingly, and this discrepancy might induce a detrimental factor in human heart.

1. Introduction

It has usually been believed in human heart and many of the experimental animals, such as dogs, that electrical systole correlates with mechanical systole, that is the end of T wave in electrocardiogram correlates with the end of mechanical systole. However, in some animals, for instance, in kangaroo, QT interval is significantly shorter than ejection time[1,2]. In kangaroo, the end of T wave occurs during mechanical systole while ventricular ejection is still proceeding[2].

It has usually been believed that tetanus occurs in skeletal muscle as in some smooth muscle, but not in myocardium. As shown in a previous study[1], however, it was found that with the occurrence of extrasystole, the myocardium in kangaroo would be stimulated to contract before relaxation was complete after a normally contracted complexes. This is considered to result in a type of incomplete totanus or summation. The disparity between the duration of ventricular refratoriness and of the left ventricular contraction explains the contracture and incomplete tetanus of kangaroo heart muscle. Kangaroo is known to be susceptible to sudden cardiac death, and this might be explained by the incomplete tetanus, mentioned above. Such behavior appears to be unique to the kangaroo for observations taken in healthy animals under normal experimental conditions. Similar findings have not been reported in normal man.

The danger of QT prolongation has been emphasized clinically, but the findings in kangaroo also suggest the danger of short QT interval. Now, the relationship between ventricular refractoriness and left ventriclar contraction in various cardiac conditions in man remains to be investigated.

The purpose of the present study is to evaluate the relationship between electrical and mechanical contraction times in the human heart.

2. Materials and Methods

Materials consisted of two groups. Group I consisted of 21 patients with chronic renal failure under hemodialysis (HD). They were 9 males and 12 females, and were 33-71 years old. They had no heart failure. Group II consisted of 6 patients with arrhythmia under the treatment by disopyramide (D). They were 2 males and 4 females, and were 25-75 years old.

In all of the patients, electrocardiograms, phonocardiograms and carotid pulse tracings were recorded in a supine position. The QT interval, as the electricial contraction time, was measured from the beginning of the Q wave to the end of the T wave, from a high fidelity electrocardiogram recorded at a paper speed of 25 mm/sec. Ejection time (ET), as the mechanical contraction time, was measured from the beginning of the upstroke to the trough of the incisural notch, from the carotid pulse tracing obtained at a paper speed of 100 mm/sec. $Q\text{-}S_2$ interval was also measuured from the beginning of the Q wave to the second heart sound from electocardiogram and phonocardiogram recorded simultaneously. The QT interval was corrected from heart rate (QTc) employing the conventional Bazzett equation, QTc = QT/ RR.

The changes of the electrical or mechanical contraction times were induced by HD in the patients of Group I, and by intravenous infusion of D 100 mg in the patients of Group II. After these interventions, the examinations were repeated again, and the contration times were measured. Serum electrolyte concentrations were measured before and after HD in the patients of Group II.

The paired t test was used for the statistical analysis. All results with a value $p<0.05$ were regarded as statistically significant.

3. Results

In Group I, after HD, the changes of QT and QTc were not significant statistically (QT and QTc prolonged with a decrease of RR interval in 6 patients, and did not prolong with no change of RR interval in 15 patients). ET showed a significant shortening in all the 21 patients (0.30 ± 0.03 sec → 0.26 ± 0.04 sec, $p<0.01$). Q-S_2 showed also a significant shortening. By HD, potassium concentration in serum decreased and calcium concentration increased.

In Group II, by D i.v., there was no significant change in RR interval, but QT and QTc prolonged significantly (QT: 0.38 ± 0.03 sec → 0.43 ± 0.04 sec, QTc: 0.41 ± 0.02 → 0.47 ± 0.02, $p<0.01$, respectively), whereas ET was unchanged.

4. Discussion

The changes of action potential are known to correlate with the mechanical events. A linear relation between time to peak force and the action potential duration has been observed by many. And clinically also the end of electrical systole is known to correlate with the end of mechanical systole.

Prolongation of electrical systole is associated with a high incidence of ventricular arrhythmia and sudden death in the patients with and without coronary artery disease[3,4]. In these patients, QT interval was found to be longer than S_2[5].

On the other hand, kangaroo has QT interval shorter than ejection time, and this discrepancy might cause sudden death in this animal[1,2].

Discrepancy between electrical and mechanical systoles has not been reported in normal man. But the relationship between these two systoles remain to be investigated in various cardiac conditions in man.

In this study, we have investigated the relationship between electrical and mechanical contraction times, when the changes of QT or ET were induced by the interventions, such as hemodialysis or disopyramide i.v. The electrical and mechanical contraction times did not change correspondingly; that is, HD induced a shortening of ET probably due to a decrease of circulating blood volume with no change or an increase of QT, and D induced a prolongation of QT with no change of ET. By these two interventions, the relationship between the two contraction times shifted to the region of rather long QT with relatively short ET. This might be rather safe, in contrast to kangaroo, in which the relationship between the two contraction times was situated in the region of rather short QT with relatively long ET and in which incomplete tetanus was induced by extrasystoles. Anyway, the discrepancies between electical and mecahnical systoles might induce a derimental factor in human heart, too. In order to clarify the meaning of the shift of the relationship between electrical and mechanical systoles, the examinations should be performed under the other interventions.

5. Conclusion

Electrical and mechanical contraction times do not change necessarily correspondingly, and this discrepancy might induce a detrimental factor in human heart.

6. References

1. M.F. O'Rourke, A.P. Avolio and W.W. Nichols. Cardiovasc Res. 20 (1986) 398.
2. Y. Sugishita, K. Iida, M.F. O'Rourke, R. Kelly, A. Avolio, D. Butcher and H. Reddacliff, Aust. N.Z.J. Med. 20 (1990) 160.
3. A. Jervell and F. Lange-Nielsen, Am. Heart J. 54 (1957) 59.
4. S. Ahme, S. Halmer, T. Lemdman, N. Rehniquist and A. Sjogren, Clin. Cardiol. 3 (1980) 303.
5. H. Boudoulas, Y.H. Sohn, W. O'Neill, R. Brown and A.M. Weissler, Am. J. Cardiol. 50 (1982) 1229.

PART V
Coronary Artery Disease: Recognition, Localization and Prognosis

LOCALIZATION OF ONE-VESSEL CORONARY ARTERY DISEASE BY EXERCISE-INDUCED ST SEGMENT CHANGES

VÍTOR GIL

ANTÓNIO VENTOSA

RICARDO SEABRA-GOMES

Department of Cardiology, Hospital de Santa Cruz
Carnaxide, 2795 Linda-a-Velha (Lisboa), Portugal

1. Introduction

The attempt to localize coronary artery disease (CAD) based on ECG changes (including ST-segment depression) in different leads is widely used. The validity of this practice has been confirmed for Q waves, T-wave inversion and ST-segment elevation[1]. However, the site of ST-segment depression during exercise correlated poorly with CAD localization[1-3], despite some previous reports suggesting the opposite[4,5]. On this study, we wanted to reevaluate with a larger series the issue of electrocardiographic localization of CAD by exercise-induced ST-segment changes, using a population of single vessel disease patients without myocardial infarction, all with ST-segment changes on a treadmill exercise test.

2. Material and methods

From our institution files, we selected all patients that had performed a coronary arteriography and a treadmill exercise test within 9 months, without major clinical events meanwhile. From that population, the inclusion criteria for this retrospective study were: 1) Absence of clinical, electrocardiographic or ventriculographic evidence of previous myocardial infarction; 2) one-vessel CAD at coronary arteriography; 3) exercise-induced ST-segment changes ≥ 1 mm on treadmill exercise test. We excluded from the study patients with conditions that made ST segment interpretation difficult, namely hypertensive response, digitalis, bundle branch block, WPW.

With those criteria, we studied 80 patients, 72 male and 8 female, 51 ± 9 years old. Diseased vessel was left anterior descending artery (LAD) in 58 patients, left circumflex artery (LCX) in 12 patients and right coronary artery (RCA) in 10 patients.

Exercise test was performed on a Quinton-3000 treadmill, using Bruce protocol with Sheffield modification. Limb electrodes were placed in the torso using a modified Mason-Likar system, with arm electrodes at midclavicular line, 2 cm below lower border of clavicles and left leg electrode on the back. Besides continuous monitoring of 3 leads, a complete 12-lead ECG was obtained at rest, at the end of each stage, at peak exercise, and also in the recovery period. Exercise was continued until maximum predicted heart rate was reached or interrupted before because of severe angina or fatigue, blood pressure fall, hypertensive response, complex cardiac arrhythmias or ST-segment depression greater than 3 mm.

Rest and peak exercise ECG were compared. Exercise-induced ST-segment depression was considered if horizontal or downsloping ≥ 1 mm or slowly ascending ≥ 1.5 mm 80 ms after J point. Exercise-induced ST-segment elevation was considered if ≥ 1 mm 40 ms after J point.

Statistical analysis used the chi-square test.

3. Results

ST-segment depression occurred in 79 patients. As shown in Table I, it was most frequent in precordial leads V5 and V6, followed by V4, for each of the vessels. ST-segment depression in V5 was significantly less common in RCA disease than with LAD or LCX diseases ($p<0.05$). In V2 or V3 ST-segment depression was less frequent, being relatively more rare in LAD patients than in LCX or RCA patients ($p<0.05$ for V2).

ST-segment depression in inferior leads was observed in more than half of patients with LAD disease, but only in one third of LCX patients and in one of ten RCA patients. This difference was quite significant ($p=0.004$).

ST-segment depression in lateral limb leads was uncommon.

TABLE I. Location of exercise-induced ST-segment depression

	n	II	III	aVF	any	I	aVL	V1	V2	V3	V4	V5	V6
LAD	(58)	57*	45*	52*	62*	3	3	-	7&	22	71	95	90
LCX	(12)	33	17	17	33	17	8	-	25	42	83	100	92
RCA	(10)	10	-	10	10	20	20	-	30	40	50	70#	70

Results: % patients within each group; n number of patients; # $p<0.05$ with LAD/LCX
* respectively $p<0.02$, $p=0.006$, $p=0.005$ and p<0004 with LCX/RCA; & $p<0.05$ with LCX/RCA;

ST-segment elevation (Table II) was found in only seven patients: in the inferior leads in one of ten patients with RCA disease, and in precordial and lateral limb leads in up to 10% of patients with LAD disease (mostly in V2 and V3).

TABLE II. Location of exercise-induced ST-segment elevation

	n	II	III	aVF	I	aVL	V1	V2	V3	V4	V5	V6
LAD	(58)	-	-	-	2	3	5	10	10	3	2	2
LCX	(12)	-	-	-	-	-	-	-	-	-	-	-
RCA	(10)	10	10	10	-	-	-	-	-	-	-	-

Results: % patients within each group; n number of patients; Differences not significant.

For the significant differences found, we derived diagnostic criteria, and analysed their accuracy. ST-segment depression in V5 was useless due to its low specificity (30%). Other criteria are shown in Table III. ST-segment depression in one of inferior leads was quite sensitive (57%) and specific (77%) for LAD identification; ST-segment depression in V2 has been highly specific (93%) in excluding LAD disease in this series, although with poor sensitivity.

Table III. Criteria for diseased vessel identification.

ST Change	Lead	Vessel	Sens	Spec	PredV
Depression	V2	LCX/RCA	27%	93%	60%
	II/III/aVF	LAD	57%	77%	87%

Sens sensitivity; Spec specificity; PredV positive predictive value; ../.. ..or..

4. Discussion

To our knowledge, this is the largest published series (79 patients) of exercise-induced ST-segment depression in one-vessel disease without previous myocardial infarction. Fuchs et al[1] and Fox et al[2] studied respectively 54 and 27 patients with one-vessel CAD and ST-segment depression on exercise test. In the study of Fuchs et al[1], almost 20% of the patients had a myocardial infarction, and ST-segment elevation occurred in almost 40% of the patients. Both studies found no significant differences between the 3 vessels in lead-by-lead prevalence of ST-depression, concluding that there is a poor correlation between the site of ST-depression on exercise ECG and the localization of CAD. We also found no significant differences between the vessels for precordial leads V3 to V6, being V5 the lead most often involved. In our series, ST-segment depression in V2 was more common for LCX or RCA disease than with LAD disease. In the study of Fox et al[2] there were no patients with ST-depression in V2, and in the study of Fuchs et al[1] it was slightly more frequent in LAD, although without significant differences. None of the three series had ST-depression in V1. ST-depression in I and aVL was uncommon in our series and in that of Fuchs et al[1] (with RCA leading in both series, but without reaching statistical significance) and did not occur in that of Fox et al[2].

ST-depression in inferior leads in isolated LAD disease has been used as an example of the poor correlation between CAD localization and ST-segment depression on exercise[1-3,6]. In the studies of Fuchs et al[1] and Fox et al[2] LAD was the vessel were ST-segment depression in inferior leads was more common (respectively 83% and 75% of LAD patients, in lead II), but it also was fairly common in LCX/RCA diseases (respectively 68% and 45% in the same lead). In our series ST-segment depression had a lower prevalence in inferior leads. Using also lead II as example, we found it in 57% of LAD patients but only in 23% of LCX/RCA patients. This difference was statistically significant. Our results suggest that ST-depression in inferior leads in isolated LAD disease may be an example of an unexpected correlation (instead of a poor correlation) between ECG and CAD localization. There are several possible explanations for this finding. ST-segment depression in inferior leads might be, in these patients reciprocal changes related to exercise-induced anterior wall motion abnormalities. However, only in a small number of these patients ST-segment depression in inferior leads was accompanied by ST-segment elevation in precordial leads. Any way it is conceivable that slight ST-segment elevation, inferior to 1 mm (and so not considerated) might have occurred in a number of additional patients. Another possible explanation assume that ST-segment depression might be caused by inferior wall ischemia in patients with a long LAD, supplying a significant portion of inferior wall. That issue was not analysed on our study. Finally, ST-segment depression in inferior leads might in fact reflect only anterior or apical ischemia in LAD patients. Papouchado et al[6] reported that placement of limb electrodes onto the torso, as used on exercise test, distorts the electrocardiogram causing significant changes in R-wave amplitude with reduction in leads I and aVL, and increase in leads II, III and aVF. They concluded that the so-called "inferior" leads on the exercise electrocardiogram are in fact modified anterior/inferior leads, since their R-waves amplitudes correlate closely with those of antero-lateral chest leads and that the inferior surface of the heart is not represented in isolation on the exercise electrocardiogram. These findings provide the best explanation for our results, were exercise-induced ST-depression in inferior leads predicted LAD disease.

In our series only 7 patients had ST-segment elevation on exercise. Although the results suggest a clear cut-off, with inferior leads predicting RCA disease, and precordial or limb lateral leads predicting LAD disease, the differences did not achieve statistic significance. Other series however agree that the site of exercise-induced ST-segment elevation predicts severe CAD localization[1,7].

In <u>conclusion</u> our results suggest that exercise-induced ST-segment depression in inferior leads in 1-vessel disease can predict LAD disease. That might be due - at least in part - to changes in ECG patterns induced by torso placement of lead limbs[6].

1. MF Fuchs, SC Aschuff, L Grunwald, FCP Yin, LSC Griffith. Circulation, **66** (1982) 1168-76.
2. RM Fox, A-H Hakki, AS Iskandrian. Am J Cardiol, **53** (1984) 1529-31.
3. RF Dunn, B Freeman, IK Bailey, RF Uren, DT Kelly. Am J Cardiol, **48** (1981) 837-43.
4. D Robertson, WJ Kostuk, SP Ahuja. Am Heart J, **91** (1976) 437-44.
5. KM Fox, A Selwyn, D Oakley, JP Shillingford. Am J Cardiol, **44** (1979) 1068-1075.
6. M Papouchado, PR Walker, MA James, LM Clarke. Eur Heart J, **8** (1987) 725-33.
7. RF Dunn, IK Bailey, R Uren, DT Kelly. Circulation, **61** (1980) 989-95.

EXERCISE-INDUCED QRS AXIS CHANGES: NEW CRITERIA FOR THE LOCALIZATION OF CORONARY ARTERY DISEASE

ANTÓNIO VENTOSA

VÍTOR GIL

RICARDO SEABRA-GOMES

Department of Cardiology, Hospital de Santa Cruz
Carnaxide, 2795 Linda-a-Velha (Lisboa), Portugal

1. Introduction

The role of exercise-induced ST-segment changes in the diagnosis of coronary artery disease (CAD) is well established. In the last decade several authors have addressed the matter of exercise-induced changes in the amplitude of the different waves of QRS complex, and its possible value in the diagnosis of CAD[1-3], but published results do not agree about the diagnostic value of such findings.

Electrocardiographic localization of CAD based on exercise ECG has been studied by us[4] and others[5,6], with emphasis on ST-segment changes. However the studies on QRS waves' amplitude changes did not analyse in general the influence of disease localization on these changes.

With the analysis of QRS axis in the present study, we intended to incorporate in one variable the potential information derived from the three waves of the QRS, in several leads. We studied exercise-induced QRS axis shifts in patients with single vessel CAD, and investigated its relation with disease localization.

2. Material and methods

From our institution files, we selected all patients that had performed a coronary arteriography and a treadmill exercise test within 9 months, without major clinical events meanwhile. From that population, we included in this retrospective study patients with one-vessel CAD and exercise-induced ST-segment changes $\geq$ 1 mm on treadmill exercise test. We excluded patients with conditions that made ST segment interpretation difficult (namely digitalis, hypertensive response, bundle branch block and WPW) and patients with enlarged QRS.

With those criteria, we studied 135 patients, 123 male and 12 female, 51 $\pm$ 9 years old. Myocardial infarction was present in 64 patients (44 anterior and 20 inferior). Three groups were studied, based on the diseased vessel: left anterior descending artery (LAD) in 97 patients, left circumflex artery (LCX) in 17 patients and right coronary artery (RCA) in 21 patients.

Exercise test was performed on a Quinton 3000 treadmill, using Bruce protocol with Sheffield modification. A complete 12-lead ECG was obtained (always with patient upright) at rest, at the end of each stage, at peak exercise, and also in the recovery period. Exercise was continued until maximum predicted heart rate was reached or interrupted because of severe angina or fatigue, blood pressure fall, hypertensive response, complex cardiac arrhythmias or ST-segment depression greater than 3 mm. Exercise-induced ST-segment depression was considered if horizontal or downsloping ≥ 1 mm or slowly ascending ≥ 1.5 mm 80 ms after J point. Exercise-induced ST-segment elevation was considered if ≥ 1 mm 40 ms after J point.

QRS axis was quantified, using the following equation that requires the measurement of the net QRS amplitude in two leads with a right-angle between them.

$$\text{Angle} = \text{Arc tan}\ \frac{QRS90°}{QRS0°} \times \frac{360}{2\pi} \quad (a)$$

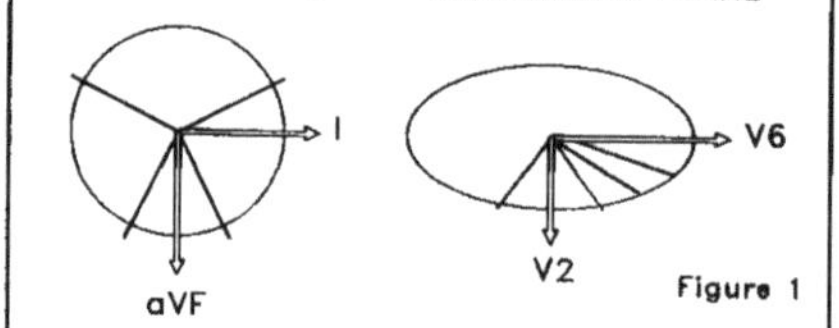

Figure 1

For the frontal plane, we used lead I as 0° and lead aVF as 90°. For the horizontal plane, we assumed lead V6 as 0° and lead V2 as 90° (Figure 1).

Measurements were performed visually on rest and peak exercise ECG's. Rest and peak exercise QRS axis and exercise-induced QRS axis changes were then calculated for both frontal and horizontal planes.

Continuous variables were studied with analysis of variance or t-test and categorical variables with chi-square test.

3. Results

Exercise test variables unrelated to QRS axis (results not shown) did not differ significantly between the three groups. Rest QRS axis was slightly more inferior and a lot more posterior in LAD group, due to the inclusion of patients with myocardial infarction (results not shown).

With exercise, QRS axis shifted inferiorly (frontal plane) and posteriorly (horizontal plane) in RCA and LCX groups while in LAD group there was almost no shift (Table I). Those differences were largely significant, and were not influenced, in each group, by the presence of myocardial infarction (Table II).

TABLE I
Exercise-induced QRS axis changes

Vessel	n	Front	Horiz
LAD	97	-4±24*	0±15**
LCX	17	+21±22	-24±27
RCA	21	+21±21	-18±19

MI myocardial infarction; Front,Horiz frontal and horizontal QRS axis changes (°); mean ± sd;
* p<0.0002 vs LCX, p<0.00005 vs RCA;
** p<0.000001 vs LCX, p<0.00001 vs RCA.

---

a) Qrs0°, Qrs90° = net QRS vector amplitudes respectively at leads 0° and 90°
When Qrs0° is (-), a 180° correction is necessary: +180° if Qrs90° (+), -180° if Qrs90° (-)

TABLE II
Exercise-induced QRS axis changes and myocardial infarction

Vessel	MI	n	Front	Horiz
LAD	-	53	0±23	+2±18
	+	44	-9±25	-2±10
LCX	-	10	+15±21	-17±22
	+	7	+28±22	-34±30
RCA	-	8	+23±17	-13±22
	+	13	+20±22	-20±17

MI myocardial infarction; Front,Horiz frontal and horizontal QRS axis changes (°); mean ± sd; differences not significant

Table III
Criteria for vessel identification

Axis Change		Sens	Spec	PredV
LAD identification				
Left	> 5°	30%	95%	94%
Anterior	> 5°	26%	92%	89%
(one of them)		46%	87%	90%
LCX/RCA identification				
Right	>20°	42%	97%	84%
Posterior	>30°	29%	99%	92%
(one of them)		53%	96%	83%

Sens sensitivity; Spec specificity;
PredV positive predictive value; ../.. ..or..

Figure 2.
Exercise-induced QRS axis changes

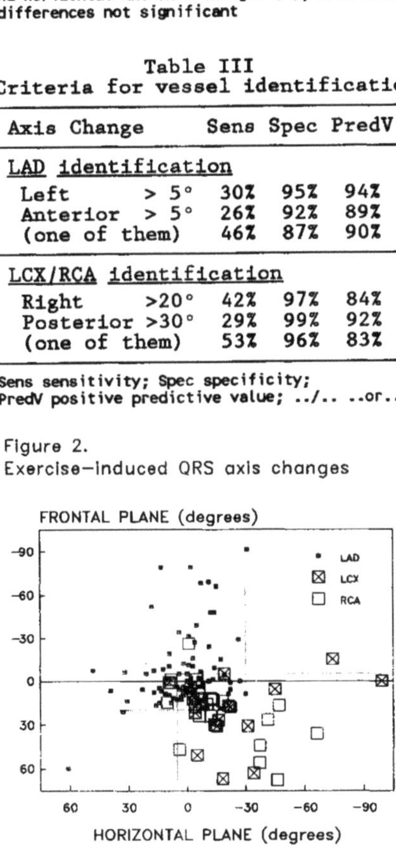

dashed lines: proposed criteria

Plotting QRS axis changes (Figure 2) it became evident that extreme values of LAD group show a left/superior or an anterior axis shift, and that extreme values of LCX and RCA groups show a right/inferior or a posterior axis shift. That distribution allowed the proposal of criteria for vessel identification, based on these results (Table III). Those criteria were highly specific for LAD identification with left and/or anterior shifts, and for LCX/RCA with right or posterior shifts.

4. Discussion

Treadmill exercise test remains a simple and unexpensive non-invasive tool which can provide important data on the individual CAD patient. ST-segment changes have been intensively studied, but other electrocardiographic and non electrocardiographic variables can also provide some additional information. Changes in the amplitude of the waves of QRS complex have been studied by several authors[1-3]. R wave amplitude changes have been related to intraventricular conduction delay[7,8]. It might, then, be expected that different localization of ischemia could affect diversely QRS in different leads. A possible association of changes of QRS waves with CAD localization has not in general been studied, except for Q wave amplitude reduction, reported as specific for LAD disease[1].

In this study, we used QRS axis with the aim of incorporating in one variable the potential information derived from the waves of QRS complex. For QRS axis estimation we used a method developed by ourselves, based on visual measurements of 4 leads (2 for each plane), allowing the study of QRS axis as a continuous variable, using the 12-lead ECG.

We investigated a population of one-vessel CAD with "positive" exercise tests. Exercise-induced QRS axis changes were analysed and related with disease localization. Both in frontal and in horizontal planes, there were no significant differences between LCX and RCA patients, but the difference between these patients and LAD patients was highly significant. The analysis of the distribution of those values revealed that extreme values in the LAD group had leftward or anterior shift, but no rightward or posterior shifts and that the opposite was true for LCX or RCA groups, allowing the proposal of criteria with excellent specificity for predicting disease localization (LAD vs LCX/RCA).

These results are consistent with ischemia-induced intramyocardial conduction delay, which has been suggested as a mechanism for R wave amplitude changes[7,8]. The axis shifts which magnitude exceeded the proposed criteria could represent in fact small, but variable degrees of fascicular block, depending on anterior or inferior localization of ischemia. Exercise-induced fascicular blocks are rare, but left anterior fascicular block has been associated with LAD disease[9], and left posterior fascicular block with RCA disease[10].

On medical literature, we found only one study relating exercise-induced QRS axis shifts and CAD localization: Ogino et al[11] studied the QRS axis on the frontal plane in 101 patients (including multivessel disease), and report that leftward shift is specific for LAD disease and that rightward shift is specific for LCX/RCA diseases. Our study, with a larger series including only 1-vessel disease, confirms those results for the frontal plane, and describes also the specificity of horizontal plane axis shifts for disease localization. The combination of the data obtained in the two planes, resulted in an improvement of sensitivity.

In <u>conclusion</u>, in this series of 1-vessel CAD with a positive treadmill stress test, exercise-induced QRS axis changes predicted the diseased vessel with an excellent specificity, in a considerable proportion of patients. These results suggest that QRS axis may be a potentially useful information to obtain from exercise test in CAD patients, deserving further investigation.

1. MA Famularo, Y Paliwal, R Redd, MH Ellestad. Am J Cardiol **51** (1983) 440-3.
2. PE Bonoris, PS Greenberg, GW Christison, MJ Castellanet, MH Ellestad. Circulation **57** (1978) 904-10.
3. JJ Glazier, S Chierchia, A Margonato, A Maseri. Am J Cardiol **59** (1987) 1295-9.
4. V Gil, A Ventosa, R Seabra-Gomes. (elsewere in this volume)
5. MF Fuchs, SC Aschuff, L Grunwald, FCP Yin, LSC Griffith. Circulation **66** (1982) 1168-76.
6. RM Fox, A-H Hakki, AS Iskandrian. Am J Cardiol **53** (1984) 1529-31.
7. D David, M Naito, E Michelson, et al. Circulation **65** (1982) 161-7.
8. K Ikeda, I Kubota, M Yamaki, et al. J Electrocardiol **21** (1988) 39-44.
9. RA Oliveros, J Seaworth, FL Weiland, CA Boucher. Chest **72** (1977) 492-4.
10. P Bobba, JA Salerno, A Casari. Circulation **46** (1972) 931-8.
11. K Ogino, M Fukugi, S Hirai, et al. Clin Cardiol **11** (1988) 101-4.

REST AND STRESS ECG FOR THE DIAGNOSIS OF THE ASSOCIATED CORONARY ARTERY DISEASE AFTER THROMBOLYSIS FOR ACUTE MYOCARDIAL INFARCTION

Pedro Abreu, Victor Gil, Aniceto Silvae
R. Seabra-Gomes

Department of Cardiology - Santa Cruz Hospital
Carnaxide - Portugal

1.INTRODUCTION

It is clearly accepted that thrombolysis is the first choice treatment in acute myocardial infarction providing there are no contra-indications.(1,2).

As several studies have suggested, prevention of reinfarction should be the main concern after the first episode of myocardial infarction,because it might decrease mortality.(3).

Considering the progressive course of coronary artery disease (CAD), and its longterm prognosis,it becames of the utmost importance to identify a multivessel disease.

Ideally all the patients treated with thrombolysis during acute myocardial infarction should be submited to coronariography, but in practice this is not possible in the majority of hospitals.(4).

It is accepted that the sub-maximal stress test has an important role in selecting patients for coronariography.(3).But,can the analysis of rest ECG be also useful?

2.MAIN PURPOSE

To identify electrocardiographyc patterns using pre-thrombolysis ECG,24 hours ECG and stress test before discharge,to determine associated disease in the other arteries in patients with acute myocardial infarction.

3.MATERIAL AND METHODS

We studied 52 patients(3 females and 49 males)with mean age of 53.9 years.All had had first Q wave myocardial infarction.

We analysed the 12 leads rest ECG,pre-thrombolysis(+/- 3.5 hours after pain onset), 24 hours ECG and the stress test before discharge,limited by symptoms or ECG changes.In both we analysed the ST changes in the "Q zone" and in "contralateral leads",assumption that ST changes (downslope)in contralateral leads mean associated disease.

We also performed selective coronariography (Judkins/Sones) before discharge and we saw the involved vessels (>70%),the infarct related artery and the presence of associated disease.

The patients were divided in two groups:A and B,respectivelly with anterior and inferior myocardial infarction.Both had 26 patients.

4.RESULTS

Results concerning the involved vessels were:In group A (AMI),sixteen patients had one vessel disease (always left anterior descending artery (LAD)),six patients two vessels (LAD plus Circunflex (CX) in 4 and LAD plus Rigth coronary artery (RCA) in 2) and four patients had three vessels disease.In group B eigthteen patients had one vessel disease (RCA in 13 and CX in 5),seven patients two vessels (RCA plus CX in 3,RCA plus LAD in 3 and CX plus LAD in 1) and finally one patient had three vessel disease.

When we analysed the ST changes in group A,assessing the ST depression in inferior leads for the diagnosis of associated disease of the CX or RCA,the results were (see table I): 1- Sensitivity (S) is 60% both for the rest ECG and for the stress test; 2- The highest specificity (E) was obtained on the 24 hours ECG -91%-; 3- The simultaneous presence of ST depression at the rest ECG and at the stress test has a higth specificity -87%-,but a low sensitivity -45%-. For the group B,and also assessing the presence of ST depression in contralateral leads for the diagnosis of associated disease to the infarct related artery,the results were: (see table II)
1- ST depression in anterior leads in the acute phase ECG has a sensitivity of 100%,but specificity of 0% (all patients had ST depression in anterior leads at the acute phase ECG); 2- If ST depression is still present in the 24 hours ECG it has a sensitivity of 60%,specificity of 92% and a positive and negative predictive value of 75% and 86% respectivelly; 3- ST depression at the stress test identifies 75% of patients with associated disease; 4-The persistence of ST depression in contralateral leads at the 24 hours ECG and the development of ST depression in the same localization at the stress test,has a sensitivity of 100% and a specificity of 91%.Positive and negative predictive value was 67% and 100% respectivelly.

ST DEPRESSION IN CONTRALATERAL LEADS - ASSOC. DISEASE

	Sens	Spec	PPV	NPV
GROUP A - AMI				
PRE-THROMBOLYSIS	62.5%	50%	62.5%	45%
24 HOURS	60%	91%	75%	88%
STRESS TEST	60%	87.5%	75%	77.5%
24H + S.TEST	50%	93%	75%	81%
GROUP B - IMI				
PRE-THROMBOLYSIS	100%	0%	100%	0%
24 HOURS	60%	92%	75%	86%
STRESS TEST	75%	66%	50%	85%
24H + S.TEST	100%	91%	67%	100%

5.DISCUSSION

The importance of the ECG analysis to the diagnosis of the infarct related artery,and the localization of the lesion in it has already been established.(5-7).

Nevertheless,contralateral lead ST changes may have further meaning concerning the diagnosis of infarct coronary artery associated disease.(8).

ST depression present in more than half of patients with inferior myocardial infarction has been associated to a more extensive infarct and a worse longterm prognosis.(8,9).The controversy rises on wether this fenomenon is only an electrical event -mirror image- ,or if it means ischemia at a distance, and therefore,associated disease.(9-11).

The results we acheived are more in favour of an electrical fenomenon,because it is present in all inferior infarction patients and in 2/3 of anterior infarction patients. So,the analysis of acute phase ECG is not very useful to our purpose,but the study of the 24 hours ECG,if it shows ST depression in contralateral leads,can give us a high degree of suspicion concernig the presence of associated disease.(12).The sensitivity of this method varies from 60% to 93%,and the specificity is always superior to 90% (91% to anterior infarction and 92% to inferior infarction).

The stress test appears to be decisive in determining the seriousness of residual ischemia.Its ability to identify the involved vessels is much lower.In one study of our group(13),among others,there is reference to ischemia in inferior wall leads, because of isolated anterior descending artery disease. Perhaps this can explain some of the discouraging results of our study.

But we wish to underline the important diagnostic role of the simultaneous analysis of 24 hours ECG plus stress test in inferior infarction patients.

In these patients the persistence of ST depression in contralateral leads in the 24 hours ECG and evidence of distance ischemia in stress test,give us 100% sensibility with a high specificity -91%- for the diagnosis of associated disease.

6.CONCLUSIONS

Although this study was performed in a small number of patients,careful analysis of the 24 hours ECG, and the stress test at the time of discharge,identifies patients with inferior myocardial infarction with high prevalence of associated disease of the left coronary artery,to whom a more agressive diagnostic and therapeutic approach should be applied.

7.BIBLIOGRAPHY

1-Final report of the Gissi study-The Lancet-Saturday 17 October 1987;

2-(ASSET)--The Lancet-Saturday 3 September 1988;

3-A.Moss,J.Benhorin. N.Engl.J.Med. 322 11-(743-753);

4-R.Seabra-Gomes.Rev.Port.Cardiol. 8(2):83-85,1989;

5-C.Bairey,P.Shah,A.Lew,S.Hulte. Am. J. Cardiol. 1987:60 456-459;

6-Fuchs ,Ashuff S.C.,Grunwald B.A.,Yin P.,Griffith C. Circulation 66:1168-1982;

7-Lew.A.,Maddahij,Shah.Am.J.Cardiol..1985;55:893-98;

8-J.Salcedo,M.Bird,R.Chambers,D.Bealauds. Am.J.Cardiol 48:1003-1009;

9-H.Goldeberg,J.Boer,J.Jucobstein. Am.J.Cardiol. 48.1009-1015;

10-D.Fergusson , N.Padian , M. Kiochon M.Marcus , C. White. Am.J.Cardiol. 1984 ; 53: 55-62;

11-P.F.Abreu,V.Gil,J.A.Silva,R.Seabra-Gomes. Rev. Esp. Cardiol. 43. supl.3 1990;30.82;

12-A.Ventosa,V.Gil,F.Morgado,M.Adao,A.Aleixo,Seabra-Gomes Rev.Port.Cardiol. 1989; 8 supl.1:166.

INFLUENCE OF MYOCARDIAL INFARCTION SIZE ON TERMINAL VENTRICULAR ACTIVATION: STUDY WITH ECG MAPPING, VCG AND VENTRICULAR LATE POTENTIALS

Slavomíra FILIPOVA, Stanislav CAGÁŇ

Department of Internal Medicine IV, School of Medicine, Comenius University, Bratislava, Czechoslovakia

In the course of the last 10 years high-resolution electrocardiography has emerged as a promising, noninvasive technique apt to stratify the risk in patients suffering from acute myocardial infarction (MI). This diagnostic value of the method is based on the hypothesis that MI region causes the lenghtening of excitation pathway, the slowing of the conduction velocity and these result in the derangements of ventricular activation fronts. Late potentials (LP) on bodysurface appear to be the manifestation of this fragmented and delayed activation of myocardial muscle. Several experimental and clinical studies have shown that these ecg manifestations may indicate the presence of the substrate for reentry in the myocardium.

The aim of the study was to observe the relation between the terminal QRS complex parameters (according to VCG QRS loops and ECG-mapping of QRS) and the values of ventricular LPs in patients suffering from acute MI. We were trying to find the parameters of QRS loop differentiating the patients with normal LPs from the patients with acute MI with abnormal values of high-resolution electrocardiography.

We have examined the group of 20 healthy persons (group H) and 65 patients with completely clinically documented acute MI (33 patients had anterior and 32 ones had inferior MI). All examination were made in acute phase of MI (3 - 20 day). MI patients were divided according to the presence of abnormal LP parameters into group N (normal LPs) and group P (positive=abnormal LPs). VCG and high-resolution ECG were recorded with the equipment CASE 15 (fy Marquette Electronics, U.S.A.). Ventricular LPs were evaluated after the filtration of XYZ leads using 40 Hz high-pass bidirectional filtering.

The borders of normal and abnormal values of ventricular LPs have not yet been standardized. We have used the recomended criteria for normal limits (according to Gomez et al., 1987 and Breithardt et al., 1991): 1) fQRSd: the filtered QRS complex duration is not longer than 114 msec; 2) LAS40: the terminal low amplitude complex remains below 40 uV shorter than 39 msec; 3) RMS40: root mean square voltage of signals in the last 40 msec of filtered QRS complex are above 20 uV.

It was used the 30-lead limited system for total surface ECG-mapping (equipment Kardio-SMEP 01, ČSFR).

Results.

We have found no statistically significant relations between the abnormal ventricular LP values and size of MI lesions determined according to integral QRS and ST-T maps, according to echocardiographic wall motion abnormalities and maximal levels of serum creatinkinase.

The LP abnormality manifests itself (Fig. 1) in the long duration of fQRSd, the long LAS40 and low voltages of RMS40 in the group P (P_A-with anterior MI; P_i - with inferior MI).

The maximal circumferential (MC) velocity of QRS loop in horizontal plane has a wide range of variability in the group H and in patients with MI, too. If the value of MC velocity in the groups N and P is expressed as a % of the same value in the group H, we can see that this parameter

Fig. 1

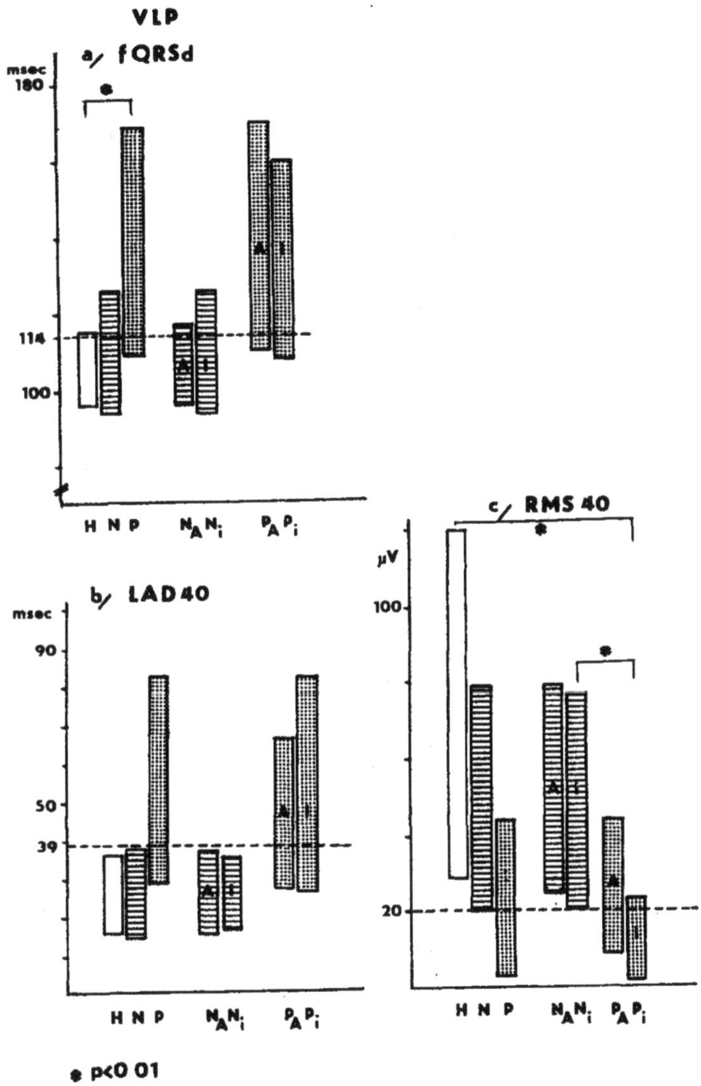

is slowed in patients with anterior MI (N_A and P_A, too); and it remains almost unchanged in patients with inferior MI (groups N_i and P_i).

Terminal circumferential (TC) velocity (Fig. 2) has been calculated from the last 32 msec of nonfiltered QRS

Fig. 2

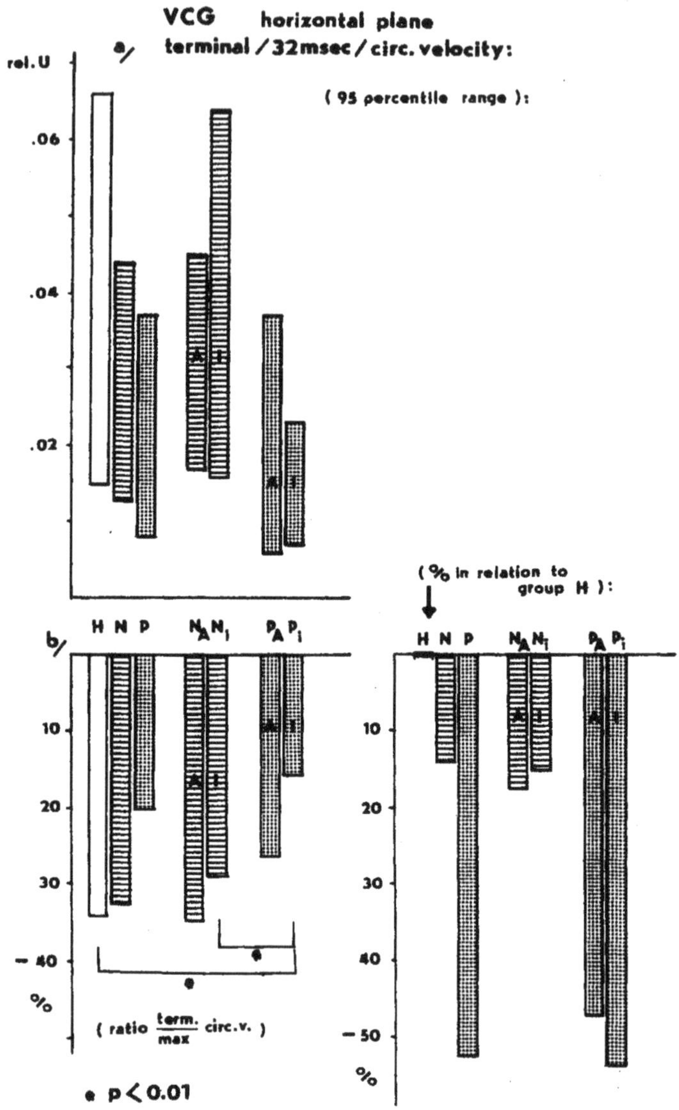

loop. TC velocity decreases gradually in the group H, the group N and P. On account of the wide interindividual variability of both measured velocities (MC and TC), we have calculating the % of slowing of circumferential velocity as the ratio of TC/MC velocity; and especially, we have expressed the % of slowing with respect to the group H. The slowing is the most obvious in MI patients P_A and P_i. There is the significant difference between the group H and the group P, especially the group P_i.

Results.

We have found the significant relation between the terminal QRS loop parameters (TC velocity, the slowing in relation to MC velocity) and the presence of abnormal values of high- resolution ECG. Terminal part of QRS loop predicts most sensitively the presence of abnormal LPs during the acute inferior MI. We assume that the parameters of the terminal QRS loop part are related not only to the locality of inferior MI, but also to the fact, that the slowed MC velocity has not been registered in all inferior MI patients (N_i and P_i).

According to the VCG analysis of QRS loop concerned with its terminal part, we can select patients with acute MI, increasingly threatened with the risk of spontaneous sustained ventricular tachycardia or sudden cardiac death and further we can decide for early indication of high-resolution electrocardiography, 24-hour Holter monitoring and echocardiographic examination and finally subsequent therapeutic procedures.

MULTIPOLAR IMAGE OF THE HEART IN CARDIAC ISCHAEMIA AND AFTER INFARCTION

TERESA ŚWIDERSKA-BŁOŃSKA

Department of Pathophysiology Medical Academy of Wrocław, Marcinkowskiego 1, 50-368 Wrocław, Poland

ABSTRACT

This paper submits the results of the investigation into 135 cases of cardiac ischaemia, including 92 post-infarction cases and 43 with post-effort angina pectoris. The patients who had sustained infarction were divided as regards electrocardiographic location.The groups of subjects were submitted to multipolar electrocardiographic recording from chest surface by means of a multi-electrode network (diamentoid), introduced to vectocardiography by the Kowrzyks. The QRS complex, divided into 8 components, served as the basis for calculating, among other things, the nondipolarity index (Km) and its graphical representation.
The course of the curve makes the groups of the patents distinct.The nondipolarity index tends to be especially high in those who sustained recurrent and large infarction.Also angina pectoris exhibits its increase.

Multipolar studies in people having sustained heart infarction and those with conduction disturbances imply a high percentage of occurrence of nondipolar effects.

The studies the present paper submits are aimed at discriminating the degree of cardiac electric field nondipolarity in patients after çardiac infarction and with angina pectoris, as well as at investigating into information contents in multipolar recording, the information to be used in electrocardiographic diagnostics in the above-cited pathological conditions of the heart. Our hitherto multipolar studies imply that it seems purposeful to first analyse the quadrupolar, then octupolar and hexadecapolar fields. These studies turn out to be useful when differentiating the locations of cardiac infarctions sustained.

This research was focussed on a group of 135 patients with documented stenocardia, including 92 patients after cardiac infarction and 43 with effort angina pectoris.

The reference group was made up by 40 health individuals.

The subjects were patients of the Clinic for Cardiology, Wrocław Medical Academy and the Consulting Unit of Wrocław General Hospital.

The clinical diagnosis was arrived at on the grounds of the clinical image. The majority of the patients (65% of the cases) had a USG test performed, while in the case of angina pectoris - electrocardiographic effort test.Some of the patients underwent a coronarography at The Clinic for Cardiac Surgery, W.M.A. The research referred to the patients 3 weeks to 2 years after the infarction.

The patients who had sustained cardiac infarction were subdivided into those who suffered from their first (single) documented cardiac infarction and the group after 2 or 3 times recurring infarction of different locations.
Table 1 displays the patients as regards their clinical diagnosis and cardiac infarction location.

Table 1

Diagnosis	ECG location	number	age	average
Cardiac infarction	anterior wall	19	34-75	51.7
	inferior wall	30	32-70	51.8
	antero-septal	9	39-73	54.2
	antero-lateral	11	51-70	59.0
	antero-inferior	8	49-65	57.2
	subendocardial	15	32-62	52.3
Angina pectoris		43	33-61	45.6

The reference group was made up by 40 healthy individuals aged 21-35, 27.8 on the average. The terminology applied was suggested by the Polish Cardiological Society. The groups of patients mentioned were submitted to multipolar electrocardiological recording. Registered were heart potentials taken from above the chest by means of multielectrode lead network, referred to as diamentoid,introduced to vectography by the Kowarzyks. In order that we might present the multipolar values in time, the QRS complex was, following Pipberger's suggestion, divided into 8 equal sections, 10 ms each. For each of the groups calculated were mean values of the multipoles and their standard deviations, nondipolarity-to-dipole index. This index was calculated from quadrupole (L2), octupole (L3) and hexadecapole (L4) components.

The nondipolarity index was defined as the multipole (L1,L2,L3)-to-dipole ratio.

When referred to QRS complex time, the course of the curve clearly distinguishes the groups of subjects. In inferior wall infarction, the highest nondipolarity index occurs at 60,70 and 80 msec. In anterior wall infarction, it tends to increase at 40 msec already.In subendocardial infarction,the nondipolar remainder increases as early as 40 msec of the QRS complex.The group of multiple concurrent infarctions, the electrographic location of which being more difficult to be univocally assessed, exhibit a still more interesting course of the curve. Nearly all of those groups display a high nondipolarity index at the QRS on set,dropping at 30 and 40 msec and re-increasing much at the QRS outset.

The results of own research we submit were compared with results from other recording systems and models (Harumi et al.,Hatala et al.,Drska et al.).Good cohesion was pointed out on considerably greater material of ours.

CONCLUSIONS

1. Nondipolarity growth is characteristic or cardiac infarction sustained and is distinctive of its location.
2. Nondipolarity growth goes together with infarction extent and defficient contractility of the heart seen in cardiac usg tests.
3. In angina pectoris, the changes revealed might prove there exists cardiac ischaemia (nondipolarity growth at 40 msec of QRS).
4. Ischaemic changes in the heart due to numerous and large infarctions stay invisible in conventional dipolar acg recordings, being revealed by multipolar recordings.

REFERENCES

1. Drska Z.,Malkova A.,Polankova M.,Valova D.: Non dipolar residue in BSPM and IEFT Ventricular Wall Motion Abnormality in Ischemic Heart Disease. 16th International Congress on Electrocardiology,Budapest,1989,33.
2. Harumi K.,Tsunakawa H.,Kanesaka S.,Nishlyama G.: In: van Dam R. and van Osteroom A.: Electrocardiographic Body Surface Mapping Martinus Nijhoff Publ.Dordrecht, 1986,pp.283-288.
3. Hatala R.,Maco M.:In: Abstracts of 14th International Congress on Electrocardiology,Berlin,1987.
4. Jagielski J.,Świderska-Błońska T.,Górnicki M.: Non-dipolarity analysis of the Estimation of Myocardial Infarction. 1989 Elsevier Science Publishers B.V. Electrocardiology 1988, 81-84.

HOLTER MONITORING-USEFULNESS IN DIAGNOSIS OF SILENT ISCHEMIA

MARTA NEGRUSZ-KAWECKA
Clinic of Cardiology, Medical Academy of Wrocław, ul. Pasteura 4, Poland

JOANNA MOSZCZYŃSKA-STULIN, PIOTR SALOMON
Clinic of Cardiology, Medical Academy of Wrocław, ul. Pasteura 4, Poland

1. Introduction

Previous studies have shown that in about 20% of patients with proven coronary artery disease silent ischemic episodes can be detected by Holter monitoring during everyday activities. The mortality in this group of patients is higher than in patients with symptomatic myocardial ischemia [1,2,3,4].

The patients with silent myocardial ischemia were classified by Cohn [5] into three clinical subgroups. Type 1 consists of totally asymptomatic patients. Type 2 consists of postmyocardial infarction patients with silent myocardial ischemia. Type 3 consists of patients with both painful and silent ischemia.

Various investigators [4,6] suggest the role of beta-endorphin in the pathogenesis of silent myocardial ischemia.

The aim of this study was to determine the frequency of silent ischemic episodes in patients with previous myocardial infarction. Additionally, the beta-endorphine plasma levels were measured to prove their relationship to the perception of the chest pain in patients with silent myocardial ischemia [4,6].

2. Patients and Methods

In the study 48 men with previous myocardial infarction (with in last 12 months) were included. 15 men with coronary artery disease without previous myocardial infarction and 12 healthy men-volunteers were as the control. All patients were of similar age. Patients with valvular heart disease, cardiomyopathy, left bundle branch block, left ventricular strain, digitalis therapy and electrolytes imbalance were excluded.

No medications, except sublinqual nitroglycerin in case of anginal pain were administred during all examination. In all patients Holter monitoring was carried out during 24-hours while the patients performed their usual everyday activities. Holter were obtained using Oxford-Medilog 3000 analyser. The ECG-recordings reviewed by two independent investigators who performed visual analysis of the monitoring periods. The patients were asked to maintain a written diary of symptoms and activities during the monitoring period. The Holter leads used corresponded to V1 and V5 of the electrocardiogram.

ST-depression was diagnosed as ischemic if there was an ST-segment depression (horizontal or downsloping) of > 1 mm, persisting 80 ms after the J point, lasting 30 seconds and returning to baseline thereafter.

Submaximal bicycle exercise test was performed in all patients. The beta-endorphine plasma levels were measured by the means of radioimmunoassay (N.E.N. Research Products E.I. Du pont de Nemorus and Co., (Inc.) Medical Products Departament). Blood samples for endorphine analysis were obtained during the rest, at the peak of the exercise and 5 minutes after exercise during the recovery period.

3. Results

In 48 patients with previous myocardial infarction 24-hours Holter monitoring detected 129 transient episodes of ST depression during daily activities. 85 episodes were silent and 44 were symptomatic.

Of the 48 patients, 23 had only silent episodes and 25 only symptomatic episodes. There were no statistically significant differences between silent and symptomatic episodes as to the mean duration and mean maximal ST depression However the heart rate was significantly slower in the silent-episode patients.

In 15 patients with coronary disease without infarction 61 episodes of ST depression were detected. 39 episodes were silent and 22 were symptomatic. The characteristics of silent and symptomatic episodes in these patients were similar to the patients with infarction. In the group of 12 healthy men no episodes of significant ST depression were detected.

In the study of the circadian rhytm of myocardial ischemia we considered the total ischemic burden (silent and painful episodes) was maximal in the hours of maximal physical and psychical activity (i.e. 6:00 - 8:00 A.M., 12:00 - 4:00 P.M., 6:00 - 8:00 P.M.) followed by maximal catecholamine release (Fig. 1).

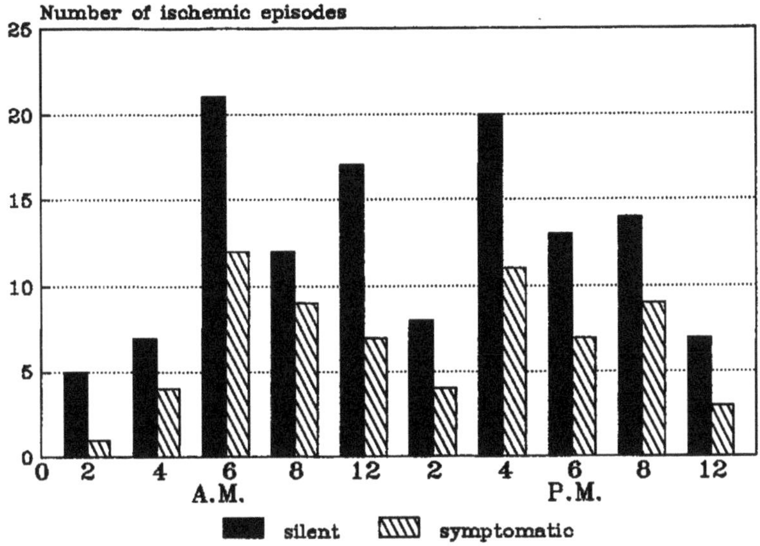

Figure 1. Circadian rhytm of ischemia in holter monitoring.

The results showed that beta-endorphin plasma levels in all investigated men significantly increased during submaximal treadmill stress test. The mean postexercise level of beta-endorphin plasma level was significantly higher in the silent-episode patients than in symptomatic episode patients and healthy men (Table 1).

Table 1. The beta-endorphine plasma levels (pg/l) in patients with coronary artery disease and previous myocardial infarction with silent and symptomatic episodes of ischemia during submaximal treadmill stress test.

	Patients with previous myocardial infarction			healthy volunteers
type o ischemia	silent (n=23)	silent and symptomatic (n=15)	symptomatic (n=13)	
at rest	x=19.26 SD=3.3	x=19.3 SD=2.76	x=12.95 SD=3.6	x=11.55 SD=7.41
peak of exercise	x=30.8 SD=7.0	x=27.09 SD=4.81	x=17.2 SD=5.6	x=16.4 SD=9.1
5 minutes after exercise	x=20.9 SD=4.4	x=23.02 SD=4.9	x=14.05 SD=3.65	x=14.7 SD=9.04

4. Conclusions

The characteristics of silent and symptomatic episodes of ischemia in patients with coronary artery disease and with previous myocardial infarction and without the infarction were comparable.

There were no significant differences between silent and symptomatic episodes as to the mean duration and mean maximal ST-depression.

The heart rate was significantly slower in the silent episodes of ischemia.

The frequency of silent and symptomatic episodes was maximal in the hours of maximal physical and psychical activity followed by increased catecholamine release and disturbances of regional coronary blood flow.

There is good evidence that the ST-segment depression during daily activities even without symptoms indicates the transient imbalance between oxygen supply and demand. Holter monitoring is useful in detection all symptomatic and silent ischemia episodes during daily life and may help to establish the proper treatment and improve the prognosis of patients with coronary artery disease.

The role of beta-endorphines in perception of the chest pain is not clear yet and needs to be studied further.

6. References

1. Kennedy H.I. et al., *Ambulatory (Holter) electrocardiography and myocardial ischemia.* Am Heart J 1989, 117,164.
2. Savage H.R. et al., *Analysis of ambulatory electrocardiograms in 14 patients who experienced sudden cardiac death during monitoring.* Clin Cardiol 1987, 10, 621.
3. Sharma B. et al., *Demonstration of exercise-induced painless myocardial ischemia in survivors of out-of-hospital ventricular fibrillation.* Am J Cardiol 1987, 59, 740.
4. Sheps D.S. et al., *Sudden death and silent myocardial ischemia.* Am Heart J 1989, 117, 177.
5. Cohn et al., *Prognostic significance of asymptomatic coronary artery disease.* Am J Cardiol 1986, 58, 51B.
6. Sheps D. S. et al., *Endorphines are related to pain perception in coronary artery disease.* Am J Cardiol 1987, 39, 523.

BICYCLE TESTS IN PATIENTS WITH ACUTE MYOCARDIAL INFARCTION ASSOCIATED WITH SILENT MYOCARDIAL ISCHEMIA

GULMIRA Z.KUDAIBERDIEVA*, ERKIN M. MIRRAKHIMOV**, NATALIYA L. TSOY*, TOKTOSUN A. AMATOV*, AIZHAMAL N. DANIYAROVA**, TASHPOLOT B. BALTABAEV*.

* Department of Emergency Cardiology, Kirghiz Institute of Cardiology, Bishkek, 720361, USSR.

** N1 Department of Internal Diseases, Kirghiz Medical Institute, Bishkek, 720061, USSR.

ABSTRACT

To assess exercise capacity of the patients, with acute myocardial infarction associated with silent myocardial ischaemia bicycle test was performed ; threshold capacity, heart rate/systolic pressure product (RPP), number of metabolic units were estimated. By the results of 24-hour ECG monitoring the patients were divided into 3 groups. All the patients were performed coronary angiography. In gr. 1 subjects threshold capacity was 98.4±7.4 W, gr.2 - 72.9±7.8 W, gr.3 - 71.9±7.8 W (p1-3 <0.05). In gr.1 RPP was 214.2±1 ,3, gr.2 - 164.5±10.5, gr.3 - 159.1±13.8 (p1-3<0.008). There also were significant differences between groups 1 and 3 in the number of metabolic units: 5.3±0.4 versus 3.6±0.5 (p<0.01). Gr.2 subjects had an intermediate number of metabolic units (4.2±0.3) The number of injured coronary arteries did not differ significantly in gr.2 and 3 (2.7±0.2 and 2.9±0.1, respectively), whereas in gr.1 the number of injured arteries was 2.1±0.2 (p1-3<0.05).

1. INTRODUCTION

Silent myocardial ischaemia has an important clinical and prognostic value in patients with coronary heart disease [1,2]. It is known that 24-hour ECG monitoring and exercise tests allow to reveal episodes of silent myocardial ischaemia (SMI) in survivors of myocardial infarction [3,4].

This study was aimed at the assessment of exercise capacity in patients with acute myocardial infarction, depending on the frequency of SMI episodes.

2. PATIENTS AND METHODS

Forty eight males with primary Q wave myocardial infarction were studied according to the WHO criteria (1970).

On the 7th day of the disease all the patients were performed 24-hour ECG monitoring with recording of modified V1 and V5 ECG leads, using cardiocomplex "Lenta MT" (USSR). We assessed the frequency of SMI episodes (lasting at least one minute) with ST depression of 1 mm or more and ST elevation of 2 mm or more in 0.08sec after "j" point.During ECG monitoring the patients kept a detailed diary.

Bicycle test was performed on the 23rd±1 day of the disease. Initial exercise was 25 W, the duration of each step was 3 minutes. Conventional criteria for the cessation of the test were used. We assessed threshold exercise capacity, heart rate/systolic pressure product (RPP) during maximal exercise, total work load performed (TWLP), number of metabolic units (MET), duration of exercise, and mean number of leads in which ischaemia was recorded.

Multipositional coronary angiography was performed on 21±1 day of disease, according to the method of Judkins (1967), using Digitron-3 (Siemens, Germany). As injured were regarded the arteries with stenosis above 50%, and the mean number of injured arteries was determined.

3. RESULTS

Depending on the frequency of SMI episodes by 24-hour ECG monitoring, the patients were divided into 3 groups. In gr.1 patients (n=20) the frequency of SMI per day did not exceed 3 episodes; in gr. 2 patients (n=14) SMI frequency ranged from 4 to 6 episodes, and in gr.3 (n=14) - more than 6 episodes.

Threshold exercise capacity was 98.4±7.4W, 72.9±7.8W, 71.9±7.8 W in groups 1,2,3, respectively ($p1-3 < 0.05$); RPP achieved 214.2±14.3, 164.5±10.5, 159.1±13.8, respectively ($p1- 3<0.008$). The number of metabolic units differed significantly between gr.1 and 3 (5.2±0.4 and 3.6±0.5,respectively, $p<0.05$). Gr.2 subjects had an intermediate number of MET (4.5±0.5). The duration of exercise was 625.0±50.9 sec in gr.1, 470.0±69.6 sec in gr.2, and 435.0±65.3 sec in gr.3($p1-3<0.03$). There also were significant differences between groups 1 and 3 in the mean number of leads in which ischaemia was recorded (3.2±0.4 versus 4.4 ±0.3, $p<0.04$). In gr.2 this parameter was 3.9±0.2. TWLP in gr.1 was 39.6±5.9 kJ, in gr.2 - 22.2±7.9 kJ, and in gr.3 - 21.9±5.4 (p 1-3 <0.03)(see Table).

Table. Results of the bicycle test.

Parameters	Groups			p 1-3
	1 (n=20)	2 (n=14)	3 (n=14)	
Threshold exercise capacity, W	98.4± 7.4	72.9±7.8	71.9±7.8	< 0.04
RPP	214.2±14.3	164.5±10.5	159.1±13.8	<0.008
MET (units)	5.2± 0.4	4.2±0.3	3.6±0.5	<0.01
Duration of exercise, sec	625.0±50.9	470.0±69.6	435.0±65.3	<0.03
Mean number of leads showing ischaemia	3.2± 0.4	3.8±0.2	4.4±0.3	<0.04
TWLP, kJ	39.6± 5.9	22.2±7.9	21.9±5.4	<0.05

The number of injured coronary arteries by multipositional coronary angiography in gr.2 and 3 did not differ significantly (2.7±0.2 and 2.9±0.3, respectively), whereas in gr.1 it was 2.1±0.2 (p1-3<0.05).

4. DISCUSSION

It is known that silent myocardial ischaemia is a frequent event in ischaemic heart disease patients[5]. In patients with stable and unstable angina pectoris[6,7,8] and MI survivors[3,9]. SMI produce an unfavourable effect on clinical course and prognosis of the disease. Some authors[4,10] demonstrated that in patients who survived MI, bicycle test did not reveal any differences between patients with overt and silent ST-segment depression as far as prognosis was concerned. Others[11] revealed that MI survivors with overt and silent myocardial ischemia did not differ on bicycle test parameters, extent and severity of coronary vascular injury.

However, the prognostic value of working capacity in AMI patients with manifestations of SMI, depending on frequency of myocardial ischaemia episodes needs further researches.

We revealed that patients with more than 6 SMI episodes per day have lower threshold exercise capacity, lower RPP and number of MET units. In the latter group of patients exercise duration was significantly less than in the group with SMI frequency < 3 episodes per day. In patients with frequent episodes, myocardial ischaemia was registered in a greater number of ECG leads. TWLP also significantly differed between groups 1 and 3. Such differences in work capacity are evidently related to the extent of coronary vascular injury, because coronary angiography demonstrated more pronounced coronary injures in patients with more frequent SMI episodes.

Thus, patients with acute myocardial infarction and frequent (more than 6) episodes of silent myocardial ischaemia have a low exercise tolerance and a more severe injury of coronary arteries.

5. REFERENCES

1. V.N.Golyakov, Yu.V.Zimin Kardiologya (USSR),5,(1987), p.27.
2. Yu.A.Karpov, V.V.Shibleva, I.N.Merculova et al. Klinicheskaya Meditsina (USSR), 4, (1991), p.40.
3. P.Ouang, N.C.Chandra, S.O.Gottlieb Am.J.Cardiol., 65, (1990), p.267.
4. D.A.Weiner, T.J.Ryan, C.H.McCabe et al.Am.J.Cardiol., 62,(1988), p.1155.
5. B.N.Singh Am.J.Cardiol., 58, (1986), p.1B.
6. P.C.Deedwania and E.V.Carbajal Circulation,81, (1990), p.748.
7. S.O.Gottlieb, M.L.Weisfeldt, P.Ouang et al. J.Am.Coll. Cardiol., 10,(1987), p.756.
8. K.Nademanee, V.Intarachot, M.A.Josephson et al. J.Am. Coll.Cardiol. 10,(1987),p.1.
9. D.Tzivoni, A.Gavish, D.Zin et al. Am.J.Cardiol.,62, (1988), p.661.
10. P.Theroux, D.Waters, C.Halphen et al. N.Engl.J.Med., 301,(1979), p.341.
11. P.Ouang, E.P.Shapiro, N.C.Chandra Am.J.Cardiol.,59, (1987), p.730.

SIGNIFICANCE OF STRESS TEST ST ELEVATION IN PATIENTS WITH MYOCARDIAL INFARCTION

Carvalho M, Cantinho G, Lacerda AP, Dionísio I, Costa BB, Alves M, Pádua F and Macieira-Coelho E

Med IV (Direct.: Prof. F. de Pádua) and I. Med. Nuclear LA3, INIC - St. Mary University Hospital, Lisbon - Portugal

Introduction

In patients (pts) with previous myocardial infarction (MI) the clinical significance of ST-segment elevation during exercise in leads with Q-Wave is controversial.

The purpose of this study was to correlate exercise ST-segment elevation with coronary artery anatomy, ventricular wall motion abnormalities and perfusion thallium myocardial defects, in order to evaluate the clinical significance of this electrocardiographic change.

Material and Methods

Fifty two, 49 M and 3 F, aged 56 $\pm$ 7 years were studied. All pts had a 1st myocardial infarction $\bar{3}$ months before the study. All pts were submitted to stress test (Bruce protocol), exercise thallium-201 scintigraphy (201-Tl), and coronariography. Radionuclide ventriculography with technetium (99m-Tc) was performed in 61% of pts.

Results

Pts were divided in 2 groups, according to the presence or absence of ST-segment elevation during exercise: Group I (↑ ST) - 15 pts; Group II (without ↑ ST) - 37 pts. All pts had ↑ ST in Q-wave leads. <u>Thallium-201 scanning</u> - In Group I (↑ ST) 5 (33%) of the 15 pts had reversible perinecrosis defects, and 10 (67%) only reversible defects outside the infarct area. In Group II, 28 pts (71%) had reversible perinecrosis defects (Fig. 1). <u>Radionuclide ventriculography</u> - All pts with ↑ ST (Group I) had ventricular wall motion abnormalities (VWA), according to the ST leads abnormalities: 2 had ventricular aneurysm (20%), 2 (20%) areas of akynesia/diskynesia and 6 (60%) hypokynetic segments. The ejection fraction was 35.6 $\pm$ 10.2. In Group II, 4 pts (18%) had important VWA. The ejection fraction was 50.1 $\pm$ 10.1 ($p < 0.001$) (Fig. 2). <u>Coronary arteriography</u> - In

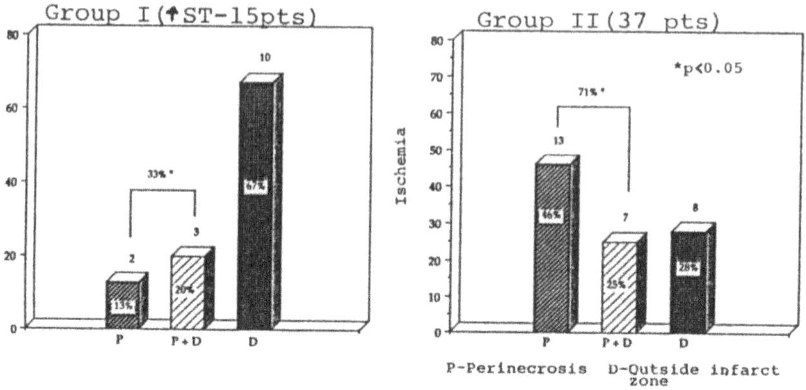

Fig. 1- Results of the 201-Tl

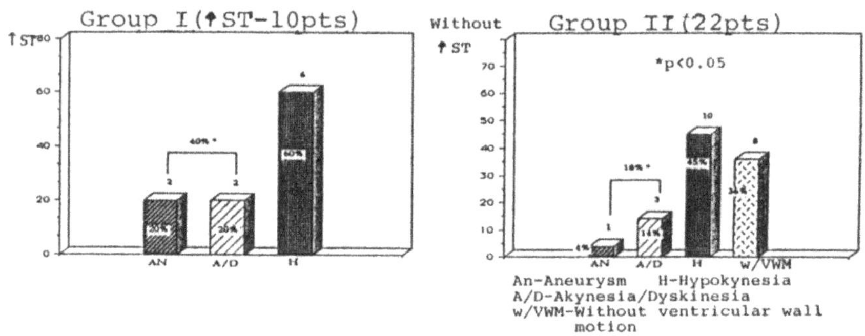

Fig. 2- Results of the 99-mTc

Group I (↑ ST), the coronariography showed obstructive lesions of 1 vessel (V) in 5 pts (33%), of 2V in 5 pts (33%) and of 3V in 5 pts (33%). The left anterior descending artery (LAD) was occluded in 14 pts (93%): 4 pts with 1V disease, and 10 pts with 2 or 3V disease. Of the 14 pts with LAD disease, 10 (71%) had critical lesions (> 90%) localized to in the 1/3 proximal of the artery (Fig. 3). In Group II, the coronariography showed obstructive lesions of 1V in 10 pts (27%), 2V in 11 pts (30%), and 3V in 16 pts (43%). Of the 37 pts of this Group, 28 (76%) had LAD disease. In 7 pts (25%) the obstructive lesions was critical (> 90%) and localized in the 1/3 proximal of the artery (**Fig. 3**)

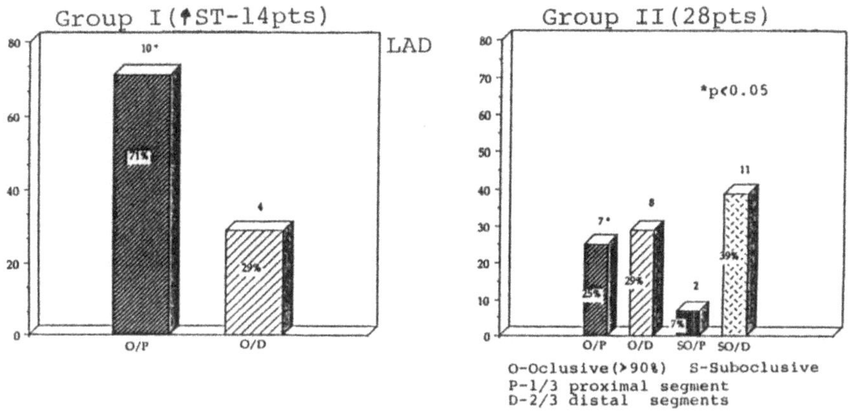

Fig. 3- Results of the Coronariography

Discussion and conclusions

Exercise ST-segment elevation in Q-Wave leads was admitted to reflect either severe myocardial ischemia, abnormal ventricular wall motion or reciprocal electrical phenomena (1-3), and patients with this electrocardiographic abnormality appear to have a poor prognosis (4).

In the present study, pts with ST-segment elevation showed low ejection fraction and 60% had important ventricular wall motion disturbances (aneurysm, akynesia, diskynesia), correlated with the leads with ST-elevation. In 93% of the pts, the left anterior descending artery was responsible for the perfusion defects corresponding to wall motion abnormalities. Of these pts, 71% showed proximal obstructive lesions $> 90\%$. On the other hand, Thallium perfusion defects showed perinfarction ischemia in only 5 (33%) of the 14 pts with LAD disease.

From the results of the present study we may conclude that exercise ST-elevation in patients with myocardial infarction is associated with proximal occluded lesions of LAD, leading to important wall motion abnormalities.

References

1) Nobration FJ, Froelicher VF. Am J Cardiol 1989; 63:986-988.
2) Dunn RF, Bailey IK, Uren R, Kelly D. Circulation 1980; 61:989-995.
3) Anora R, Ioachim L, Mtaza D, Horowitz SF. Clin Cardiol 1988; 11:127-139.
4) Bruce RA, Fisher CD, Pettinger M, et al. Circulation 1988; 77:897-905.

ASSESSMENT OF RESIDUAL ISCHEMIA AFTER ACUTE MYOCARDIAL INFARCTION - USEFULNESS OF THE FIRST 12 LEADS ECG

Carvalho M, Lacerda AP, Dionísio I, Cantinho G, Pádua F and Lopes MG

UCIM, Medicine IV and I. Med. Nuclear - LA3, CCUL-INIC, St. Mary University Hospital, Lisbon - Portugal

Introduction

During the acute phase of a myocardial infarction some times ST segment depression can be found in the ECG leads opposite to the infarcted area with ST segment elevation. The genesis of this electrocardiographic abnormality is controversial, being related to a "reciprocal" projection of the ST segment vector, to a more extensive myocardial necrosis, or be caused by distant ischemia.

The purpose of the present study was to evaluate the clinical significance of the "reciprocal" ST-T changes during the acute phase of myocardial infarction, correlating these findings with myocardial perfusion defects.

Material and Methods

Twenty eight patients (pts), 25 males and 3 females, with a mean age of 56 $\pm$ 6 years, were studied. All pts had a first Q-Wave myocardial infarction diagnosed by clinical, electrocardiographic and enzymatic methods. Thirteen pts had anterior myocardial infarction and 15 inferior myocardial infarction.

A twelve leads ECG was recorded at admission to the coronary care unit. "Reciprocal" ST-T abnormalities were considered in the presence of horizontal or downsloping depressed ($\geqslant$ 1 mm) ST segment, 0.08 s after J point, in two or more contiguous leads, or in the presence of a negative T-wave $\geqslant$ 0.5 mV. All patients were submitted to an exercise Thalium-201 stress test, 3 months after the myocardial infarction. Myocardial perfusion scanning begun 5' after the intravenous administration of 74 MBq (2 mCi) of Thallium-201. Thomographic images were collected 5 minutes and 3-4 hours (redistribution images) after peak exercise. Thallium defects were classified as either reversible (ischemia) or irreversible (necrosis) considering perfusion or non-perfusion during redistribution phase of non-perfused areas, at peak exercise.

Results

Of the 13 pts with anterior myocardial infarction 11 had "reciprocal" ST-T abnormalities in inferior leads. All these pts had residual ischemic areas: one pt had reversible perinecrosis defect and 10 pts both reversible perfusion defects in inferior and perinecrosis area **(Fig. 1)**. The 2 pts with anterior MI, without inferior ST-T changes, didn't show residual ischemia.

Of the 15 pts with inferior myocardial infarction, 9 (60%) had "reciprocal" ST-T abnormalities. Of these pts, 3 had only irreversible perfusion inferior defects, and 6 (67%) reversible perfusion defects in anterior and perinecrosis segments **(Fig. 2)**.

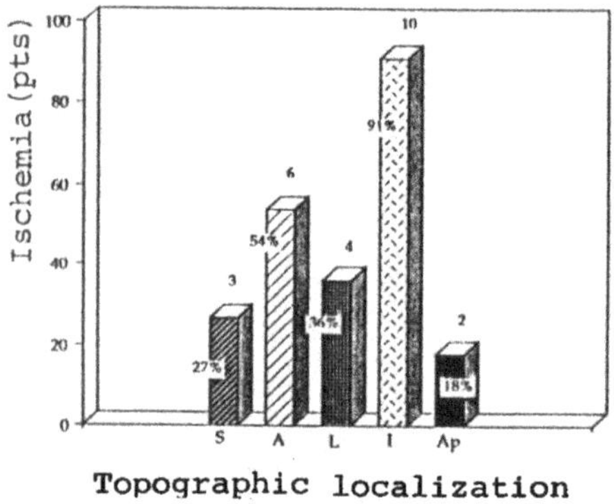

Fig. 1- Ischemia in pts with Anterior MI and Inferior ST-T abnormalities

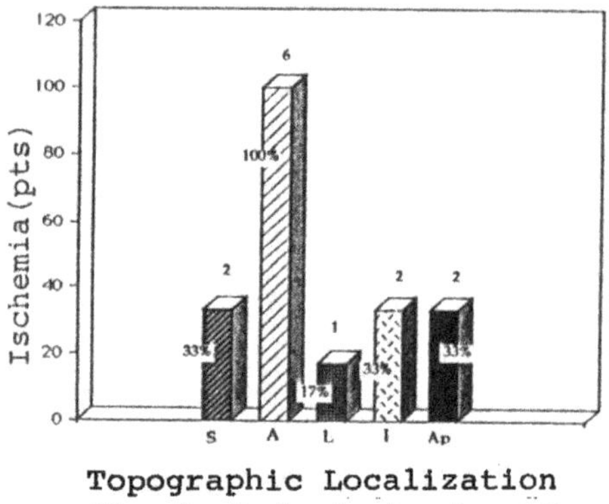

Fig. 2- Ischemia in pts with Inferior MI and Anterior ST-T abnormalities

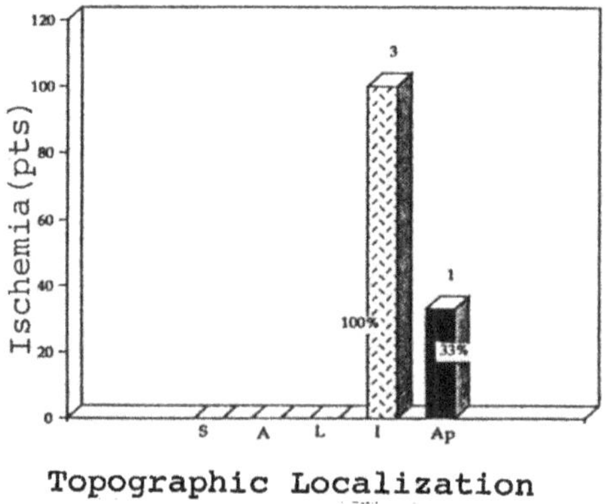

Fig. 3- Ischemia in pts with Inferior MI and without ST-T Anterior abnormalities

Of the 6 pts with inferior myocardial infarction without ST-T reciprocal changes, 3 had irreversible inferior perfusion defects, and 3 had reversible perfusion defects localized to the inferior leads **(Fig. 3)**.

Discussion

The genesis of ST-T "reciprocal" abnormalities in the acute phase of myocardial infarction is controversial. Previous studies related this electrocardiographic change to either reciprocal projection of the ST-segment vector, to more extensive myocardial necrosis, or to concomitant contralateral ischemia.[1-3] However, the prevalence of multivessel disease is thought to be higher, and these pts have been reported to have more extensive left ventricular dysfunction and worse clinical prognosis.[4]

In the present study, 91% of pts with anterior MI and ST-T inferior abnormalities had inferior myocardial ischemia. In pts with inferior MI and anterior ST-T abnormalities, 67% had anterior myocardial ischemia. Patients without "reciprocal" ECG abnormalities had only necrosis or perinecrosis ischemia.

We conclude that ST-T changes remote to the area of infarction, detected in the first ECG, identify patients with higher risk for late remote ischemia at that level. In these pts more agressive diagnostic and therapeutic attitudes are justifiable.

References

1) Boden W, Spodiek D. Am J Cardiol 1989; 63:358-86.
2) Berger P, Ryan T. Circulation 1990; 81:401-411.
3) Lew A, Hod H, Cercek B et al. JACC 1987; 10:519-526.
4) Willems Y, Willems R, Willems G, et al. Circulation 1990; 82:1147-1158.

THALLIUM-201 SCANNING IN T-WAVE PSEUDONORMALIZATION DURING EXERCISE

A.P. Lacerda, M. Carvalho, Z.C. Silva, J. Madeira, G. Cantinho, C.C. França, C. Vinha, F. de Pádua and M.G. Lopes

UCIM/Medicina IV (Hosp. Santa Maria), Inst. Medicina Nuclear (Fac. Medicina de Lisboa), LA3, CCUL-INIC, Instituto Nacional de Cardiologia Preventiva, Lisbon, Portugal

ABSTRACT

The significance of the evolution of previous inverted T waves at rest to an upright T wave during exercise - "pseudonormalization" (Tw-/+) was studied, analysing myocardial perfusion (x201 Tl) at peak exercise and at rest 4 hours later. Seventeen patients (pts) in which Tw-/+ was the only abnormality in stress test, were submitted to x201 Tl. Eight pts had previous myocardial infarction (Group A) and 9 pts were considered to have angina (Group B).

Results: Sixteen pts (94%) had reversible perfusion defects compatible with ischemia (I) in x201 Tl. All the pts of Group A showed a 100% segmentar correlation ECG/x201 Tl in the areas of necrosis. Correlation of I segments was found in 6/8 pts. In Group B, 8/9 pts had I in x201 Tl, with a 100% correlation ECG/x201 Tl in inferior segments. In anterior/ant-lateral Tw-/+, most x201 Tl segments were found in inferior or inf/dorsal areas.

Conclusions: 1) Exercise Tw -/+ should be recognized as an important criteria of ischemia in pts with known or suspected coronary artery disease. **2)** In pts with previous myocardial infarction Tw -/+ remote to the infarcted area is associated with the presence of ischemia in that area. **3)** Segmental correlation ECG Tw -/+ with ischemic areas must be assessed with further studies, namely coronary arteriography.

INTRODUCTION

The clinical significance of normalization of previously inverted primary T waves, in the rest ECG, induced by exercise stress testing, is still under discussion. It is not an uncommon finding in stress test laboratories, and it is allways difficult to interpret the fenomenon, because there are no definite criteria concerning this abnormality. Is it "nonspecific"? Some authors consider nevertheless that it can occur due to myocardial ischemia or abnormal wall motion, corresponding to the affected ECG lead zones. Some other investigators think it may be a reciprocal ECG response to events occurring in the opposite ventricular wall. The purpose of this study was to evaluate the clinical significance of previous primary inverted T wave presenting with "pseudonormalization" (Tw -/+) during exercise treadmill testing, without ST segment deviation.

PATIENTS AND METHODS

1) Population

Patients (pts) were picked up from a population with known or suspected coronary artery disease who underwent a treadmill stress test, during a six months period. They were not taking digitals or other antiarrhytmic therapy.

Patients with secondary ST-T wave abnormalities on resting ECG, and ischemic exercise ST segment depression were excluded. We also rejected (after the Echo study) cases of right or left ventricular hypertrophy, mitral valve prolapse or other valvulopaties as well as hypertrophic cardiomiopathy.

Seventeen pts met the criteria for inclusion in the study (13M, 4F, mean age: 56 years) as the only abnormality in stress test was previously inverted T wave at rest that became upright during exercise (Tw -/+). Eight pts had a previous Q wave myocardial infarction (MI) - Group A, and 9 pts had anginal symptoms - Group B.

2) Protocol

The study included: 1) Finding of Tw -/+ during treadmill maximum stress test (Bruce protocol); 2) Evaluation of myocardial perfusion with Thallium-201 imaging. The pts exercised by supine bicycle ergometry (Astrand protocol). Three ECG leads were continuously monitored and a standard 12- lead ECG was recorded every minute. Maximum stress tests were terminated by marked fatigue, chest disconfort/pain and/or disrhytmia (there were no other ECG abnormalities besides Tw -/+). A single dose of 2.2 mCi of Thallium-201 (201 Tl), was injected IV at peak exercise, and exercise was continued for 1 minute thereafter. Tomographic 201-Tl scans were initiated within 5 minutes after exercise, and redistribution images were obtained 4 hours later. Thallium imaging was considered either normal or with perfusion defects: irreversible (corresponding to necrotic areas) or reversible perfusion defects (ischemia). The scans were studied analysing 5 different segments: septal, anterior, lateral, inferior and apical.

RESULTS

Sixteen of the 17 pts (94%) had a positive 201-Tl scan with reversible perfusion defects, revealing the existence of ischemic areas. One patient (from Group B) had a normal 201-Tl scan.

All Group A (previous MI) pts showed a 100% segmentar correlation between ECG Q wave leads and 201 Tl irreversible perfusion defects. Correlation of ischemic segments was found in 6 of the 8 pts. In these 6 pts Tw -/+ was recognised in leads remote to the infarcted area, and indeed the topographic correlation with the ischemic segments in 201 Tl scans was excellent. In the other 2 pts T w-/+ coincided with Q wave leads (anterior wall) and 201 Tl scans revealed the presence of inferior ischemia.

Considering Group B pts (angina), 8 of 9 pts had reversible perfusion defects in 201 Tl scans. Topographic correlation between Tw -/+ ECG leads and 201 Tl segments was excellent when ischemia was found in the inferior wall (3/3). Nevertheless when the fenomenon was found in anterior/antero-lateral ECG leads, most (5/6) reversible defects in 201 Tl scans were found in inferior or infero-dorsal segments.

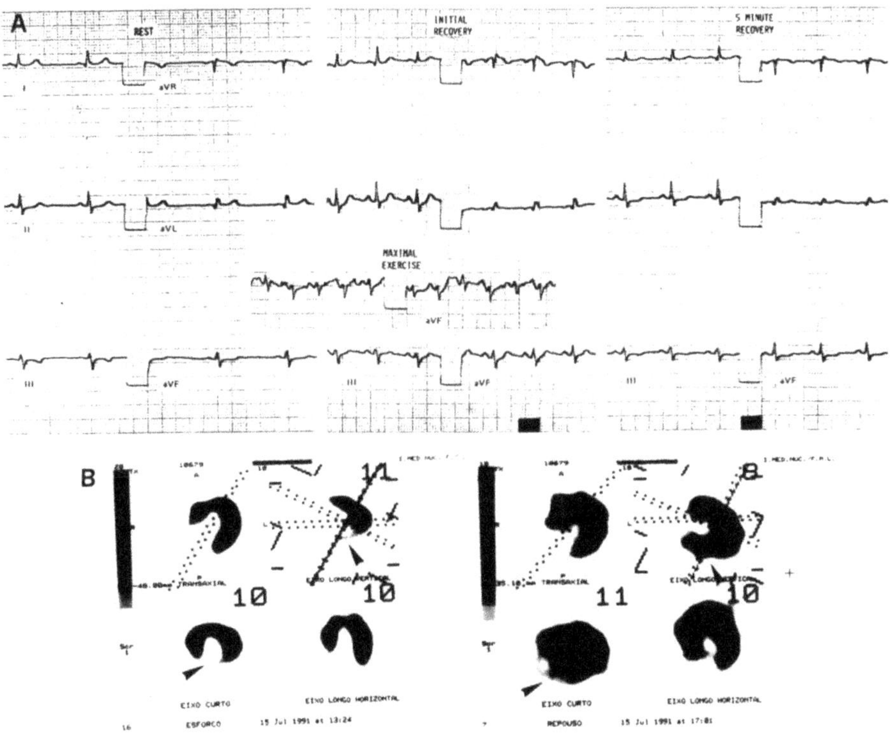

Fig. 1.A) Exercise stress test (Bruce prot.) of a 50 years old man with chest pain. Rest ECG showed inverted T waves in leads III and avF which turned upright at maximal exercise (9', asymptomatic) and during the inicial period of recovery, becaming negative again at 5' recovery.
B) Tomographic Thallium 201 scans taken after maximal exercise (left) and 4 hours later (right) revealed the presence of a reversible perfusion defect in inferior segments, coincident with the ECG leads with T wave "pseudonormalization".

DISCUSSION AND CONCLUSIONS

In a similar study of 45 pts, JJ Marin et al (1) concluded that in pts with a high prevalence of coronary artery disease Tw -/+ was highly specific for the presence of the disease, representing predominantly either previous injury or exercise induced ischemia in myocardial segments corresponding to the afected ECG leads.

Carl J. Lavie et al (2) could show with radionuclide angiography, in a study of 23 pts, that Tw -/+ was more sensitive but less specific than a "classical" positive exercise test, for predicting new wall motion abnormalities or a decrease in the ejection fraction with exercise, in populations with a high prevalence of ischemic heart disease.

Recently T. Ogawa et al (3) could demonstrate, in pts with prevous MI, that Tw -/+ in the infarcted area was a sensitive marker of abnormal wall motion (with the same clinical significance as ST elevation).

From our study we can conclude that: **1)** Exercise T wave "pseudonormalization" should be recognised as an important criterion of ischemia in patients with known or suspected coronary artery disease, recommending more agressive studies; **2)** In patients with previous myocardial infarction, T wave "pseudonormalization" remote to the infarcted area is associated with the presence of ischemia in that area; **3)** Segmental correlation between ECG leads with T wave "pseudonormalization" and ischemic areas must be assessed with further studies, namely coronary arteriography.

REFERENCES

1) J.J. Marin, M.K. Heng, R. Sevrin and V.N. Udhoji, Am Heart J 114 (1987) 1342.
2) CJ Lavie, JK Oh, HT Mankin, IP Clments, ER Giuliani and RJ Gibbons, Chest 94 (1988) 512.
3) T. Ogawa, M Ishii, K Iida, R Ajisaka, I. Yamaguchi, Y Sugishita and I Ito, Am. J. cardiol. 65 (1990) 962.

EFFECTS OF CORINFAR ON DURATION OF CORRECTED Q–T INTERVAL IN PATIENTS WITH VASOSPASTIC ANGINA PECTORIS

NAILYA T. DAVYDOVA

Laboratory of Functional Diagnosis, Kirghiz Institute of Cardiology, Bishkek, 720361, USSR

TILEKBEK S. MEIMANALIEV, AIZHAMAL N. DANIYAROVA, ERKIN M. MIRRAKHIMOV

Kirghiz Medical Institute, Bishkek, 720061, USSR

1. PATIENTS AND METHODS

Hyperventilation tests were performed in 65 patients with the episodes of vasospastic angina pectoris (mean age 44.4+1.3 years). These tests provoked vasospastic angina pectoris in 45 patients (69.2%).

2. RESULTS AND DISCUSSION

Hyperventilation tests were accompanied by the development of anginal attacks and ECG changes of ischemic type manifested in ST segment elevation 1 mm or more in one or several leads. Antianginal effect of corinfar was assessed in 15 patients with vasospastic angina pectoris by paired 5-minute hyperventilation test [1,2]. On the next day after the initial test, under similar conditions repeated hyperventilation tests were performed after sublingual intake of 20 mg of corinfar. In fourteen of 15 patients total antianginal effect was observed(the absence of vasospasm and ECG ischemic changes). In one patient pain duration and ST segment elevation were reduced from 15 to 7 minutes.

After corinfar administration systolic and diastolic arterial pressure decreased. Hyperventilation affected further reduction of arterial pressure, with diastolic pressure reducing by 10.9% ($p<0.05$). During corinfar treatment hyperventilation test decreased corrected Q-T interval from 0.42±0.01 to 0.41±0.008 ($p>0.05$).

Thus, corinfar, being an antianginal drug, positively affects the ventricular electric systole in patients with vasospastic angina pectoris. Changes of corrected Q-T interval during hyperventilation tests may serve as an additional criteria for the estimation of myocardium.

3. REFERENCES

1. Girotti L.A., Crosatto J.R., Messuti H. et al. Amer. J. Cardiol. 49(1982)834.
2. Yasue H. Chest 78(1980)2165.

CARDIOVASCULAR SYSTEM'S REACTIONS IN ENDURANCE TRAINED ATHLETES UNDER HYPOKINESIA AND PHYSICAL EXERCISE WITH CHRONIC HYPERHYDRATION

Yan G. Zorbas
Hypokinetic Physiology Laboratory
European Institute of Environmental Cybernetics
GR-162 32 Athens, Greece

ABSTRACT

Studies were performed on 18 long-distance runners during 364 days of hypokinesia (decreased number of steps/day) in order to examine the effects of a daily intake of fluid and salt supplementation (FSS) and intensive physical exrcise (PE) on cardiovascular system's reactions during physical loads. For the simulation of the hypokinetic effect the athletes were kept under an average of 1000 steps/day. The subjects were divided into three equal groups of 6: 6 underwent a normal ambulatory life (control subjects), 6 were placed under hypokinesia (HK) and intensive PE (trained subjects)and the remaining 6 were subjected to HK and intensive PE and consumed daily FSS (water 26 ml/kg body wt and NaCl 0.10 mg/kg body wt) (hyperhydrated subjects). During the performance of physical loads were recorded the tacho-oscillograms of the branchial artery, sphygmograms of the femoral artery, kinetocardiograms of the left (region of the upex beat) and right (4th intecostal space of the right, near the sternum) heart and the arterial pressure. Significant changes were observed in both trained and hyperhydrated subjects during physical loads. However, the cardiovascular stystem's reactions during physical loads were more pronounced in trained than hyperhydrated subjects. It was concluded that a chronic hyperhydration may be used to counteract effectively cardiovascular system's changes in highly trained subjects during prolonged restriction of activity.

1. Introduction

Data were obtained under the influence of HK indicative of significant changes in cardiovascular system during the performance of physical loading tests (1). These phenomena were related primarely to the development of signs of deconditioning of cardiovascular system during exposure to HK (1). At the present time the overall reaction of cardiovascular system to physical loading tests during HK, as a result of application of computation and automation in industry and housekeeping facilities and utilization of transporation by modern man, does not differ essentially from the reactions of cardiovascular system of people who are not at the present time subjected to HK; however, there are data available which suggest that people will exhibit a sequence of significant changes including cardiovascular reactions and reduction in endurance to physical load tests as the level of restriction of motor activity increases (2). Asthenization of the functional state of cardiovascular system is the basic factor in the development of symptomatology of "hypokinetic syndrome" and "hypokinetic disorders" (2). Thus, the aim of this study was to evaluate the effect of a daily FSS intake and intensive PE on cardiovascular system's reactions of endurance athletes during physical load tests and under the influence of HK.

2. Materials and Methods

Experiments were performed on 18 male long distance runners who were engaged in regular endurance exercise training and were on an average of 30,000 steps/day. Subjects aged from 19 to 24 years, weighed from 69 to 74 kg, and had an average VO_2 max of 68 ml/kg body/min. The nature and the procedures of the study were explained to each subject and the study had previously been approved by the University Ethical Committee. Each subject gave written inform consent.

For the isimulation of the hypokinetic effect the number of steps taken per day by the volunteers restricted to an average of 1000, for 364 days (prior to exposure to HK all subjects were on an average of 30,000 steps/day),while they were allowed to remain in a clinostatic position for about 10h/day that included sleeping and resting time and in an orthostatic position for about 14h/day that included different activities, including PE, so that the study would be approximately like the normal life style of a non-active sedentary person. The number of steps taken per day by the volunteers averaged to 1000 and were calculated using a pedometer.

The subjects were on a diet consisting of freshly prepared foods. The caloric value of the diet ranged from 2500 to 2800 kcal/day, with 50% complex carbohydrates, 30% fat and 20% protein, 8.6 mg sodium chloride (NaCl) and 3350 ml water.

All volunteers were divided into three equal groups: Six volunteers underwent a normal ambulatory life (control subjects); six volunteers were subjected to intensive PE and HK and six volunteers were also subjected to intensive PE and HK but consumed daily FSS in small divided doses (water

26 ml/kg body wt and NaCl 0.10 mg/kg body wt) and served as hyperhydrated subjects. Intensive PE consisted of a 20 min warm-up period and an exercising period of 60 to 65 min, twice a day, on a 6 day cycle, that is 5 days of training plus 1 day of active rest, performed on a bicycle ergometer in a seated position as well as a combination of athletic exercises that involved the main muscle groups. The calories expended on the set of intensive PE ranged from 500-600 kcal/h.

Physical load tests with graded PE, which consisted of 3750 kg-m, within 5-min of pedaling at a mean rate of 750 kgm/min and speed of 60 r/min,were performed. The graded PE load actually was fluctuated on different days of HK from 3010-4050 kg-m, that is, it was on the level of average load. The volunteers were tested on a bicycle ergometer, with a pedaling force of 750 kg-m/min for 5 minutes.

During graded PE tests, which were performed several times during the prehypokinetic and hypokinetic periods, were determined the tachooscillograms of the branchial artery, sphygmograms of the femoral artery, kinetocardiograms of the left (region of the upex beat) and right (4th intercostal space on the right, near sternum) heart and arterial pressure in the arm cuff using a Polinom-2M equipment. We analyzed the significance ($P < 0.05$) of differences between the two periods of the study by the ANOVA method.

3. Results and Discussion

During HK all volunteers were maximaly comfortable and had not complained of any discomfort. However, three trained volunteers experienced chest pain, heartburn,headaches, dyspepsias and some other symptoms inherent to HK (1), which either disappeared spontaneously or disappeared after the administration of an additional FSS (2). Some of the volunteers also displayed a lack of interest in performing any kind of physical activities (1).

By the end of HK the trained volunteers lost weight, while the hyperhydrated volunteers gained weight which exceeded the prehypokinetic period values, Maximum oxygen uptake was, on the average, decreased in trained subjects, while increased in the hyperhydrated subjects. The increase of body weight in the hyperhydrated volunteers may be indicative of the possibilities of compensation and even exceeding metabolic losses with chronic hyperhydration and adequate food allowance, provided a good appetite was retained due to gustatory qualities of rations.

The results obtained revealed that during the initial stages of HK heart rate (HR) exhibited a tendency toward a reduction and at the later stages manifested a tendency toward an increase in both trained and hyperhydrated volunteers. The changes in the phase structure of the cardiac cycle were usually characterized by shortening of phases of isometric contraction and relaxation, extension of period of ejection and accelerated filling. Rheographic recordings were determined a tendency toward increased minute volume (MV) during HK, in comparison to prehypokinetic period values, and significant increase of stroke volume (SV)during the initial stages of HK. Blood pressure (BP) was not demonstrated any change, or else, manifested a tendency toward a reduction (with exception of systolic pressure). Specific peripheral resistance and its relation to nominal values was decreased, while the rate of propagation of the wave in the aorta, on the contrary, increased, without manifesting any distinct dependence on the duration of HK.

An analysis of the results obtained with the use of electrocardiographic recordings revealed that the demonstrated changes in cardiovascular system were not pathological in nature but they were had an effect on both the examined hemodynamic parameters and the physical fitness of trained and hyperhydrated subjects during HK.

Functional tests with graded PE during HK also revealed a number of differences in both trained and hyperhydrated subjects, as compared to the results obtained during physical load tests in the course of the prehypokinetic period. The changes in the parameters of hemodynamics and phase structure of the cardiac cycle consisted on the following characteristics: the heart rate during HK was higher than during the prehypokinetic period in the course of graded PE tests in both trained and hyperhydrated subjects,and in spite of the fact that there was a reduction in the physical load being performed. After the graded PE tests,there was a more pronounced reduction of absolute duration of phases of isometric contraction and relaxation, more marked shortening of absolute duration of ejection period, greater increase in intrasystolic index and more marked shortening of phase of rapid filling. During graded PE tests minute volume increased and stroke volume decreased. Arterial blood pressure and peripheral resistance were increased but to a less extent. Absolute rate of propagation of the pulse wave over the aorta was increased.

It was concluded that the demonstrated changes in the cardiovascular system of subjects during graded PE tests and during HK were indicative of the presence of hypokinetic overt phenomena of physical deconditioning, while at the same time it was revealed that intensive PE and chronic hyperhydration cannot be used to prevent cardiovascular system changes in endurance athletes during prolonged HK.

4. References

1. Ye.A.Kovalenko and N. N. Gurovskiy, Hypokinesia, (Meditsina, Moscow, 1980) p 319
2. I. V. Fedorov, Metabolism Under Hypodynamic Conditions (Izdatel'stvo Nauka, Moscow, 1982) p 254

PART VI
Arrythmias: Diagnostic and Clinical Problems

THE DIFFERENT HORIZONS OF TEMPORALITY IN THE CARDIAC ELECTRIC FIELD

ERNST SCHUBERT
Institute of Physiology, Humboldt-University,
Hessische Straße 3/4, 0-1040 Berlin, FRG

ABSTRACT

The cardiac electric field contains diagnostically well investigated information about the spatial distribution of excitation in the heart. Further kinds of information concern the temporal behaviour of the process of spreading of the excitation within one beat, of the dynamics of the serial generation of the cardiac electric field measured by heart rate and of three different spectral components of heart rate variability over a longer time range. The means of evaluation of these various temporal aspects are demonstrated and their results are interpreted for the argumentation about excitation conduction in the heart, influences upon the frequency of the heart beat and the autonomic determinants of the heart rhythmicity.

1. Spatiality and temporality of the cardiac electric field

The electrophysiological events of the excitation process of the heart generate an electrical field within the body which follows the physical algorithms of time-space problems. The distribution of potentials and the flow of currents within this field are determined by the conductivity conditions of the space of the body and the distribution and borderlines of the organs with differing electrical properties. From these the spatial configuration of the field pattern at the body surface can be derived by the way of the foreward solution of the cardiac electric field. Its main components are spatial properties and many important diagnostic informations are the results of the spatial behaviour of the excitation cycle in the spacious configuration of the heart. The only temporal aspect of these problems is the course of the cardiac excitation cycle which influences or causes the diagnostic assertions. The scientific content of this corpus of electrocardiology may be considered as well established throughout the many decades of biophysical, physiological and clinical research in electrocardiology.

Meanwhile clinical as well as theoretical improvements in methodology, knowledge and data processing abilities provoked the interest in a widened and integrated analysis of the various approaches to the temporal behaviour of the cardiac electric field.

2. The 3 temporal aspects of the behaviour of the cardiac electric field

2.1 The dynamics of the excitation cycle

The normal excitation cycle of the heart follows a fixed pathway beginning at the sinus node. After the activation of the atria the ventricular myocardium becomes excited. Afterwards recovery of the myocardium takes place, expressing the repolarization. All the steps of this sequence normally have well determined durations. Thus within the interval of the electrical activation of the heart the cardiac electric field exhibits dynamic changes in its configuration reflected in characteristic shifts and intensity changes of its extrema i. e. maximum and minimum, and the line or area of zero potential. The registration of the cardiac electric field throughout one whole cycle represents a series of pictures containing the sequence of moving potential distributions, with various speed of the shifting and differing velocities of increase or diminution. The main aspect of the temporal character of this phenomenon can be visualized in the record of the pathway of the maximum and minium as presented in the hodogram.

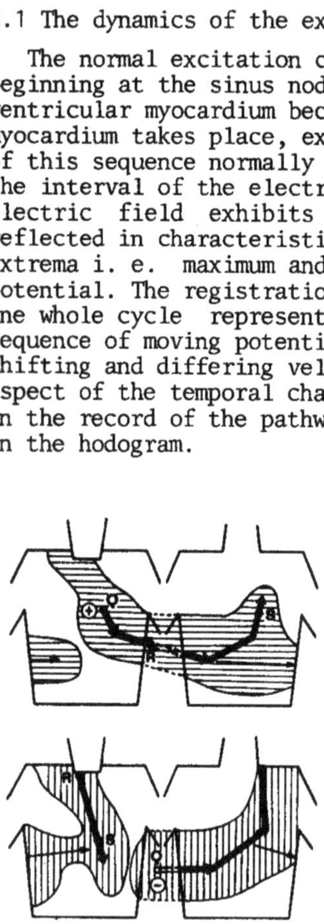

Fig. 1 Hodogram of the QRS-complex after data of Taccardi

Thus fig. 1 shows the path of the maximum area in the QRS-interval (upper part) beginning precordially with a downward shift to the left and to the back side of the thorax till to the end of S. In some cases S max is situated at the right scapula, in other cases it surrounds the thorax at the right side. The pathway of the minimum area (fig. 1, lower part) is longer and runs with a higher speed. It starts at the left side with Q, ascends at the back to the right shoulder till to R and goes down on the front to the precordial region at S. In some cases it surrounds the thorax under the right shoulder. For the atrial activation and the repolarization of the ventricles corresponding hodograms appear with differing velocities and potentials. The hodogram from P through QRS till T reflects the main movement of the cardiac electric field within one beat.

Connection and distance between maximum and minimum reflect the position and magnitude of the representative integral vector. The dynamics of its temporal changes can be recorded also by the vectorcardiogram. The potential changes in one point or between two points in the field are the content of the leading off from one or two electrodes, by which method the standard elctrocardiogram is derived. All these phenomenons are completed within the time interval of one beat, i. e. within time the of about 1 s, thus giving the shortest temporal horizon of the behaviour of the cardiac electric field.

2.2. The dynamics of the rhythmical generation of the field

The one beat cycle of the cardiac activation is repeated rhythmically caused by the oscillating activity of the sinus node as the normal pacemaker of the heart. That is an autochthonous electrical function of the myocardium underlying the controlling influences of the vegetative nervous system. Thus the counteraction of the separate cardiac automaticity and the nervous influences can be observed by the study of the sequence of the generation of the cardiac electric field.

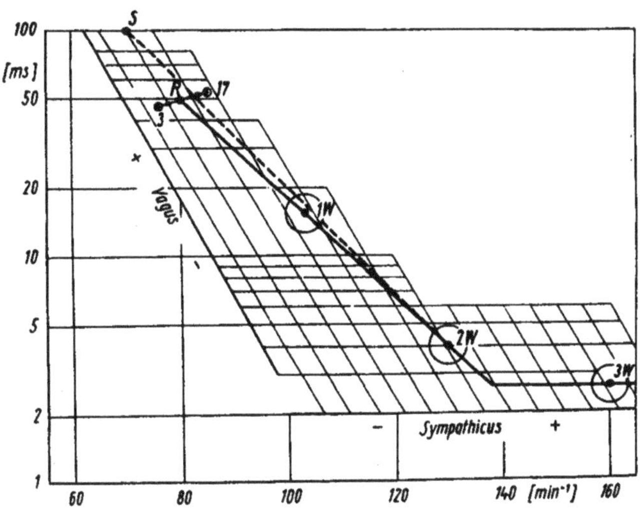

Fig. 2 Rhythm diagram of the heart beat (after Schubert[3]) (s. text)

Measurements of this phenomenon depict heart rate as the parameter characterizing the frequency of the repetitive field generation. Its values are assembled in a well defined narrow range between 60 and 80 repetitions per min in resting individuals depending on age. During physical and mental activity increases of heart rate occur in a well known relation to the intensity of the load. The load dependency is ascribed mainly to the sympathetic drive of the heart. More detailed observations result in the fact of an oscillating of heart rate about its mean value in a large part related to the respiratory frequency. This phenomenon is called sinusarrhythmia. It diminishes with increasing load intensity and has proved to reflect the strengh of the parasympathetic tone of the heart (see Eckberg[2]). Loading effects as well as influences of physical training or of the diurnal rhythmicity in the vegetativ cardiac innervation can be visualized in the rhythm diagram of heart rate in min^{-1} vs. sinusarrhythmia in ms as shown in fig. 2. The different combinations of the two parameters under the different physical load intensities of 1, 2 or 3 W/kg body weight, in the different times of the day at 3 and 17 h (3, 17) and for trained sportsmen (S) and untrained people (R) in rest are indicated.

These informations about the setting of the autochthonous cardiac activation and its interplay with regulatory influences under different conditions for the generation of the cardiac electric field need the evaluation of heart rate and its variability measured as sinusarrhythmia. That is possible within a temporal horizon up to 1 min, characterizing the second part of temporality of the cardiac electric field and its informational content.

2.3. The components of the rhythmicity of the field

In longer records of heart rate during stationary phases within a time of about 10 min the variability of the heart beat demonstrates longer oscillations in different rhythms. This rhythmicity can be analyzed by the help of the Fast Fourier Transformation. That leads to the spectral analysis of heart rate variability, which makes evident 3 components. The highest rhythm C is related to respiratory frequency and usually situated at a frequency band between 0,15 and 0,5 Hz. A middle fraction B appears at 0,05 to 0,15 Hz

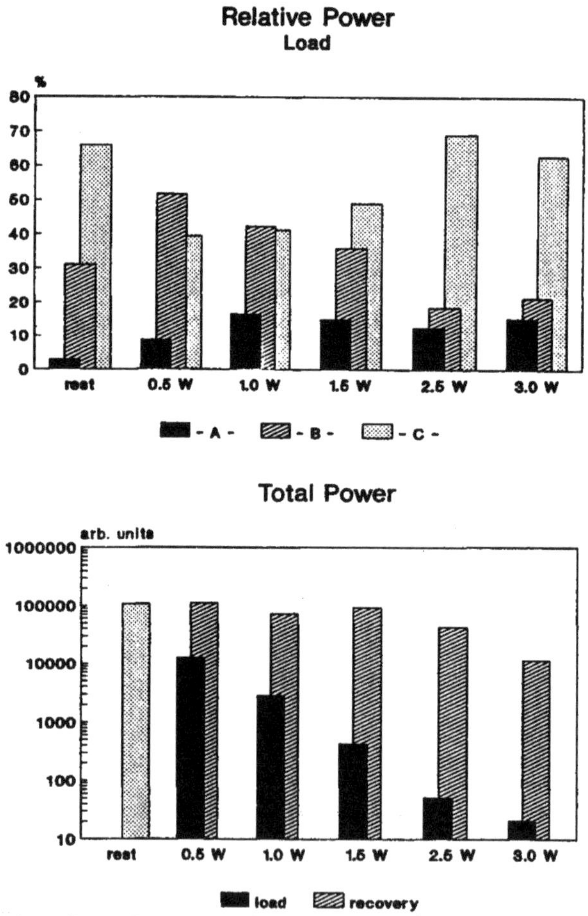

Fig. 3 Relative and total power in spectral density (s. text)

in relation to the blood pressure oscillations and the lowest component A lies at 0,033 to 0,05 Hz in connection to peripheral vascular reactions referring to thermoregulatory activities. The correspondence to different regulatory influences can be proved experimentally and relays for B and C mainly to parasympathetic and for A also to sympathetic control mechanisms (see Akselrot[4]). Normally these components contribute with different relative power to the total power of the spectral density as shown in fig. 3. The new information out of this evaluation of the cardiac electric field is the contribution of the different components, containing less than 5 % for A, about 30 % for B and 65 % for the respiratory part C in resting conditions. Under physical load characteristic changes occur as a strong diminution of total power depending on load intensity and fully repairing within a 5 min recovery period of rest. During the decrease of total power also the partizipation of the different components changes indicating a relative increase in the contribution of the sympathetic influences expressed by component A and a biphasic behaviour of the blood pressure control influences of component B.

The observation of the long term horizon of the cardiac electric field expressed in the rhythmicity of its generation in this way opens the diagnostic approach to the single regulatory influences upon the heart.

3. The meaning of the temporal horizons of the field

Whereas the temporo-spatial problems of the cardiac cycle are well investigated the larger ranges of a temporal analysis are able to deliver new information. The analysis starts from the investigation of the serial events of the generation of the cardiac electric field measured by heart rate and of the exactness of the setting of heart rate in relation to loads of different origin expressed by sinusarrhythmia. The combination of these parameters needs for its measurement a series of heart beats thus presenting a temporal horizon in the order of 1 min. Within this intervall the opportunity of a quantitative estimation of the compound strength of the controlling influences of vagus and sympathicus and an evaluation of their reactions on functional loads has proved to become meaningful. Modern analyzing techniques deliver the last step of investigative information in the temporal horizon of about 10 min. Here components with an origin from different regulatory system can be discriminated. Expressions of such influences within one cardiac cycle are very small thus inducing high technical expenses and a great uncertainty of the whereas resulting information the analysis of spectral power and its components deliver high resultion, abilities.

4. References

1. B. Taccardi, Circ. Res. **12** (1963) 341-352
2. D. L. Eckberg, J. Appl. Physiol. **54** (1983) 961-966
3. E. Schubert, Bull. Acad. Méd. Bel. **13** (1981) 195-206
4. A. Akselrod et al., Science **213** (1981) 220-222 and
   Am. J. Physiol. **249** (1985) H 867- H 875

DISOHOMOGENEITY OF VENTRICULAR REPOLARIZATION IN NON-ISCHEMIC PATIENTS WITH MALIGNANT VENTRICULAR ARRHYTHMIAS

LUIGI DE AMBROGGI, M. SILVIA NEGRONI, CATHERINE KLERSY, TITO BERTONI
Centro E. Malan, San Donato Hospital, University of Milan, San Donato, Italy.

To identify markers of ventricular repolarization disparities in patients with malignant ventricular arrhythmias, we recorded surface potential maps from 117 chest leads in 10 patients (group I), aged 39±16 years, with malignant ventricular arrhythmias (sustained and non sustained ventricular tachycardia, ventricular fibrillation) and in 30 healthy subjects, aged 26±7 years (group II). Four patients had mild arrhythmogenic right ventricular disease, one patient mild dilated cardiomyopathy; in 5 patients no cardiac disease was documented. Maps of the integral values of the QRST interval were obtained by calculating at each lead point the algebraic sum of all instantaneous potentials multiplied by the sampling interval (2 msec). Moreover all 117 ST-T waveforms were analyzed in each subject; by applying principal components analysis, we computed a "similarity index" which represents to what extent (in %) one fundamental pattern of ST-T reproduces all the recorded waveforms. A low value of similarity index indicates a large variety of ST-T waves, likely to reflect the disparity of ventricular repolarization. The mean value of similarity index was significantly lower in group I patients than in group II (62±12% vs 77±8%, p=0.004). In group I 6 patients presented a similarity index lower than 69% (1 SD below the mean for group II). In no case a multipolar distribution of the QRST integral maps was observed.
The lower values of similarity index observed in patients with ventricular arrhythmias suggests a greater then normal dispersion of the ventricular repolarization times. This condition may enhance the vulnerability to malignant ventricular arrhythmias.

A correlation between electrical disparities of the ventricular repolarization and vulnerability to ventricular arrhythmias has been demonstrated by experimental studies[1].
The detection of repolarization disparities from the body surface presents difficulties and several methods have been proposed[2-6].

The aim of our study was to identify signs of ventricular repolarization disparities in patients with malignant ventricular arrhythmias by analyzing body surface potential maps.

Study population

Body surface maps were recorded from 10 patients, 5 males and 5 females, (group I), aged 39±16 years, with malignant ventricular arrhythmias: sustained

(1 patient) and non sustained (7 patients) ventricular tachycardia, ventricular fibrillation (2 patients). Four patients had mild arrhythmogenic right ventricular disease, one patient mild dilated cardiomyopathy; in 5 patients no cardiac disease was documented. Thirty healthy subjects, 15 males and 15 females, (group II), aged 26±7 years, were also studied as controls.

Methods

117 ECG leads were recorded from the anterior and posterior chest and converted in a digital format with a sampling rate of 500 Hz per channel. The data were then processed on a IBM AT computer.

In the present study only QRST integral maps and the similarity index were considered.

The **QRST integral maps** were obtained by calculating at each lead point the algebraic sum of all instantaneous potentials multiplied by the sampling interval (2 msec). The values in uV x sec were transferred to a diagram representing the thoracic surface; then isointegral contour lines were drawn.

The procedure for obtaining the **similarity index** has been described in previous papers[7]. Briefly, in each subject the morphology of all ST-T waveforms was analyzed. The ST-T wave was divided into successive 20 msec intervals and the mean potential value of each interval was considered. Thus, each ST-T wave is represented by a discrete series of 15-20 values. In each subject we performed a "principal components analysis" [8] of the original 117 sets of values. This analysis allowed the identification of one set of values, corresponding to the first principal component, which better represents, by mean of appropriate multiplication factors, the majority of the 117 sets of values recorded in that subject.

Therefore, we define as similarity index, expressed in percent, the ratio between the information content of the first principal component and the total information of the original data. Actually, a high value of similarity index indicates a great similarity of all waveforms to one fundamental waveform, i.e. a great similarity of all waveforms to each other. On the contrary, a low value of similarity index indicates a large variety of ST-T waves, and this is considered a marker of repolarization disparities.

Results

The mean value of similarity index was significantly lower in patients with arrhythmias than in control subjects (62±12% vs 77±8%, p=0.004).

Considering as cut-off point a value of 69%, that corresponds to the mean value for the control group minus 1 SD, we found that 6 out of 10 patients had a lower value, whereas only 3 out of 30 controls had a value below this threshold.

As concerns the QRST integral maps, in no case a multipolar distribution was observed, which is considered a marker of gross electrical inequalities. In 7 patients the distribution of the QRST integral values was within normal limits. In the 3 remaining patients the distribution was bipolar, but a negative area larger than normal was present on the anterior thorax. In these 3 cases similarity index was definitely low.

Conclusion

The similarity index appears more sensitive than the multipolar distribution of QRST integral maps in detecting abnormalities of repolarization, which can be related to electrical disomogeneity of the ventricular recovery process.

The lower values of similarity index observed in patients with ventricular arrhythmias suggest a greater than normal dispersion of the ventricular repolarization times. This condition, favoring the reentry phenomena, may enhance the vulnerability to malignant ventricular arrhythmias.

References

1. M.J. Janse, A.L. Wit, *Physiol. Rev.,* **69** (1989) 1049.
2. J.A. Abildskov, L.S. Green, R.L. Lux, in *Cardiac Electrophysiology and Arrhythmias,* eds D.P. Zipes, J. Jalife (Grune and Stratton, Orlando, 1985).
3. M.J. Gardner, T.J. Montague, C.S. Armstrong, B.M. Horacek, E.R. Smith, *Circulation* **73** (1986) 684.
4. S. Yasamura, I. Kubota, K. Ikeda, K. Tsuiki, S. Yasui, *J. Electrocardiol* **20** (1987) 114.
5. T. Bertoni, M.L. Breghi, M. Marconi, G. Bonifaccio, L. De Ambroggi, in *Electrocardiology '87,* eds E. Schubert (Akademie Verlag, Berlin, 1988).
6. K. Harumi, H. Tsunakawa, G. Nishiyama, S. Kanesaka, in *Electrocardiology '87,* eds E. Schubert (Akademie Verlag, Berlin, 1988).
7. L. De Ambroggi, M. S. Negroni, E. Monza, T. Bertoni, P.J. Schwartz, *Am. J. Cardiol* (1991) in press.
8. D.G. Kleinbaum, L.L. Kupper, *Applied Regression Analysis and Other Multivariable Methods* (Duxbury Press, Boston, 1978) .

USE OF DELAYED POTENTIALS IN THE PREVENTION OF SUDDEN DEATH WITH IMPLANTABLE CARDIAC DEFIBRILLATORS OR AMIODARONE IN PATIENTS WITH MALIGNANT HYPERKINETIC VENTRICULAR ARRHYTHMIAS

L. Chiodi, D. Rossi, A. Fazi, R. Idini, C. Gremigni, R. Vergassola

Department of Cardiology
Ospedale S.M. Annunziata
Florence, Italy

ABSTRACT

The high, short-term mortality among patients with malignant hyperkinetic ventricular arrhythmia treated with empirical drugs has made it necessary to evaluate electrical instability and verify the effectiveness of pharmacological treatments by means of more or less invasive procedures. In recent years electrophysiological studies have assumed a fundamental role in the diagnosis and treatment of malignant HVA. Doubts still remain concerning possibilities of generalized use because the tests are invasive. Our study aims at evaluating whether the presence of delayed potentials in patients with malignant HVA is a reliable marker for arrhythmic risk and whether there are parameters capable of predicting possible pharmacological protection or the need for surgery. We studied 18 patients with malignant HVA who, during amdiodaronic treatment also underwent high-resolution ECG and EPS. A comparison of the test results showed that positivity of delayed potentials with a 40-250 Hz filter is a parameter that can predict the ineffectiveness of amiodarone treatment. This finding, however, requires confirmation by further and broader studies.

INTRODUCTION

Among patients with malignant hyperkinetic ventricular arrhythmia (MHVA), that is sustained ventricular tachycardia (SVT) accompanied by dyspnea, angor or syncope, or cardiac arrest secondary to ventricular tachycardia, or ventricular fibrillation, who receive empirical antiarrhythmic treatment, the mortality rate after 1-2 years due to recurrent arrhythmia is 30%-40%. For this reason, modern treatment must be guided by instrumental tests capable of verifying the effectiveness of the elected treatment.

METHODS AND RESULTS

We studied 18 patients (14 males and 4 females), mean age 61.7 ±9.8 years. The underlying cardiac disease was post-infarctual ischemic heart disease in 12 patients, primary dilatative cardiomyopathy in 2 patients and congenital cardiopathy in 1 patient. No cardiac disease was ascertained in the last patient. All the patients' histories were positive for documented episodes of MHVA non secondary to reversible causes (electrolyte imbalance, toxic drugs, acute myocardial infarction, etc.). All the patients were subjected to dynamic ECG according to Holter and high-resolution ECG. In addition, 14 patients underwent electrophysiological study and 9 had ventriculocoronariographies (Table 1).

The high-resolution ECG was performed according to Simson with 25-250 Hz and 40-250 Hz filters. The following parameters were analyzed: duration of filtered QRS, duration of terminal filtered QRS with voltage under 40 uV (LAS40), root-mean-square voltage of the last 40 msec of the filtered QRS (RMS40).

EPS was performed according to the following protocol: ventricular stimulation in steps with a rising number of extrastimuli, from 1 to 3 on 8-drive beats with increasing stimulation frequency (100-130-150 beats/min) at two different stimulation sites (apex and eflux section of the right ventricle); stimulation duration was 2 msec and the amplitude was twice the threshold value.

Cardiac defibrillators (ICD) were implanted in 12 patients (Group I: 9 males, 3 females, age 65.5 ±0.7, 11 IC, 1 DCM). Of this group 4 had presented episodes of MHVA during chronic amiodarone treatment and the other 8 because unstable SVT or VF had been induced in 6 and 2 patients, respectively during the EPS after loading with amiodarone (15 mg/kg per os for 15 days).

In the remaining 6 patients (Group II: 5 males, 1 female, age 54.0 ±11.1, 3 CI, 1 DCM, 2 HCM) in whom neither SVT nor VF could be induced at the EPS during amiodarone treatment, chronic therapy was undertaken with this drug.

High resolution ECG revealed a significant difference between the two groups with 40-250 Hz filters for the parameters RMS40 (5.4 ±4.0 vs 24.6 ±12.0 $P < 0.01$) and LAS40 (73.6 ±18.9 vs 43.5 ±38.8 $P < 0.05$). Considering RMS40 $<$ 25.0 uV + LAS40 $>$ 40.0 msec with 40-250 Hz filters as the criterion for positivity, we found delayed potentials in 12/12 patients in Group I and 1/6 patients in Group II ($P < 0.01$).

PATIENTS WITH MALIGNANT HYPERKINECTIC VENTRICULAR ARRHYTHMIAS

PATIENT	SEX	AGE	BASE CP	EF%	E.P.S.	INDUCED ARR.
1. A.G.	M	60	PIIC	(14)	+	VT
2. B.O.	F	75	PIIC	20	n.eff.	
3. B.R.	F	63	PIIC	45	+	VF
4. C.E.	M	59	PIIC	38	+	VT
5. E.D.	M	58	DCM	(26)	+	VF
6. F.C.	M	63	PIIC	19	n.eff.	
7. G.O.	M	74	PIIC	(15)	n.eff.	
8. L.A.	M	68	PIIC	(28)	+	VT
9. L.R.	M	63	PIIC	25	+	VT
10. M.A.	M	68	PIIC	23	+	VT
11. S.D.	F	77	PIIC	(23)	+	VT
12. V.D.	M	65	PIIC	(18)	n.eff.	
13. B.B.	M	56	PIIC	50	-	
14. C.R.	M	50	HCM	(45)	-	
15. F.B.	M	72	CON	(38)	-	
16. G.G.	M	46	DCM	52	-	
17. P.L.	F	62	NI	(33)	-	
18. P.A.	M	41	HCM	36	-	

The first 12 patients received automatic defibrillator implants.
The last 6 were treated with drugs.
PIIC: post-infarction ischemic cardiopathy
DCM: dilatative cardiomyopathy
CMI: hypertrophic cardiomyopathy
CON: congenital
NI : no ascertained cardiopathy
EF : ejection fraction as per ventrilography (the data in parentheses were obtained from echocardiograms)

At the subsequent follow-up (10.9 ±7.9 months) there had been no deaths. Shocks had been reported in 10/12 patients with AICD. None of the patients without AICD reported any episodes of dyspnea, angor or syncope, and only one had reported palpitations.

CONCLUSIONS

Even if this survey is limited in scope, preliminary follow-up results confirm the superiority of treatments guided by EPS and similar techniques over empirical treatments in the prevention of MI in patients with MHVA.

Even though in our study high resolution ECG seems capable of distinguishing patients who required automatic defibrillator implants from those who can be managed with drugs, as of this writing, it should be considered complementary to EPS. As a method it still requires further confirmation regarding its validity as the sole instrumental criterion for AICD implants.

REFERENCES

1) D. Zipes et. al., Guidelines for Clinical Intracardiac Electrophysiologic Studies. A report of the ACC/AHA, JACC 1989:1827-42.
2) L. Dreifuss et.al., Guidelines for Implantation of Cardiac Pacemakers and Antiarrhythmia Devices. A report of ACC/AHA, JACC 1991:1-13.
3) M. Schoenfeld, The Cardiac Arrest Survivor: Lessons from the Electrophysiology Laboratory, JACC, 1988:979-81.
4) A. Raviele et al., Aritmie ipercinetiche ventricolari letali: valutazione diagnostica-prognostica. G.It.Card. 1989.19:1035-48.
5) M.B. Simson et al., Detection of delayed ventricular activation on the body surface in dogs, Am.J.Physio. 1981,241:H363.
6) R.A. Freedman et al., Signal-averaged electrocardiograms in patients with nonischemic congestive cardiomyopathy: relationship to sustained ventricular tachyarrhythmias. Circulation 1985,72-1038
7) R.A. Denniss et al., Correlation between signal-averaged electrocardiogram and programmed stimulation in patients with and without spontaenous ventricular tachyarrhythmias, Am.J.Cardio. 1987,59:586.
8) R.A. Winkle et al., Long)term Outcome With the Automatic Implantable Cardioverter-Defibrillator, JACC, 1989:1353-61.
9) Kim G. Soo, Management of Survivors of Cardiac Arrest: Is Electro physiologica Testing Obsolete in the Era of Implantable Defibrillators? JACC. 1990:756:62

VENTRICULAR TACHYCARDIA AND HYPERTROPHIC CARDIOMYOPATHY HOLTER AND SIGNAL-AVERAGED ECG EVALUATIONS PRELIMINARY RESULTS

R. Idini, D. Rossi, L. Chiodi, F. Bandini, A. Florian, M. Masini, C. Gremigni, R. Vergassola

Department of Cardiology
Ospedale S.M.Annunziata
Florence, Italy

ABSTRACT

In post-MIA, DP is a commonly accepted predictive marker for significant arrhthymic events. Due to is electrophysiological characteristics HCM lends itself readily to correlation with DP. The aim of this study is to find DP in patients with HCM diagnosed by ECG, ECO M-Mode, "D", Doppler, Color Doppler and 48 hour dynamic ECG. We examined 16 patients (9 males, 7 females, aged from 50-60 years). To exclude ischemic cardiopathy we subjected all 16 patients to cycloergometric stress tests and ECO-dipyridamole. We did not find any positive DP in the patients even though 2 did present sustained VT during the Holter test. We can, therefore, conclude in accordance with other data reported in the literature that there is no correlation between HCM (independently of VT) and DP.

The positive correlation between delayed potentials (DP) and ventricular tachycardia in the post-infarction stage is certain. However, the relationship between DP and VT in other cardiopathies such as hypertrophic cardiomyopathy, dilatative cardiomyopathy, arrhythmogenic disease of the right ventricle is not certain. The histopathological picture of HCM is characterized by miofibrillar disarray, site of important compromission of refraction and of the decremental conduction in a non-homogenous yet still vital cellular fabric. This outlines the potential geometry of the intraventricular return circuits which constitute the background of high ventricular irritability and the lethal nature of major arrhythmias (Bettini and

Furlanello, 1990). The association between VT and HCM has already been reported in the literature. The incidence of sudden death in HCM, in the studies on non-selected patient groups varies from 2% to 3% yearly. The search for markers to identify sub-groups with unfavorable prognoses is one of the main objectives in studies of patients with HCM. The aim of this study is to compare the results of high-resolution ECG in patients with or without episodes of VT documented by dynamic, Holter ECG. We did not, at this point in the study, consider it necessary to subdivide the cases of HCM according to the site and extent of the hyptertrophy and whether or not there is significant obstruction of eflux.

We examined 16 patients (9 males, 7 females, age 57.1 ±11.9) with HCM, document by ECO M-mode, B-mode, and Color Doppler. The patients underwent dynamic ECG for 48 hours and high resolution ECG (time dominion analysis according to Simson with low-pass 250 Hz filters and high pass filters at 25 and 40 Hz). We also subjected all the patients to diprydamol ECG following the generally accepted protocol and that is, with two doses (0.56 mg/kg and then, after 4', 0.28 mg/kg as the second dose). We did not encounter any echocardiographic modifications of the base segmentary kinetics, nor any ECG modifications. There were no significant side effects. All the patients were given aminoophyline at the end of the provocative test. On the basis of the patient histories and Holter recordings, patients were divided into two groups: GROUP I (5 patients: 4 males, 1 female; age 51.4 ±7.6) with sustained VT (2 patients) and non-sustained (3 patients); GROUP II (11 patients, 5 males, 6 females, age 59.7 ±12.8) without VT. None of the parameters taken into consideration (duration of filtered QRS, duration of filtered terminal QRS with voltage under RO uV, root-mean-square voltage of the last 40 msec of the filtered QRS) showed any statistically significant differences between the two groups.

The small number of cases in the study do not, at this time, allow any conclusions to be drawn. It is our intention to broaden the study and then evaluate any relationships between the site and extent of myocardial hypertrophy, VT documented by Holter tests and the presence of DP.

TABLE 1: PATIENTS EXAMINED

INITIALS	SEX	AGE	SVT	NSVT	DP	ECO
1. B.G.	M	64	N	N	N	Ng
2. C.R.	M	50	N	N	N	Ng
3. D.G.	M	70	Y	N	N	Ng
4. G.M.	M	74	N	Y	N	Ng
5. P.P.	M	50	N	Y	N	Ng
6. P.A	M	41	Y	N	N	Ng
7. R.M.	M	39	N	N	N	Ng
8. T.R.	M	62	N	Y	N	Ng
9. T.M.	M	70	N	N	N	Ng
10. Z.A.	F	55	N	N	N	Ng
11. Z.R.	F	49	N	N	N	Ng
12. Z.S.	F	69	N	N	N	Ng
13. A.N.	M	62	N	N	N	Ng
14. C.L.	F	58	N	N	N	Ng
15. G.C.	F	69	N	N	N	Ng
16. C.G.	M	50	N	N	N	Ng

LEGEND
M = male
F = female
N = no
Y = yes
Ng= negative

REFERENCES

1) K. Iida, K. Yukisada, Y. Sugishita et al., Impaired left ventricular rapid filling during exercise in patients with hypertrophic cardiomyopathy. Clin.Cardio. 10:147,1987.

2) E.G. Rovelli, F. Parenti, S. Devizzi S., Apical Hypertrophic Cardiomyopathy of Japanese Type Am.J.Cardio. 57:358, 1986.

3) E.G. Olsen, Myocardial disarray revisited. Br.Med.J. 285:991 1982

4)W.J. McKenna, Arrhythmia and prognosis in Hypertrophic Cardiomyopathy, Eur Heart J. 4:225 1983

5) W. McKenna, P.J. Counihan, T. Chikenas, Identification of high risk patients with hypertrophic cardiomyopathy, New Trends Arrhyth. VI, 1/2, 745, 1990.

THE VENTRICULAR ARRHYTHMIAS IN MITRAL VALVE PROLAPSE

K.Kulczuga-Kaczmarek, K.Łoboz-Grudzień,
A.Kostecka-Pokryszko, A.Kowalska,
T.Hirnle, C.Kucfir

Dept. of Cardiology of T. Marciniak, A. Falkiewicz
and Dept. of Cardiosurgery M.A. of Wrocław, Poland

ABSTRACT

The ventricular arrhythmias (VA) were examined in 80 pts with mitral valve prolapse (MVP) - mean age 38 years - using ECG at rest, the exercise test and 24h Holter monitoring during daily activity. In 45 pts the mitral regurgitation (MR) was detected. VA occured in 40% pts in ECG at rest, vs 74% pts during 24h Holter monitoring vs 88% pts during exercise test. VA occured in 78% pts with MR vs 63% without MR (NS).The Lown grades 4A occured in 18%, 4B in 4,5% with MR but in none without MR (p 0,001). VA in pts with MR were more frequent than in pts without MR. Exercise test increased frequency of VA in pts with MVP.

The ventricular arrhythmias (VA) is important clinical problem in mitral valve prolapse (MVP). The mechanism of VA is still unknown (1,2). Lately the authors suggest the influence of mitral regurgitation (MR) on VA in pts with MVP (2,3).

METHODS

The study consisted of 80 pts with MVP in age from 16 to 60 years (mean age 38 years). Ratio men/female was 1:3. MVP confirmed by 2D Echocardiography. In 45 pts MR was detected by pulsed Doppler Echocardiography and was qualified as mild (+), moderate (++), and severe (+++). VA were examined in ECG at rest, during exercise test and in 24h Holter monitoring during daily activity.

The degree of VA was evaluated using Lown grades classification. The influence of MR on VA was determined.

RESULTS

Frequency of VA were compared in ECG at rest, in 24h Holter monitoring and during the exercise test (table 1) VA occured in the ECG at rest only in 30%pts, in 24h Holter monitoring in 74% pts but the exercise test showed VA in 88% pts with MVP.

Tab. 1

Frequency of VA in the ECG at rest, in 24 h Holter monitoring during daily activity and during the exercise test

n = 80

	ECG at the rest	24 h Holter monitoring	the exercise test
VA	24 30%	52 74%	69 88%

The table 2 presents the frequency of VA in MVP depending on MR. VA occured in 35% pts (75%) with MR vs 63% without MR (NS).

Tab. 2

VA in relation to MR presence

n = 80

	MR absent n = 35	MR present n = 45
Ventricular Arrhythmias (VA)	22 63%	35 75%

The frequency of VA and Lown grades classification in relation to presence and severity of MR are shown in table 3 and 4.

Tab. 3

The Lown grades of VA in relation to MR

		Lown classification 1-2	3	4A	4B
		VPCs	multiform	couples	VA
MVP	with MR n=45	24	2	8	1
	without MR n=35	31		1	

Tab. 4

The Lown grades of VA in relation to degree of MR

		Lown classification 1-2	3	4A	4B
		VPCs	multiform	couples	VT
MVP	mild (+) n=17	88 %		12 %	
	moderate (++) n=13	70 %	15 %	15 %	
	severe (+++) n=5			× 80 %	20 %

× $P < 0,01$

With the presence and increasing of MR severity the higher Lown grades of VA 4A or 4B were detected.

DISCUSSION:

The presence of complex VA: multiform, couplets, and VT may have a risk of sudden death (1,2,4). Our study showed the pts with MVP with MR have higher risk of VA in compare to those without MR. The ours results are similar to others authors (3,4,5). It suggests the influence of MR on VA occurence. We showed that the exercise test increased frequency of VA in pts with MVP. The authors consider that the exercise test in pts with MVP may have important to set up right indications to individuality treatment of complex VA mostly those dangers of life (2,6).

CONCLUSION:

1) VA in pts with MVP with MR were more frequent than in pts without MR
2) With increasing of MR severity the higher Lown grades of VA 4A or 4B were detected
3) Exercise test increased frequency of VA in pts with MVP

REFERENCES

1. Chesler E., Edwards JE: Mitral valve prolapse and sudden death. Primary Cardiology, 1984, 75
2. Brandenburg R. et al. Cardiology, Year Book Medical Publishers, 1987, p. 817
3. Kligfield P. et al : Complex arrhythmias in mitral regurgitation with and without mitral valve prolapse: contrast to arrhythmias in mitral valve prolapse without mitral regurgitation. Am.J.Cardiol.1985:55: 1545-1549
4. Kligfield P. et al : Arrhythmias and sudden death in mitral valve prolapse. Am. Heart J. 1987:113: 1298-1307
5. Panidis I.P. et al: Prevalence and severity of mitral regurgitation in the mitral valve prolapse syndrome: a Doppler echocardiographic study of 80 patients. J.Am.Cardiol. 1986:7:975-81
6. Perlof J.K. et al. Clinical and epidemiologic issues in mitral valve prolapse. Overview and perspective. Am.Heart J. 1987:113:1324-1332

MECHANISMS OF ATRIAL FIBRILLATION IN PACED PATIENTS

J. SNOECK
Dept. of Cardiology, University Hospital Antwerp,
Wilrijkstraat 10, 2650 Edegem,
Belgium.

H. DECOSTER, C. VRINTS, M. VERHERSTRAETEN, H. HEUTEN, M. BERKHOF, X. MARCHAND*, J.C. KAHN*.
Dept. of Cardiology, University Hospital Antwerp,
Wilrijkstraat 10, 2650 Edegem,
Belgium.
* CHI Poissy, France.

Abstract :
The aim of the study was to determine the mechanisms responsible for the increased incidence of atrial fibrillation in VVI paced patients.
For this purpose P-wave parameters derived from the 12-lead surface ECG were studied in a population of 285 VVI paced patients up to five years after pacemaker implantation.
The study of the P-wave characteristics showed significant changes after pacemaker implantation that are indicative for the presence of a progressive atrial disease. P-wave duration parameters were significantly more prolonged in patients with evolution to atrial fibrillation then in the patients who remained in sinus rhythm .The occurrence of atrial fibrillation could be correlated with the incidence of VVI pacing and also with the incidence of retrograde AV conduction. A high incidence of retrograde conduction resulted in a five-fold increase of the occurrence of atrial fibrillation.
P wave duration parameters at implantation have a predictive value for the development of atrial fibrillation.

Introduction :
Left atrial abnormalities as they can be detected on the surface ECG have been described in many diseases affecting the left heart [1,2]. It was recently reported that VVI pacing may also lead to the development of P wave abnormalities [3]. The development of Atrial Fibrillation (A.F.) is another manifestation of atrial disease. A higher incidence of A.F.is observed in patients with VVI pacing both for AtrioVentricular Block (VVI-AVB) and for Sick Sinus Syndrome (VVI-SSS). Several studies suggest that this increased incidence may be causally related to the use of VVI pacing [4,5,6].

Methods :
A consecutive series of 285 patients paced for symptomatic AVB or SSS was studied. The incidence of A.F. during a follow-up of five years after implantation was registered. A set of P wave measurements was performed at four moments during the follow-up : at implantation and respectively at one, three and five years after implantation. This set consisted of : duration parameters and amplitude parameters

(DII and V1), combined parameters (P.T.F. & P.I.F.) and two measurements related to pacing and derived from careful examination of all ECG tracings :

- pacing incidence (U) : an index of the time the patient is using the pacemaker, expressed in three increasing degrees (U1<U2<U3).
- incidence of retrograde atrial conduction (RC), also expressed in three increasing degrees (RC1< RC2<RC3)

Results :

Incidence of Atrial Fibrillation : the incidence in VVI paced patients 5 years after implantation is 32 % and 11 % in the DDD group ; in the VVI paced patients the incidence varies with the pacing indication: 27 % in the VVI-AVB subgroup versus 46 % in the VVI-SSS subgroup. The important differences between these two subgroups are already significant two years after implantation.

In the results of the P-wave measurements a statistically significant increase is noted after each interval, for several parameters. This increase is most marked for those parameters that reflect left atrial involvement. Some parameters that are indicative for right atrial involvement also show a significant increase, although less marked and less homogeneous.(Fig. 1) These results show the electrocardiographic expression of a progressive atrial disease.
The P-wave duration parameters V1, DII and -Ph of the group of patients with evolution to A.F. are significantly higher than those of the group that remain in sinus rhythm during follow-up. (Fig. 2)

Associated diseases :
In fig. 3 the P wave measurements at implantation are considered into two groups of the total population: group A without and group B with associated diseases. These groups were each further divided in two subgroups : A1 and B1 are the patients with A.F. after 5 years and A2 and B2 are those still in sinus rhythm after 5 years. The comparison of these four subgroups shows a significant difference between A1 and A2 and also between B1 and B2. There is however no significant difference between A1 and B1 nor between A2 and B2.
The incidence of atrial fibrillation at five years after implantation is however significantly higher in the population with associated pathology (41 % vs 19 % ; $p < 0.05$).
It appears therefore that associated pathology facilitates the occurrence of A.F.

Pacing incidence and Atrial Fibrillation : the more the pacemaker is used the higher is the incidence of A.F. after 5 years : U1 = 0 % . ; U2 = 17 % . ; U3 = 45% .
Paired T-test : U1 vs U2 $p < 0.05$, U2 vs U3 $p < 0.005$, U1 vs U3 $p \leq 0.001$.

Retrograde conduction and Atrial Fibrillation :
A low degree of retrograde conduction (RC1) is observed in 82 % of the VVI-AVB population and the incidence of A.F.in these patients is 14 %. In the VVI-SSS population RC1 is observed in 70 % of the patients and the incidence of A.F. is 28 %. There is no significant difference in the incidence of A.F. between the patients with AVB and SSS. A high degree of retrograde conduction (RC3) is observed in 8 % of the VVI-AVB population and in 14 % of the VVI-SSS population ; the incidences of A.F in the patients with RC3 of these two subgroups are 89 % and 100 %. There is thus also no significant difference in the incidence of A.F. between these patients with AVB and SSS.

Comparing the incidences of A.F. in the RC1 group with those in the RC3 group it can be observed that the incidence of A.F. is five times higher in the RC3 group both in the SSS and in the AVB subgroups.
These results indicate that retrograde conduction is a very important factor in the genesis of A.F. in AVB as well as in SSS and it is furthermore important to note that retrograde conduction is more frequently observed in SSS.

Conclusions :
The most important contributing factors for atrial fibrillation in VVI pacing that can be derived from this study are :
1. The consequences of the ventricular pacing itself.
2. The values of P wave duration parameters at implantation.
3. The presence of associated heart diseases.
4. The incidence of retrograde conduction.

References :
1. Snoeck J.et al., *Progress in Electrocardiology,* Ed. P.W. Macfarlane (Pitman Medical Publishing Co Ltd, 1979) p. 289-295.
2. Hopkins C., Barett O. *J. Electrocardiol.*, **22** (1989) 359.
3. Snoeck J. et al. *PACE*, **13** (1990) 2091.
4. Rosenqvist M.et al. *Am. Heart J.*, **116** (1988) 16.
5. Markewitz A. et al. *PACE*, **9** (1986) 115.
6. Santini M.et al. *Am. J. Cardiol.*, **65** (1990) 729.

	0 vs 1 year	0 vs 3 years	0 vs 5 years	1 vs 3 years	1 vs 5 years	3 vs 5 years
V1	≤ 0.0001	≤ 0.0001	≤ 0.0001	≤ 0.0001	≤ 0.0001	≤ 0.0001
-Ph	≤ 0.0001	≤ 0.0001	≤ 0.0001	≤ 0.0001	≤ 0.0001	≤ 0.0001
+Ph	NS	< 0.001	< 0.005	NS	NS	N S
-A	≤ 0.0001	≤ 0.0001	≤ 0.0001	< 0.001	< 0.005	N S
+A	< 0.005	≤ 0.0001	≤ 0.0001	< 0.05	< 0.005	NS
DII	≤ 0.0001	≤ 0.0001	≤ 0.0001	≤ 0.0001	≤ 0.0001	≤ 0.0001
P.T.F.	≤ 0.0001	≤ 0.0001	≤ 0.0001	≤ 0.0001	≤ 0.0001	< 0.0001
P.I.F.	< 0.01	< 0.0005	< 0.0005	< 0.05	< 0.001	N S

Fig.1: Table of significances of the evolution of P-wave parameters after the six intervals post-implantation in the VVI population. (Paired t-test).
V1 :duration V1 ; -Ph : duration negative phase V1 ; + Ph : duration positive phase V1 ; +A : amplitude +Ph ; -A : amplitude -Ph ; DII : duration DII ; P.T.F. : (-A) x (-Ph) ; P.I.F. : (+A) x (+Ph).

P wave duration parameters at implantation

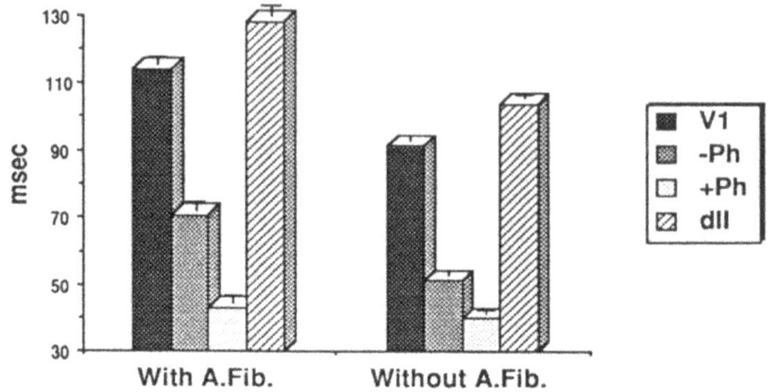

ANOVA: V1 $p \leq 0.0001$ dII $p \leq 0.0001$
-Ph $p \leq 0.0001$ +Ph NS

Fig.2: The importance of the P wave duration parameters at implantation in relation to the occurrence of atrial fibrillation

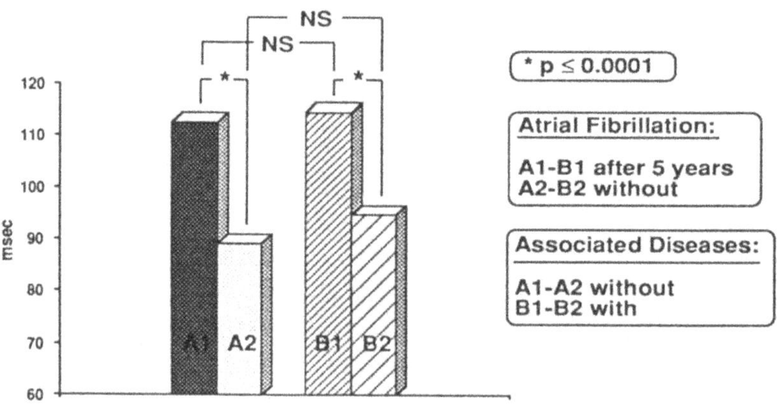

Fig.3: The importance of P wave duration in V1 at implantation in relation to the occurrence of atrial fibrillation in the subgroups with and without associated diseases.

A STUDY OF ATRIAL VOLUME IN THE PATIENTS WITH ATRIAL FIBRILLATION USING COMPUTED TOMOGRAPHY

FUMITAKE INOMATA, MD.

Department of Cardiology, Kikuna Memorial Hopital, 4-4-27, Kikuna, Kohoku-ku, Yokohama-shi, Kanagawa-ken, 222, Japan

ABSTRACT:

To test the relationship between atrial fibrillation(AF) and accurate atrial volume(AV) using ultrafast computed tomography(UFCT). We performed ECG-triggered and enhanced UFCT on 95 patients (pts)(63 males and 32 female). They were divided into 3 groups:53 pts with sinus rhythm(RSR) (group I), 34 pts with chronic AF(group II) and 8 pts with paroxysmal AF (PAF)(group III). The volume of right and left atrium were as follows; group I:70.0±24.8, 78.9±22.7, groupII:157.3±38.7. 174.0±46.0, group III:73.2±19.5, 77.8±23.7(ml), respectively. Pts with Af have larger AV than pts. with RSR and AF, significantly (p=0.0001). There was no significant difference of AV between pts with RSR and PAF. There was no correlation with AV on duration of AF and groupII. Conclusion: 1) There is no significant difference in the atrial volume between RSR and PAF group. 2) There is no need of increased atrial volume for the generation of AF. 3) Chronic AF is accompanied with the increased left and right atrial volume. 4) This increased volume may be necessary for the maintenance of AF.

PURPOSE OF THIS STUDY:

I examined the relationship of atrial volume between in the patients with sinus rhythm and chronic atrial fibrillation and examined the hypothesis that increased atrial volume is necessary to maintain atrial fibrillation.

Method:

Ultrafast computed tomography (Imatron C-100) was used to the patients at supine position putted in ECG. ECG-triggered scanning enhanced film, at the time of 80% of mean R-R interval-diastollic phase, was took and covered with overall the whole heart by 100 msec photographic time on each 1 to 2 beat using non-ionized contrast medium from 1 to 2 ml per second, intravenously. I traced 8 to 20 left and right atrail silhouettes, manually. Right and left atrial volume were calculated from sum of these traced data.

Patient Classification:

I divided the patients into 3 groups to examine whether there is relation between the genesis of atrial fibrillation and atrial volume or not and that there is relation of atrial volume between the patients with regular sinus rhythm(RSR) and chronic atrial fibrillation(AF). Patients classification were as follows:

Group I: patients with regular sinus rhythm (RSR)

Group II: patients with chronic atrial fibrillation (AF)

Group III: patients with paraxysmal atrial fibrillation (PAF)

Patient characteristics: (Table):

There was no significant difference in body surface area (BSA), right atrial pressure (RAP), and pulmonary capillary wedge pressure (PCP) which affect atrial volume 3 groups. But only difference is the age that younger generation was pointed out in group III.

Results:

Right atrial volume were as follows:Group I: 70.0 $\pm$ 24.8 ml , Group II: 157.3$\pm$38.7 ml , Group III:73.2 $\pm$ 19.5 ml . Left atrial volumes were as follows; Group I:78.9$\pm$22.7 ml, Group II:174.0$\pm$46.0 ml , Group III:77.8$\pm$23.7 ml. Each atrial volumes of group II were larger than group I and group III, significantly (p=0.0001). And there was no difference of each atrial volume between group I and group III.

Discussion:

Now that I can say as follows; 1) There is no significant difference in the atrial volume between group of regular sinus rhythm and paraxysmal atrila fibrillation. 2) Then, there is no need for increased atrial volume for the generation of atrial fibrillation. 3) But in chronic atrial fibillation group, there is increased atrial volume. It is difficult to conclude whether increased atrial volume is the cause or the result of atrial fibrillation.

Duration of chronic atrial fibrillation versus atrial volume: (Figure)

To examine that increased atrial volume is the result or chronic atrial fibrillation, I examined the correlation of atrial volume and duration of chronicatrial fibrillation in 25 patients with lone atrial fibrillation in the patients group II of chronic atrial fibrillation. There is no carrelation between duration and atrial volume in the patients with lone atrial fibrillation. That is to say, there was no fact there is longer duration of atrial fibrillation , more increased atrial volume.

Conclusion:

1) Chronic atrial fibrillation is accompanied with increased left and right atrial volume.

2)From the result of duration of chronic atrial fibrillation versus atrial volume,there is no correlation between duration and atrial volume in the patients with lone atrial fibrillation.
Thus this increased atrial volume may be necessary for the maintenance of atrial fibrillation.

Table

Patient characteristics

	RSR	*AF*	PAF	*Pvalue*
N	53	34	8	
Age	63	65	47	.003
BSA(M²)	1.6	1.6	1.7	.195
RAP(mmHg)	5.0	3.9	0.5	.247
PCP(mmHg)	7.8	10.9	4.5	.071

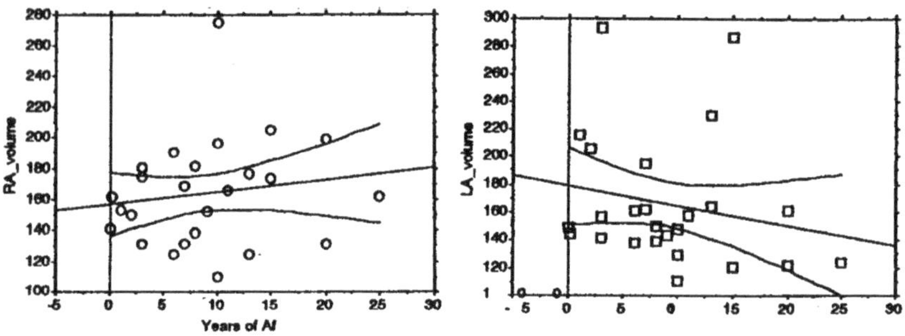

Figure

Af interval vs atrial volume

References:

1)Lyons, R.H.,Farah%A.,Moe,G.K,. and Abildkov, J.A.:Circulation (1959), 20:451
2)Garrey,W.E.: J.Physiol. (1914), 33:397
3)Inomata,K., J.Tokyo Medical College (1961), 19:2087

REGISTRATION OF PRE-ATRIAL AND ATRIAL ACTIVITY BY SIGNAL AVERAGED ELECTROCARDIOGRAM IN HEALTHY SUBJECTS AND PATIENTS WITH SICK SINUS SYNDROME

MACIEJ KUCZBORSKI
Clinic of Cardiology, Institute of Cardiology, Medical Academy, Sterlinga 1/3, Lodz/Poland

and

HALINA PRACKA, SLAWOMIR WOJCZUK
Clinic of Cardiology, Institute of Cardiology, Medical Academy, Sterlinga 1/3, Lodz/Poland

The aim of study was analysis of preatrial (pre-P) and atrial activity (AP) recorded by signal averaged electrocardiogram (SA-ECG), obtained from the body surface in 32 healthy subjects (H), 22 patients with severe sinus bradycardia (SB group) and 35 patients with bradycardia-tachycardia syndrome and frequent atrial fibrillation (BTS group). Significant differences between parameters of pre-P and AP in healthy subjects and patiens with sick sinus syndrome were observed. SA-ECG is very useful method for diagnosis the sick sinus syndrome, especially for identifying patients at risk of atrial fibrillation.

Analysis of signal averaged atrial activity recorded from the body surface has been used to predict the risk of atrial arrythmias (1-3). Recently invasive and noninvasive methods of registration of sino-atrial (SA) node activity were performed (4-5). Kao and al. recorded SA node electrogramms from a bipolar esophageal electrode (5). The aim of our study was analysis of pre-P and atrial potentials (AP) recorded by signal averaged electrocardiogram (SA-ECG) from the body surface in healthy subjects (H) and patients with sick sinus syndrome (SSS).

Methods

The system of the data storage and analysis was built on the base of low noise amplifiers of the ECG signal working in Frank's orthogonal system connected with 12 bit analog- to- digital converter in microcomputer PC-AT. Recordings were made in 20 series in X,Y and Z orthogonal leads. To eliminate noise and fluctuations about 100 P waves were averaged. Then averaged signal was filtered using 25 Hz or 40 Hz high-pass Butterworth digital filters. The amplitude of pre-P (A pre-P), duration (D pre-P), amplitude of atrial potentials (A-AP), duration AP (D-AP) and duration of baseline (BL) from the end of AP to the beginning or the QRS complex in SA-ECG were measured.

The statistical analysis concerning parameters in 3 groups of patients was made.

Materials

SA-ECG were recorded in 32 healthy subjects (H), in 22 patients with severe sinus bradycardia (SB group) and 35 patients with bradycardia-tachycardia syndrome and frequent atrial fibrillation (BTS group).

Results

Analysis of pre-P recordings

The mean values of A pre-P and D pre-P in 3 groups of patients are presented in table I.

TABLE I

	H	SB	BTS
A pre-P (uV)	19,8±11,9	8,2±4,5	16,5±5,1
D pre-P (ms)	118,6±19,9	94,9±43,0	120,7±35,5
A-AP	31,5±11,0	21,1±8,7	30,6±11,0
D-AP	139,2±13,1	150,6±15,9	154,3±16,0
BL (ms)	22,7±12,3	32,4±28,3	11,1±15,3

The most significant differences in pre-P parameters were observed in SB group in comparison with H and BTS group. Respectively pre-P parameters were:

A pre-P: H>SB $p<0,001$, BTS>SB $p<0,01$ and H>BTS NS;

D pre-P: H>SB $p<0,01$, BTS>SB $p<0,01$ and H<BTS NS.

The representative pre-P recordings are shown in figure 1.

Analysis of AP recordings

The mean values of A-AP, D-AP and BL are presented in table I. As may be seen (table I and figure 2) there are considerable differences in A-AP between H and SB group. The A-AP was significantly lower in SB group in comparison with

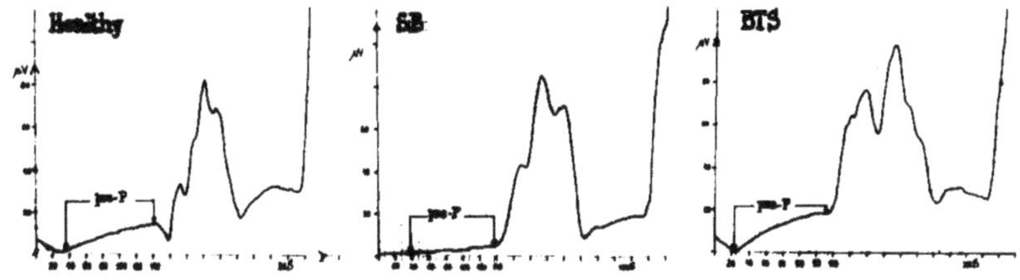

Fig. 1: pre-P potenrials in H, SB and BTS group.
Note lov A pre-P in SB group.

H (SB<H p<0,0005) and BTS group (SB<BTS p<0,001). There were non statistical between H and BTS group. The D-AP was prolonged both in SB and BTS in comparison with H group (H<SB p<0,005, H<BTS p<0,0001). There were no statistical differences in SB and BTS group. We observed marked differences in BL duration between BTS and other two groups (H>BTS p<0,002; SB>BTS p<0,0005; SB>H NS). The representative AP recordings are shown in figure 2.

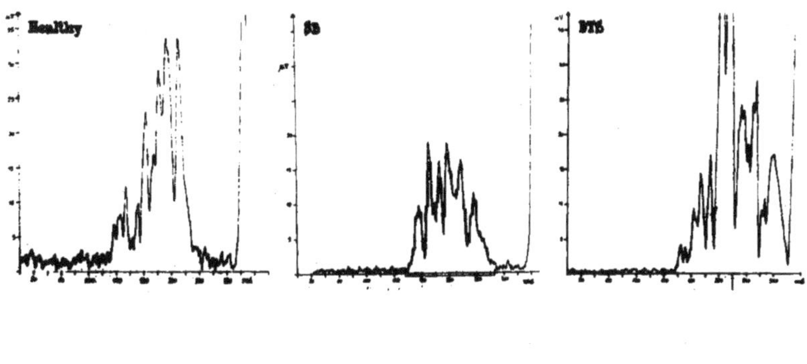

Fig. 2: AP in H,SB and BTS patients. Note the lowest A-AP in SB group and lack of BL in BTS group.

Discussion

The exact source of pre-atrial potentials registered in our study has not been definitely established, but we consider them to originate from SA node region. We observed marked differences in amplitude and duration of pre-P between healthy subjects and patients with various forms of SSS. However the exact significance of the morphology of pre-P needs further studies, it seems that SA-ECG from the body surface can be useful method for registration of sino atrial activity.

The analysis of atrial potentials showed the significant differences in AP parameters in healthy subjects and patients with SSS. We think that on the base of our studies we can distinguish defined picture of SA-ECG in H group-high amplitude of pre-P and AP, non prolonged D-AP and present BL; in SB group very low A pre-P and A-AP, prolonged D-AP. In BTS group most characterized is lack or very short BL. We conclude that SA-ECG is very useful method for diagnosis the sick sinus syndrome, especially for identifying patients at risk of atrial fibrillation.

References

1. T. Yamada, M. Fukunami, M. Ohmori, *Clinical significance of atrial signal averaged electrocardiogram for detection of patients with paroxysmal atrial fibrillation*, Circulation 80(4)(1989)II-636.
2. Y. Yamaguchi, K. Kuga, Y. Sugishita, *The signal averaged electrocardiogram as a screening test for the occurrence of paroxysmal atrial fibrillation*, J. Am. Coll Cardiol 11(2)(1988) 116A.
3. T. R. Engel, N. Vallone, J. Windle, *The signal averaged electrogram in patients with atrial fibrillation or flutter*, AM Heart J. 115(1988)592.
4. M. J. Stopczyk, W. Wajszczuk, R. Zochowski, *Pre-P(sino atrial node region) activity recording from the right atrial cavity by signal averaging*, PACE 2(1979)156
5. T. Kao, B. C. Yu, C. W. Kong, C. Y. Chen, B. N. Chiang, *A noninvasive pre-atrial activity recording by signal averaging using esophageal electrode*, PACE 11(1988)1168.

THERAPY OF RECURRENT ATRIOVENTRICULAR NODAL REENTRANT TACHYCARDIA USING RADIOFREQUENCY CURRENT [#]

Włodzimierz J.Musiał[*], Heinz F.Pitschner[**], Jorg Neutzner[**]

[*] *I Medical Clinic, Medical Academy Łódź, Poland, 93-113 Łódź, Milionowa 14*
[**] *Kerckhoff-Klinik, Bad Nauheim, FRG 6350 Bad Nauheim, Beneckestrasse 2-8*

ABSTRACT

Preliminary clinical results of modification of antegrade conduction in 5 patients with recurrent atrioventricular nodal tachycardia were presented. Radiofrequency current was used. It was possible to titrate the amount of energy by changing the power and the time of application. The modification procedure was repeated several times since PQ interval increased more than 50% with the noninductibility of tachycardia. The therapeutic effect correlated with prolongation of atrio-ventricular nodal conduction (AH interval). No changes of HV time were noted. The precise localisation of the electrode was of primary importance, since the RF current produced much smaller leasions than DC shock. Endocardial mapping allowed to find the optimal modification place. The procedure was safe and well tolerated without general anesthesia.

Electrical ablation introduced for treatment of refractory cardiac arrhythmias at the beginning of eighties is now an established alternative for surgical procedure.[1] The conventional technique of ablation using direct current (DC) defibrillation to achieve complete heart block has now decreasing clinical value.[2] There has been however a growing interest in modification of atrioventricular (AV) conduction to prevent arrhythmias and to avoid implantation of a pacemaker. A new energy source used to create partial AV block is the radiofrequency (RF) current[3,4].

It is the purpose of this paper to present our preliminary results using this method in 5 patients with recurrent AV nodal reentrant tachycardia (AVNRT).

RF current used for ablation causes low power coagulation

[#]The study was done during Dr. Musiał's training as a Alexander von Humboldt scholarship holder.

without sparking. The electrode which is in a good contact with the tissue allows to flow the current directly from the catheter into the low resistant and moist tissue. As the result heat arises and slowly drives extra and intracellular water out of the tissue. Because of the risk of perforation produced temperature should never exceed $100^{\circ}C$. Commercially available RF generators like HAT 100 device (produced by Ing. P. Osypka FRG), used by us, deliver a 300 kHz or greater unmodulated sinusoidal waveform in the bipolar or unipolar output mode[3,4]. The unipolar output was used in our patients. In spite of large current the maximum voltage is low. In contrast to the high voltage DC-defibrilation the RF desiccation does not cause barotraumatic effect. In adition general anesthesia can be omitted, because high frequency RF current does not stimulate neuromuscular fibers. RF pulses do not affect catheter's integrity[3,4].The precise localisation of the electrode is of primary importance since the RF current produces much smaller and more discrete lesion, than DC shock[3,4]. The second requirement is the stability of the catheter necessary to ensue good tissue contact. These are the drawbacks of the technique which makes the procedure time consuming. Fig. 1. shows the typical position of the electrodes during modification.

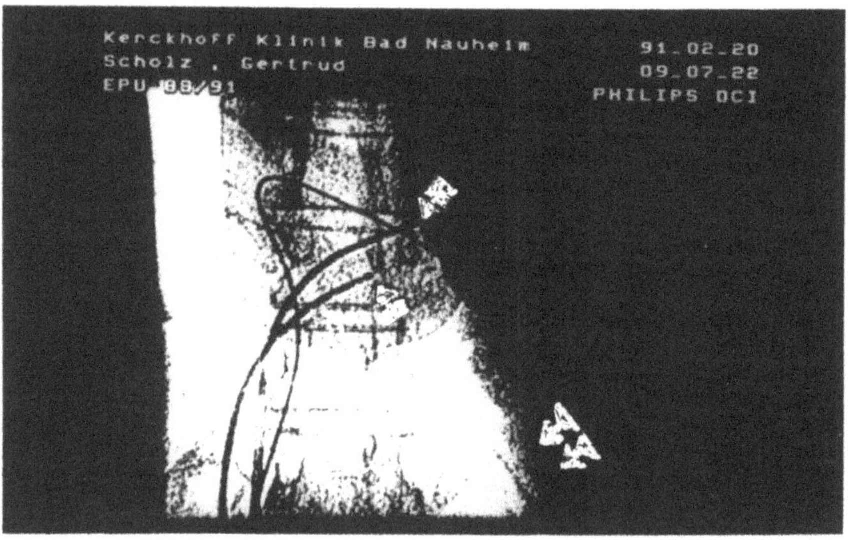

Fig. 1
Position of the catheters during modificaton procedure. Two quadripolar electrodes introduced through the femoral vein were positioned in the His bundle region. The upper one (light arrow) was used as a radiological and electrical reference point (see also fig.2). The lower one (dark arrow) positioned near the distal bipole of the reference electrode served for modification. It was connected

with the RF generator. The third bipolar electrode placed in the right apex was used for pacing and recording (two arrows).

We usually placed catheters in AV region until a relatively large atrial potential with only barely visible His bundle deflection was obtained. During AVNRT the place of the earliest retrograde atrial depolarization was searched for - Fig. 2.

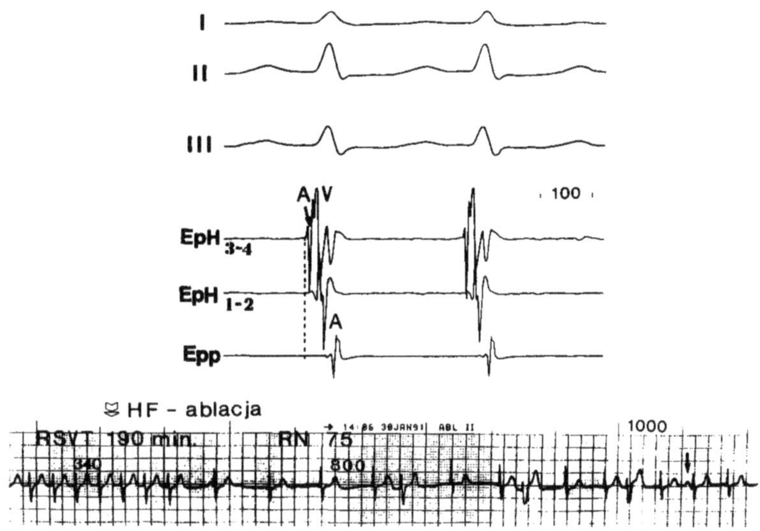

Fig.2.
Upper tracing: endocardial mapping during AVRNT. The recording leads are ECG leads I, II, III, aVR and bipolar electrograms from a quadripolar catheter positioned in the His bundle region (EpH). The earliest atrial activation (A) during tachycardia(arrow)became evident in the His bundle region through the distal pair of electrodes (EpH_{3-4}). This bipole was used as a reference point for modification. Lower tracing: ECG recording during modification. At the beginning AVRNT 190/min was present. The application of RF energy (indicated by arrow) caused termination of the tachycardia with the appearance of accelerated junctional rhythm 75/min. Premature ventricular beats were also seen. This phenomenon suggested the proper placement of the ablation catheter and was a good predictor of successful modification.

Changing the power and the time of application it was possible to titrate the amount of energy to achieve the desired effect. Current and voltage were monitored during the procedure. We repeated the modification several times since PQ interval increased >50% with noninductibility of the tachycardia. The therapeutic effect correlated with modification of antegrade AV conduction as demonstrated by AH interval prolongation. No prolongation of HV time was noted - Fig. 3. These changes allowed to avoid the induction of AVNRT despite the persistence of 1:1 AV conduction.

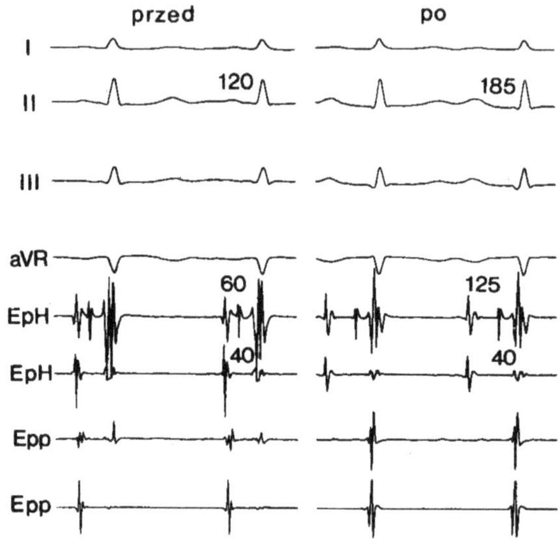

Fig. 3.
Electrocardiograms and His bundle recordings before (left) and after (right) RF modification. Before modification short PQ (120 ms) and AH (60 ms) interval was seen. Application of RF energy caused prolongation of PQ to 185 ms and AH to 125 ms. No changes of HV time were noted. Epp-high right atrial electrogram, EpH-His bundle electrogram.

RF modification offered several advantages over the use of DC-ablation. No malignant ventricular arrythmia, hypotension or myocardial perforation were seen, all of which were reported after DC-ablation.[1] The procedure was safe and generally well tolerated, however slight chest pain during energy application was sporadically noted. So the first results of our study are positive and we think that RF modification of AV conduction will be a useful technique to treat patients with recurrent AVNRT refractory to pharmacologic therapy. The technique is a promising alternative to the DC ablation.

REFERENCES

1. G.T. Evans and al., *Pace* **11** (1988) 1621
2. M.M. Scheinman, *Circulation* **83** (1991) 1489
3. S.K.S. Huang, *Pace* **14** (1991) 28
4. N.G. Tullo, H. An and S. Saksena, *Electrical therapy for cardiac arrrhythmias* (Saunders Comp. Philadelphia, 1988) p. 684

USEFULNESS OF NONINVASIVE STUDIES IN ASSESSMENT OF ACCESSORY PATHWAY IN PATIENTS WITH WOLFF-PARKINSON-WHITE SYNDROME

JAN RUTA
Department of Electrophysiologic Studies, Institute of Cardiology, Medical Academy, Sterlinga 1/3, Lodz /Poland

and

M. ZIELIŃSKA, S. CERANKA, J. K. WRANICZ, M. WIERZBICKA, H. BOLIŃSKA, H. PRACKA
Department of Electrophysiologic Studies and Cardiology Clinic, Institute of Cardiology, Medical Academy, Sterlinga 1/3, Lodz /Poland

The aim of the study was the comparative estimation of the value of noninvasive methods in the definition of anterograde effective refractory period of the accessory pathway (ERP AP) in patients with Wolff-Parkinson-White syndrome (WPW). The studies including esophageal atrial pacing, treadmill exercise test and Ajmaline test were performed in 24 patients with WPW syndrome, 14 males and 10 females aged 23-45 years. According to the duration of the ERP AP patients were divided into two groups. Group I consisted of 19 patients with ERP AP > 250ms and group II included 5 patients with ERP AP ≤ 250 ms. In all patients the disappearance of the WPW morphology was estimated during our studies. In group I the narrowing of the QRS complex was observed during: exercise test in 12 patients and Ajmaline test in all patients. In group II the abolition of the preexcitation was stated: during exercise test in 1 patient and Ajmaline test in 5 patients. Basing on the performed study we consider that exercise and Ajmaline tests can be helpfull but not decisive in the estimation of the properties of the accessory pathway.

The properties of the accessory atrio-ventricular connection is most frequently investigated during invasive electrophysiologic studies and only few reports concern the results achieved with noninvasive methods (2,3).

The aim of this study was the estimation of the usefulness of noninvasive investigations in the assessment of the anterograde effective refractory period of the Kent bundle in patients with WPW syndrome.

Methods

The study population consisted of 24 patients with WPW syndrome, 14 males and 10 females aged 23-45 years, in whom ERP AP was determined during esophageal atrial pacing. In routine ecg and during Holter monitoring the preexcitation pattern was permanent in 20 patients and intermittent in 4 patients. 17 patients were classified as type A and 7 patients as type B applying Rosenbaum's classification. 18 patients suffered from recurrent paroxysmal tachycardia or/and atrial fibrillation and 6 patients were asymptomatic.

All patients underwent (Fig.1):

1. esophageal atrial pacing using single extrastimulus technique for determination of the ERP AP
2. treadmill exercise test according to Bruce protocol
3. Ajmaline test

Results

Esophageal pacing

ERP AP>250 ms was stated in 19 patients (group I) and ERP AP≤250 ms in 5 patients(group II).

Exercise test

Block in the Kent bundle developed in 12 patients with ERP AP>250ms and in 1 patient with ERP AP≤250ms. There was no strict correlation between normalisation of the QRS complexes during exercise and the length of the refractoriness of the Kent bundle.

Ajmaline test

Ajmaline blocked the anterograde conduction in the accessory pathway in all patients as well with long (260-400ms)as with short effective refractory period of the Kent bundle (240-250ms).

Combined tests

During two noninvasive methods including exercise and Ajmaline tests a disappearance of the delta wave was observed as well in patients with ERP AP>250ms (6 patients) as in those with ERP AP≤250ms (1 patient).

Discussion

In patients with WPW syndrome an identification of those at risk of ventricular fibrillation is an important problem. It is known that patients with a short anterograde

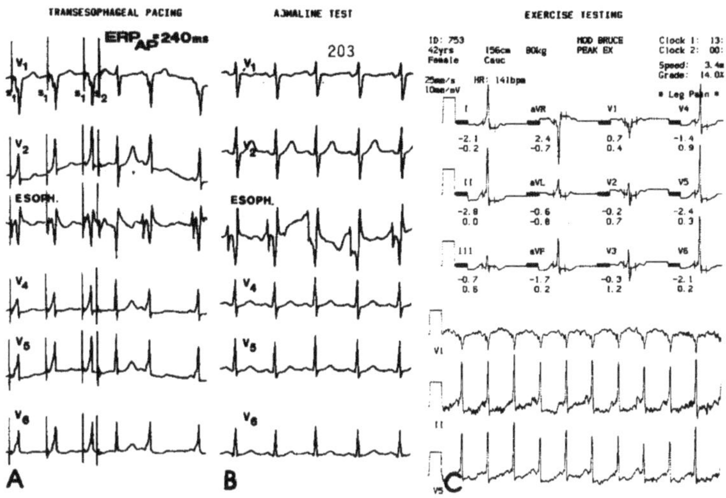

Figure 1.: **A.** The determination of the **ERP AP** during esophageal atrial pacing (S1S2=240ms), **B.** The abolition of ventricular preexitation by Ajmaline, **C.** The preexcitation pattern is not abolished during the exercise test.

effective refractory period of the accessory pathway less than 250ms may develop ventricular fibrillation during atrial fibrillation (1). The most reliable method for determination of the ERP AP is an electrophysiologic invasive investigation,but a question remains if it is necessary to perform it in each case. To assess the usefulness of noninvasive methods in the determination of the properties of the accessory atrio-ventricular connection in patients with WPW syndrome we performed comparative analysis of the results of esophageal pacing, exercise and Ajmaline tests.

Our results in opposition to other authors suggest that in individual patients Ajmaline can block the conduction not only in those with ERP AP of more than 250ms (2) but also in patients with refractoriness of the Kent bundle between 240 and 250ms. Because of this fact the Ajmaline test can not be a certain criterion for the detection of patients at risk of ventricular fibrillation.

Also the exercise test like the Ajmaline test is not able to discern patients with short refractoriness of the accessory pathway. We observed the abolition of the preexcitation both in patients with ERP AP of more than 250ms and in those with ERP AP of 250ms or less. Our results support a report of Eshchar (3) who did not find a reliable correlation between ERP AP and the conduction through the accessory atrio-ventricular connection. It seems that the behavior of the conduction in the Kent bundle depends rather on relation between properties of the accessory and normal pathway than on the absolute value of the refractoriness of both these pathways (4).

During combined exercise and Ajmaline tests we observed a disappearance of the delta wave in patients of both groups, those with a short and a long ERP AP. It suggests that also a combination of these noninvasive methods can not with certainly detect patients with a relatively short refractoriness of the Kent bundle.

Because our findings were obtained only in few patients they require further investigations in a greater population.

Conclusion

Exercise test and Ajmaline test can be helpful but not decisive in the estimation of the properties of the accessory pathway in patients with WPW syndrome.

References

1. G.J.Klein, T.M.Bashore, T.D.Sellers, E.L.C.Pritchett, W.M.Smith and J.J.Gallagher, *Ventricular fibrillation in the Wolff-Parkinson-White Syndrome*, N.Eng.J.Med. **301** (1979) 1080
2. G.Critelli, J.J.Gallagher, F.Perticone, F.Coltorti, V.Monda and M.Condorelli, *Evaluation of noninvasive tests for identifying patients with preexcitation syndrome at risk of rapid ventricular response*, Am.Heart J. **108**(1984)905
3. Y.Eshchar, B.Belhassen and S.Laniado, *Comparison of exercise testing in the Wolff-Parkinson-White syndrome*, Am.J.Cardiol. 57(1986)782
4. S.Levy, J.P.Broustet, J.Clementy, B.Vircoulon, P.Guern and H.Bricaud, *Syndrome de Wolff-Parkinson-White . Correlations entre l'exploration electrophysiologique et l'effet de l'epreuve d'effort sur l'aspect electrocardiographique de pre-exitation*, Arch.Mal.Coeur. 72(1979)634

Reduced Instantaneous and Circadian Heart Rate Variability in Sudden Arrhythmogenic Cardiac Death. A Case Report.

H.-D. Esperer
University Heart Centre, University of Erlangen-Nürnberg
D-8520 Erlangen, Germany

J. von der Emde
Head of the Department of Cardiac Surgery, University of Erlangen-Nürnberg, D-8520 Erlangen, Germany

Abstract

In five patients with sinus rhythm, who were on Holter monitoring while suffering sudden arrhythmogenic cardiac death (SACD), instantaneous as well as circadian heart rate variability (HRV) were shown to be significantly reduced as compared to age matched patients with chronic stable coronary artery disease. These findings suggest an imbalance in autonomic cardiac tone to be essentially involved in the genesis of lethal arrhythmias in patients with structural heart disease.

Introduction

Although development of potentially lethal ventricular arrhythmias is obviously due to multiple factors, a growing body of experimental and clinical evidence suggests that changes in the autonomic cardiac tone resulting in an imbalance of sympathovagal activity play a major role in their genesis[1]. Recently it has been shown that heart rate variability (HRV) is a useful tool for noninvasive assessment of cardiac vagal efferent activity[2]. The occurrence of sudden arrhythmogenic cardiac death (SACD) during Holter monitoring permits valuable insights into the context of rhythm alterations and trigger events of the terminal arrhythmia (TA). By now only a few reports have delt with changes in heart rate variability (HRV) in this setting[1,3,4]. This report describes 6 patients, who died suddenly while being Holter monitored.

Material and Methods

The study comprised 6 patients aged 56 - 74 years, four suffering from severe coronary artery disease (CAD) and two from dilated cardiomyopathy (DCM). Arrhythmia analysis was performed on a Pathfinder III (Reynolds). For HRV determination a modification of the RR-Scope software[5] was used. HRV was quantified in terms of **SDANN**[1], **rMSSD**[1], **pNN50**[2] and **CV** (= SD/NN). In one patient with atrial fibrillation HRV analysis could not be performed. The HRV indices of the SACD patients were compared with those of five age matched patients suffering from chronic stable CAD. The mean interval of Holter monitoring was 10.4 ± 8.8 hours (range: 2 hr 50 min - 22 hr 50 min) in the SACD and 18.3 ± 5.8 hours in the reference group.

Results and Discussion

Ventricular tachycardia (VT) degenerating into ventricular fibrillation (VF) was the lethal arrhythmia in all cases. The density of ventricular ectopic activity (VEA), i.e.: isolated PVCs, ventricular couplets and nonsustained VT, was significantly increased 1.5 to 2 hours before the lethal event in two patients, whereas in three patients VEA was equally distributed throughout the Holter period. Interestingly, in one case, there was a decrease in ventricular ectopic activity 85 minutes before it resumed again just prior to the onset of the terminal VT (Table I)

Table I: Clinical Features of the SACD Patients Studied

Pat.	Diagnosis	Rhythm	VEA	HR-mean	ST-Segment Shift
1	CAD	Sinus	+	no Change	-
2	CAD	Sinus	+++	Increase	-
3	CAD	Sinus	+++	Increase	Elevation
4	CAD	Sinus	+	Decrease	-
5	DCM	Sinus	+	Increase	Elevation
6	DCM	AF	++	no Change	Elevation

In 3 patients there was marked ST-segment elevation for some minutes in the period 90 to 132 minutes before TA onset.

Fig.1: HRV in SACD & Reference Patients

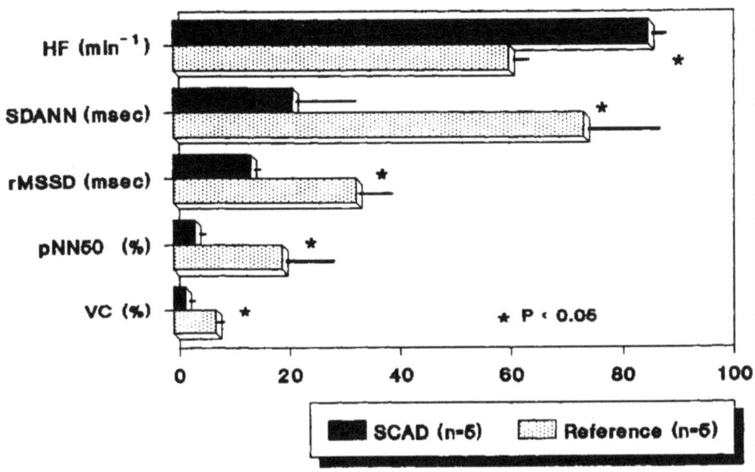

Fig.2: Instantaneous HRV prior to terminal VT

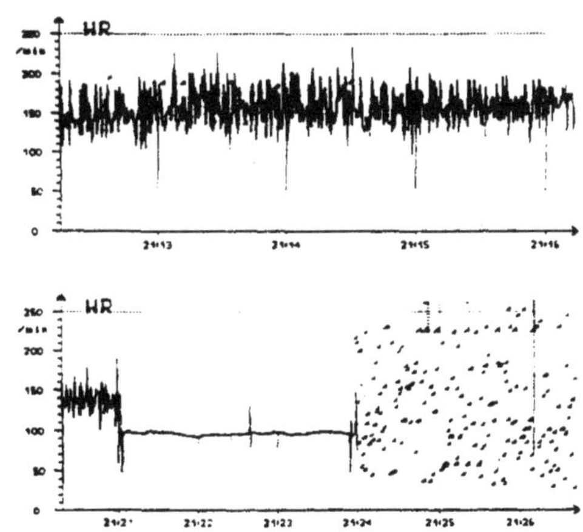

In 4 patients mean heart rate increased just prior to the onset of VT, whereas it decreased in one and did not change in another (Tab.I). The indices of heart rate variability were significantly reduced in the SACD patients as compared to the reference group (Fig.1). Whereas in the SACD group the respective mean values for SDNN, rMSSD, pNN50 and CV were 21.6 ± 11.1 msec, 14.0 ± 3.5 msec, 3.9 ± 0.9 % and 2.2 ± 0.6 %, they amounted to 74.0 ± 13.8 msec (SDNN), 33.1 ± 7.1 msec (rMSSD), 19.7 ± 11.6 % (pNN50) and 7.6 ± 1.3 % (CV) in the reference patients. Mean heart rate was significantly higher in the SACD patients than in those with stable coronary artery disease: 85.7 ± 4.6 /min (676.4 ± 43.6 msec) versus 60.7 ± 5.1 /min (996.5 ± 60.7 msec). Fig.2 shows a typical NN-interval tachogram of a patient during the last minutes before sudden cardiac death: four minutes prior to the onset of the lethal VT there was an abrupt reduction in instantaneous HRV resulting in total loss of the short-term oscillations present before. Another striking difference between each group pertains to the 24-hour profile of HRV. Whereas there was a clear cut day to night rhythmicity of the HRV indices in the reference group, with higher values during the early morning hours (0:10 h - 5:00 a.m.), the **circadian HRV pattern** was completely blunted in the SACD patients.

These results add to the findings of others[3,4] suggesting an imbalance in autonomic cardiac tone to be essentially involved in the genesis of lethal ventricular arrhythmias in structurally compromised hearts. From these data, however, it cannot be told whether reduced HRV is an epiphenomenon just indicating sympathovagal imbalance or whether HRV reduction per se is an arrhythmogenic mechanism, or both.

References

1. D.H. Singer, G.J. Martin, N. Magid et al., *Am J Cardiol* **60** (1987) S46
2. D.J. Ewing, J.M.M. Neilson, P. Travis, *Br Heart J* **52** (1984) 396
3. G.J. Martin, N.M. Magid, G. Myers, et al., *Am J Cardiol* **86** (1987) 60
4. P. Coumel, *New Trends Arrhythm* **5** (1989) 181
5. H.-D. Esperer, F.O. Mahmoud, J.von der Emde, *New Trends Arrhyth* **7** (1991) 23

ELECTROPHYSIOLOGIC EFFECTS OF SOMATOSTATIN IN MAN

ROMAN BUBIŃSKI, KONSTANTY MARKIEWICZ, WŁODZIMIERZ KUŚ

Department of Cardiology, Military Medical Academy, 113 Żeromskiego Str., 90-549 Łódź, Poland

ABSTRACT

The peptide Somatostatin (S) is present in humman cardiac tissue. We examined the electrophysiologic effects of intravenous S (8.5 ug/min) in 12 patients undergoing electrophysiologic testing.

S prolonged the mean sinus cycle length by 13%, intraatrial, sinuatrial and AV nodal conduction time by 9, 15 and 10%, respectively. Effective refractory periods of atrium , AV node and right ventricle were prolonged by 7, 8 and 7%, respectively during S infusion (all p values less than 0.01). Antegrade AV nodal Wenckebach cycle length, as well as retrograde, increased significantly (by 9 and 10%, respectively).

In 6 of 12 cases S made sustained supraventricular tachycardia (SVT) either no longer inducible or at least nonsustained. The mean cycle length of induced SVT increased by 13%.

In conclusion, S exerts marked depressive electrophysiologic effects on human heart and my be effective in the termination of SVT.

1. Introduction

Somatostatin (S), a naturally occurring peptide, was first discovered more than 20 years ago. This peptide was later found in many other tissues, including human cardiac tissue[1]. The high concentration of S were found in the sinus and AV nodes[2].

S exerts various effects on cardiovascular system. They have been described bradycardia and transient increase of systemic arterial pressure in healthy human volunteers[3], negative inotropic and chronotropic effects in experimental animals[4,5], depressive effect on the AV junction[6].

2. Purpose of the study

The purpose of the present study was a complete estimation of the effect of S on the cardiac conduction system in man during antegrade and retrograde conduction.

3. Characteristics of patients

The studied population consisted of 12 patients (pts): 5 women and 7 men, mean age 43 yrs. (range, 16 to 67). They underwent invasive electrophysiologic testing because of sudden unexplained heart palpitations. Almost all the pts had organic heart disease: 5 coronary arterial disease, 4 accessory AV pathway (2 WPW syndrome, 2 concealed AV pathway), 2 mitral valve prolapse. Only 1 pt had no organic heart disease.

All the pts were informed about the protocol of the study and all gave their written consent. The protocol was approved by the Ethics Committee of the Hospital of Military Medical Academy in Łódź.

4. Electrophysiologic testing

Electrophysiologic tests were performed in the fasting. All antiarrhythmic medications were discontinued at least 72 hours before the procedure. Under local anesthesia three multipolar elctrode catheters (USCI, Billerica, USA) were introduced percutaneously into the right and left femoral veins. Under fluoroscopic guidance the catheters were positioned high in the right atrium, in the region of His bundle, and in the ventricular apex.

The stimulation protocol used has been described in detail previously[7]. Briefly, it consisted of: incremental atrial and ventricular pacing to the paced cycle length that induced AV or ventriculoatrial (VA) Mobitz type second block, testings to determine refractory periods, programmed (using single and double exstrastimuli) atrial and ventricular stimulation for tachyarrhythmia induction, and finally burst type stimulation of the right atrium. The protocol required nearly 30 min to complete.

The following electrophysiologic variables were assessed: sinus cycle length (SCL), intraatrial (PA), intranodal (AH), His-Purkinje system (HV), and the whole AV (PV) conduction times, duration of His bundle potential (H), sinuatrial conduction time (SACT), longest sinus node recovery time ($SNRT_{max}$), corresponding heart rate-corrected sinus node recovery time ($SNRT_c$), atrial (A), AV nodal (AVN), and ventricular (V) effective refractory periods (ERP), retrograde AVN ERP (R AVN ERP), antegrade Wenckebach (W CL) and Mobitz type II cycle length (M II CL), retrograde AVN Wenckebach (RW, CL), and Mobitz type II cycle length (RM II CL), VA conduction time (VACT), SVT cycle length (SVT CL). Also the duration of QRS complex (QRS), QT interval (QT) were measured from the surface electrocardiogram in II lead. Corrected QT intrerval (QTc) was calculated accor ding to the method of Bazett.

5. Somatostatin administration

After measuring all electrophysiologic variables in the control state, each pt was given S (Stilamin, Serono, Germany) intravenously with a syringe pump at a dose of 8.5 ug/min, for about 30 min.

All the electrophysiologic measurements were repeated in the same order, beginning from the 6th min after the start of S injection.

Statistical analysis was performed using the t-test or when appropriate, the non-parametric Wilcoxon's test.

6. Results

The mean values for all electrophysiologic and electrocardiographic parameters tested are listed in the table below.

7. Discussion

S is used clinically not only as an investigative toll. Presently the drug is mainly used in the treatment of acromegaly and several forms of acute gastrointestinal disease[1,8]. However, a list of clinical indications for S and its long-acting analogue octreotide is still extending[9]. Experimental and clinical studies suggest that S acts on the cardiovascular system as a negative inotropic agent, which can reduce cardiac output, slow the heart rate, and restore sinus rhythm in pts with paroxysmal supraventricular and junctional tachycardia[3,4,5,6]. The way by which S inhibits cardiac functon is unclear. Recent reports suggest that S may exert its cardiac action via a cholinergic pathway[6].

Our data confirm the earlier observations of depressive effect of S on the AV junction. We assert that this effect is refered to the antegrade, as well as retrograde conduction. The most pronounced depressive effect we observed in the sinus and AVN function. In the half of our cases S made sustained SVT either no longer inducible or at least nonsustained. Thus, the electrophysiological properties of S allow to affirm that it may be effective in the termination of paroxysmal reentry SVT involving the sinus and AV nodes. Further studies are required to determine an appropriate antiarrhythmic dose of S.

Table
Electrophysiologic and electrocardiographic effects of intravenous Somatostatin. All values are expressed in milliseconds as mean ± SD. For explanation of the abbreviations used see the above text.

Parameter	Control	Somatostatin	p
SCL	817.2±124.9	924.3±169.2	<0.01
PA	31.3± 4.8	34.2± 5.1	<0.01
AH	91.3± 22.1	100.7± 21.4	<0.01
H	18.2± 5.6	19.1± 4.9	>0.05
HV	43.4± 13.3	45.5± 14.2	>0.05
PV	158.8± 29.7	173.2± 34.9	<0.01
SACT	132.5± 35.2	151.7± 40.3	<0.01
SNRTmax	986.2±184.0	1105.0±237.6	<0.01
SNRTc	241.2±134.0	266.7±162.3	>0.05
A ERP	207.1± 51.1	222.5± 53.8	<0.01
AVN ERP	273.3± 59.2	294.4± 63.1	<0.01
V ERP	250.8± 37.0	269.6± 36.1	<0.01
R AVN ERP	270.8± 53.0	287.5± 52.1	<0.01
W CL	392.2± 82.1	426.8± 90.3	<0.01
M II CL	340.3± 46.0	382.7± 58.3	<0.01
RW CL	498.1±164.0	550.6±175.4	<0.01
RM II CL	404.8±110.3	454.7±128.3	<0.01
VACT	238.9± 63.4	262.8± 89.3	>0.05
SVT CL	347.8± 31.4	391.9± 28.9	<0.01
QRS	82.7± 19.0	85.0± 18.8	<0.05
QT	360.0± 28.6	377.9± 30.7	<0.01
QTc	399.7± 19.3	395.5± 24.0	>0.05

8. References

1. R.Hall, M.D.Page, C.Dieguez, M.F.Scanlon, *Hormone Res.* **29** (1988) 50.
2. S.M.Day, J.Gu, J.M.Polak, S.R.Bloom, *Br.Heart J.* **53** (1985) 153.
3. S.M.Chernish, R.E.Miller, B.D.Rosenak, R.L.Brunelle, *Gastroenterology* **76** (1979) 1113.
4. R.Quirion, D.Regioli, F.Rioux, S.St-Pierre, *Br. J. Pharmacol.* **66** (1979) 251.
5. F.Rioux, R.Kerouac, S.St-Pierre, *Neuropeptides* **1** (1981) 319.
6. S.C.Webb, D.M.Krikler, W.G.Hendry, T.E.Adrian, S.R. Bloom, *Br. Heart J.* **56** (1986) 236.
7. R.Bubiński, K.Markiewicz, M.Cholewa, L.Górski, Z.Gawor, W.Kuś, *Int. J. Cardiol.* **24** (1989) 327.
8. D.H.Van Thiel, V.J.Dindzans, R.R.Schade, *Drugs of Today* **24** (1988) 743.
9. R.J.Comi, *Cleveland Clinic J. Med.* **57** (1990) 37.

IS HOLTER MONITORING USEFUL TO EVALUATE THE EFFICIENCY OF FLECAINIDE ADMINISTERED TO PATIENTS AFFECTED BY ATRIAL ECTOPIC TACHICARDIA

Stefano Tognarini,MD
Division of Cardiology
Laboratory of Electrophysiology
USL 25, Padiglione Villa Marina
Via Forlanini, 57025 -Piombino- Italy
Enrico Pardini,MD
Division of Cardiology,Laboratory of Electrophysiology
USL 25,Padiglione Villa Marina,Via Forlanini

ABSTRACT

Ten patients,with persistent Atrial Ectopic Tachycardia,were given Flecainide i.v.,that caused the arrhythmia termination; Dynamic Ecg, recorded every month during a period of 25 months,only two patients developed symptomatic arrhythmias relapse in agreement symptoms.

The aim of this study is tu evaluate the efficay of Flecainide acetate by Dinamic Ecg,in patients with ectopic atrial tachycardia.Besides the clinical examination,the ECG monitorization in radio-telemtry,the chest x-ray,the echocardiographic examination,the tyroid tests and other routine hematochemical tests,we carried out an endocavitary electrophysiologic study,followed by pharmacological test with flecainide (during electrophysiologic study). We studied ten patients (pts),6 male and 4 famale,whose average age was 64 years. They had a surface ecg pattern or dynamic ecg recording of persistent atrial ectopic tachycardia (AET),in agreement many Authors (1-3).Two pts were affected by hypertension and two pts were affected by mitral valve prolapse laflet.All pts were given Flecainide i.v.(1.5 mg/Kg in 15')that caused the arrhythmia termination followed by stable sinus rythm (SR). The pts were treated with flecainide orally (200 mg.

twice a day) from then on.
We evaluated the efficiency of this drug analyzing the dynamic ecg-recorded every month-and reading the diary bookwritten by each pts. The follow up lasted an average period of 25 months during which two pts only developed symptomatic arrhythmia relapse.Other pts were symptomatic for palpitations (diary book)but they didn't have evidence of AET at the holter recording. The ecg recorded with holter method was readen in two ways for each patient:1)watching the automatic report 2)observing the compacted printout of the whole dynamic ecg recorded (about 24 hours).

CONCLUSIONS

We have verified that the automatic report was never wrong in misdiagnostic AET.On the other way many false positive AET were recognised with automatic report.They were generally due to myopotentials.

REFERENCES

1. Goldreyer BN,Gallagher JJ,Damato AN:The electrophysiologic demonstration of atrial ectopic tachycardia in man.Am.Heart J. 1973;85:205
2. Coumel PH:Tachicardie sopraventricolari. In Krikler DM,Goodwin JF,eds. Cardiac arrhythmias. The modern electrophysiological approach.London: WB Saunders Co,1976:134-165.
3. Salerno JA,Chimienti M,Vigano' M,Bobba P: Focal supraventricular tachycardia-clinical, electrophysiological and therapeutic aspects. In:Masoni A,Alboni P eds. Cardiac Electrophysiology today. London and New York:Academic Press.1982; 203-223.

STRATEGY OF TREATMENT OF EXTRASYSTOLES IN OUTPATIENTS.

YA.S.VASILTZEV
Clinical Department, Institute of Cardiology, Tomsk, USSR.

YU.I.ZYABLOV
Scientific-consultational Department, Institute of Cardiology, Tomsk, USSR.

N.D.PLOTNIKOVA
Scientific-consultational Department, Institute of Cardiology, Tomsk, USSR.

SUMMARY.

There were two groups of patients investigated. The first group consisted of 31 patients with ischemic heart disease, the second - patients with idiopathic extrasystoles. Every patient underwent Holter monitoring of ECG, acute pharmacological test with ethacizin (at once 100 mg per os), bicycle ergometer test (submaximal load) before and after drug taking. The frequency of ventricular extrasystoles was 315,6 per hour in the first group of patients, and 210,4 per hour - in the second one. Antiarrhythmic effect of the drug was considered positive in cases of 75 and more per cent decrease of the whole extrasystolic number, absence of group and polytopous ventricular extrasystoles, runs of ventricular tachycardia, also after exercise test. Ethacizin effectivity was on the average in 66,6% cases, the arrhythmogenic effect of the drug was noticed in 5,5% cases. Drug effectivity increased to 86% in cases of spontaneous extrasystolic variability about 50%, arrthythmogenic effect was absent. 100 and more per cent increase of spontaneous extrasystolic frequency variation was accompanied with drug effect decrease to 53% and increase of cases of arrhythmogenic effect (12.5%). Thus, there existed a correlation between extrasystolic variability frequency and antiarrhythmic drug effect.

Present data concerning extrasystolic incidence among adults are not quite complete [1, 2, 3, 4]. Treatment of extrasystoles in outpatients presents frequently an empirical selection of antiarrhythmic drug and its dose without considering extrasystolic features, drug effect duration in an individual patient and possible complications. The aim of our study was to evaluate these problems.

MATERIALS AND METHODS.

Clinic-epidemiological study of extrasystolic incidence was carried out within the limits of medical registration of patients with cardiac rhythm and conduction disorder, fulfilled in Tomsk in 1987-1988. Relatively small town extension and its population (500,000 people) provided a reliability of the study. After analyzing case histories of medical institutions, data concerning outpatients with cardiac rhythm disorder and those with extrasystoles documented by electrocardiographic (ECG) record were included into specially designed registration cards.So we got an automatic data bank of patients with arrhythmias. Using the method of occasional numbers a representative group of patients with ventricular extrasystoles was formed, it contained every tenth patient.The group consisted of 143 patients (75 men and 68 women, age range 16-84). To study spontaneous extrasystolic variability rate and to maintain antiarrhythmic therapy we divided two groups of patients; the first group consisted of 71 patients with ischemic heart disease and the second - of 29 patients with idiopathic extrasystoles. Spontaneous variability rate was correlated with the mean number of circadian extrasystoles evaluated after double monitoring and presented in per cents. 68 patients under went graded submaximal bicycle ergometer test. Antiarrhythmic drug selection was done out of hospital by using acute pharmacological test. In this study we used ethacizin (a single dose 100 mg per os) with simultaneous cardiac monitor setting for the period of 24 hours. The criterion of effective drug use was considered 75 and more per cent decrease of ventricular extrasystoles and complete absence of high grade extrasystoles and runs of ventricular tachycardia. The arrhythmogenic effect was diagnosed in cases of more than twice increase of extrasystolic number and high grade extrasystoles. In cases of positive test results drug taking continued (using individual effective dose) for during 30 days with 24-hours Holter monitoring of ECG on the 7th and 30th day after its termination.

RESULTS AND DISCUSSION.

In 1988 medical census revealed 3,717 patients with various cardiac rhythm disorders, including 2,046 patients with extrasystoles (57,1% from the whole number of patients registered during this census). During two years extrasystolic incidence was on the ave rage 6,38 per 1,000 people and remained approximately similar between men and women, but in patients over 60 years it was significantly higher than in patients under 60 yr. Spontaneous extrasystolic variability rate varied from

9 to 170% in both groups. We confirmed a described in literature fact of inverse correlation between extrasystolic variability rate and its frequency, and also a trend of decrease of nocturnal extrasystolic number versus a diurnal one in both groups [5, 6]. On the whole, ethacizin effectivity during acute pharmacological test was 73,7% in patients with idiopathic extrasystoles, and 60,1% - in patients with ischemic heart disease. We revealed a correlation between a spontaneous extrasystolic variability rate and ethacizin effect in acute pharmacological test, which hadn'd been previously reported in literature. As a rule, low drug effectivity and its high arrhythmogenic effect were seen in cases of high (more 50%) spontaneous extrasystolic variability, and, on the contrary, high ethacizin effectivity (97,7%) and complete absence of arrhythmogenic effect were noticed in cases of extrasystolic changeability less 30%. There existed a correlation between the effect in acute pharmacological test and longterm treatment, especially in cases of idiopathic extrasystoles. Thus, extrasystoles restored with previous frequency, in cases of mean extrasystolic frequency about 30 per hour and spontaneous variability rate more 50% on the 10th day after course termination, that demanded further continuation of drug taking. In patients with frequent extrasystoles from 30 to 100 per hour and spontaneous variability rate of about 30% the effect was present during more than 30 days. Spontaneous variability rate appeared to influence on drug pecularities and must be considered in antiarrhythmic therapy management. The maintenance of antiarrhythmic therapy is incorrect in cases of rare extrasystoles with great circadian spontaneous variations of its frequency, because it doesn't result in desired outcome, but frequently causes clinical deterioration.

REFERENCES.

1. Nicolic S., Bishop R.Z., Singh I.B., Circulation.V1 (1982) p.175.
2. Anderson I.Z., Austr.N.Z.I.Med.V3 (1986) p.409-412.
3. Orth-Somer K., Hogsted C., Brit.Heart J.V3 (1986) p.98-105.
4. Meinertz T., Hofman T., Hasper W., Amer.J.Cardiol.V4 (1984) p.275-279.
5. Rosenberg M.I., Uretz E., Denes P., Amer.Heart J.V4 (1983) p.275-290.
6. Янушкевичус З., Забела П., Каволюнене А., Тезисы доклада 2-го с'езда кардиологов Литвы, Каунас.(1984) с.24-26.

PART VII
Late Potentials

LATE POTENTIALS RECORDING: IS IT TIME TO STANDARDIZE?

ANDRE VARENNE
Laboratoire de Cardiologie (CRECEC), CHU Pasteur
06031 Nice, France

HERVE RIX, BARBARA OFICJALSKA
Laboratoire Signaux et Systèmes,
Université de Nice-Sophia Antipolis, 06000 Nice, France

ABSTRACT

Standardization of any new measurement method requires an adequate knowledge of the phenomenon to be measured. So, is it time to standardize late potentials (LP) recording? And what do we know today about them? In fact, LP are only the easiest detectable part of the delayed inhomogeneous depolarisations (DID), low voltage fragmented signals, arising in areas of an abnormal myocardium. DID may modify the QRS signal not only beyond its normal end (LP), but also inside it, specially in bundle branch blocks (BBB), and in its begining. We know little on DID nature and their beat-to-beat changes. So, it is difficult to consider DID - even in their easiest detectable component (LP) - as a good subject for standardized recording. Despite that, there is a risk for a de facto standardization due to the devices marketed, most of them using the vector magnitude method (VMM). If VMM has given important results, it proposes arbitrary criteria of LP presence, excludes patients with BBB and may lose information. So VMM cannot be considered as the ideal one. Other signal processing methods (time-frequency analysis, wavelets, beat-to-beat recording) are under investigation. In conclusion, we think that our knowledge of the phenomena to be recorded (DID) and the recording systems are still too far from their achievement to be standardized.

Is it time to standardize late potentials recording? When we submitted this abstract, we thought this could lead to an interesting discussion. But a few days later we received the April issue of JACC[1] in which standardization was stated and approved by the European Society of Cardiology, the American Heart Association and the American College of Cardiology after consultation of many international experts. Thereby our communication could be taken either as an obsolete or a provocative one, or both...

So we were pleasantly surprised with the acceptance of this paper, which evidently implies that the debate on the subject is still wide open. Therefore, we will try to answer two questions: what is the nature of late potentials? Do we have any method ready to use for standardization?

1. Nature of late potentials.

In 1973, Boineau and Cox[2] demonstrated that electrograms from ischemic regions of the canine heart were delayed and fractionated and then could be a source of reentrant premature ventricular contractions. In 1978, these delayed inhomogeneous depolarisations (DID) were recorded the first time on man, by Fontaine et al[3] and Uther et al[4], using body surface electrodes and signal averaging. These DID, appearing as low level (microvolts) post-QRS signals were called late potentials (LP). In fact, LP are the easiest detectable part of DID, which may be also hidden inside QRS - particularly in case of bundle branch blocks (BBB), or - according to the ischemic sites - they may fragment the begining of QRS (early delayed potentials)[5,6]. In 1978, Berbari et al[7] demonstrated, using cardiac pacing, that this fragmented electrical activity was of variable duration in relation with the cardiac rate. So, the only reliable method to record such dynamic changes, which can be critical to ventricular arrhythmias, should be the beat-to-beat recording. But this technique, despite some interesting experimental results, has not entered clinical use. Moreover, time-domain analysis is not sufficient to study non-stationary transient signals as DID. The frequency-domain - and specially time-frequency analysis - provides useful informations. In conclusion, we have to admit that our knowledge of DID nature is yet to much incomplete to be the object of a standardized recording method.

2. Late potentials recording.

In fact, LP are today recorded using the sequential averaging method - which shows only their statistical mean value for a variable number of averaged beats and deletes their beat-to-beat changes. Most of LP recorders based on this technique, use the *vector magnitude method (VMM)*, proposed by Simson[8].

But these available marketed systems differ so considerably from one another that results are not comparable and make multicentric studies not homogeneous. For instance, a comparative analysis of 4 commercial devices made by Henkin[9] in 1990, has demonstrated difference in 19% in LP detection and in 23% in their duration. Obviously, a standardization is required. But the question rises: is the VMM the optimal standard?

ACC policy statement demonstrated that a consensus was obtained concerning electrodes, amplifiers and sampling. But, if the committee recognizes as a standard a bipolar XYZ orthogonal lead system, it admits that "additional studies are needed to determine the optimum lead system".

In fact, the main problem is cardiac signal processing. The analysis of the vector magnitude of the filtered QRS complex can undergo significant alterations in relation with the filtering[10] - 25 or 40Hz high pass cut off - while false positive results vary according to this bandwidth[11] as well in relation with the algorithms determining the noise level, the onset and the end of QRS[12]. Moreover, VMM is not appropriate in the presence of intraventricular conduction troubles. Thereby, paradoxically enough, by this method, infarcted patients with BBB - who have high risks of ventricular arrhythmias - can not be included into LP statistics.

In addition, drugs which notoriously increase QRS duration are able to affect the results. Moreover, VMM leads to a lack of information, as in figure 1., in which a Wolff-Parkinson-White delta wave cannot be identifiable after VMM. It was fortunate that Mrs Wolff, Parkinson and White were employing the biological neuronal computer of their own, which avoided the pitfalls of too sophisticated data processing methods!... In conclusion, we are questioning about this method which establishes chronological criteria of LP within limits of a millisecond precision[1], without duly giving inherent

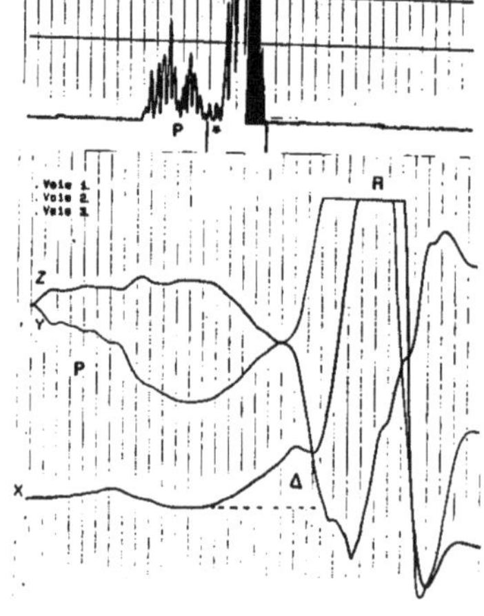

Fig.1. WPW recorded using: a) VMM (40-300Hz bidirectional filter), b) XYZ leads (80-300Hz). Delta-wave in b) is not identifiable in a).

standard deviations.* So we dare think that such definitions are a little bit arbitrary and consequently we agree with the commitee when he says "it is anticipated that further refinement and other approaches may improve the diagnostic power of the high resolution ECG".

One of these approaches is *visual identification* of LP. It was the original basis of the first experiments[2,7] and of the first clinical description[3,4,13]. Despite its subjective character, it permits easily to distinguish between a normal repolarisation and an abnormal one with LP (figure 2.)[14]. Using it, we could describe different features of LP (figure 3.) and identify them, even in presence of BBB[14]. So we think that it is important that recording devices provide a good edition of the XYZ leads - concurrently with the VMM.

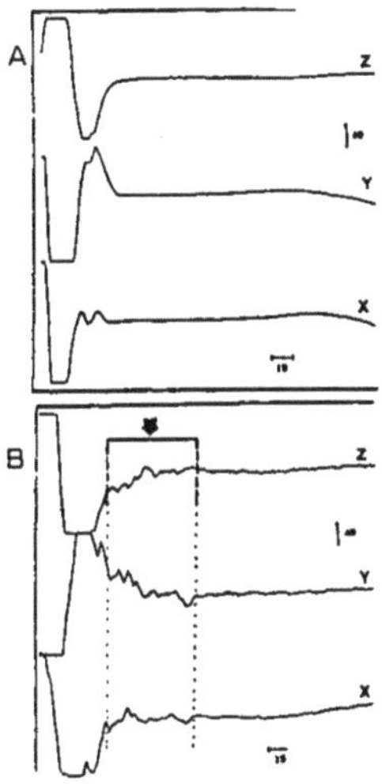

Fig.2. Visual identification of LP (80-300Hz):
a) normal, b) abnormal with LP of 60ms.

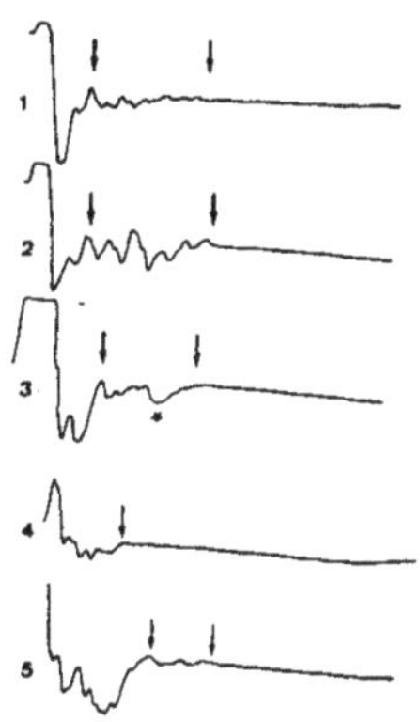

Fig.3. Different features[14] of LP in patients without (1,2,3) and with BBB (4-terminal potentials inside S, 5-terminal potentials inside S, followed by LP).

The frequency analysis methods open new promising perspectives. Fast Fourier Transform applied to the terminal part of QRS could be useful to detect LP even in BBB. Time-frequency analysis is proposed by means of appropriate transforms like short time Fourier analysis (spectrotemporal mapping[15]) or wavelet transform[16]. These approaches or others, as adaptative filtering, actually in investigation, could contribute - in addition will very low noise amplifiers, spatial averaging, and may be directional electrodes - to get the final step which is beat-to-beat recording.

In conclusion, we think that recommendations proposed by the committee concerning hardware are great of use and should be followed by companies producing high resolution ECG equipement. But we have to stress that our knowledge of the phenomena to be recorded - DID - and the present status of the recording methods are still too far from their achievement to be standardized.

In this new and fascinating field, we will agree with Cain et al[17], to say "the best is yet to come".

---

*"a LP exists[1] (using 40Hz high-pass bidirectional filtering) when 1) the filtered QRS complex is greater than 114 msec, 2) there is less than 20uV of signal in the last 40msec of the vector magnitude complex, and 3) the terminal vector magnitude complex remains below 40uV for more than 38msec."

References.

1. ACC Policy Statement, *JACC* **17** (1991) 999.
2. J.P.Boineau, J.L.Cox, *Circulation* **48** (1973) 702.
3. G.Fontaine, R.Frank, F.Gallais-Hamonno, F.Allali et al, *Arch.Mal.Coeur* **71** (1978) 854.
4. J.B.Uther, C.J.Dennett, A.Tan, *Excerpta Medica* (Amsterdam 1978) 80.
5. F.Walczak, R.Kepski, K.Peczalski, M.Stopczyk et al., *X World Congr Cardiol* (1986).
6. M.Itoh, *Circulaton* **80 suppl II** (1989) 482.
7. E.J.Berbari, B.J.Sherlag, R.R.Hope, R.Lazzara, *Am J Cardiol* 41 (1978) 697.
8. M.B.Simson, *Circulation* **64** (1981) 237.
9. R.Henkin, E.B.Caref, G.J.Kelen, N.El-Sherif, *J Electrocardiol* **22** suppl (1990) 19.
10. J.A.Gomes, S.L.Winters, D.Stewart, A.Targonski et al., *Am J Cardiol* **60** (1987) 1290.
11. S.N.Erne, H.D.Hahlbohm, J.Korsukiewitz, H.P.Lehman, *J Electrocardiol* **18** (1985) 315.
12. M.Oeff, E.R.von Leitner, R.Sthapit et al., *Eur Heart J* 7 (1986) 25.
13. G.Breithardt, R.Becker, L.Seipel, R.R.Abendroth et al., *Eur Heart J* 2 (1981) 1.
14. A.Varenne, P.Blanc, J.P.Camous, L.Grangier et al., *Arch Mal Coeur* **11** (1986) 1971.
15. P.Lander, D.E.Albert, E.J.Berbari, *J Electrocardiol* **22** (1990) 95.
16. O.Meste, H.Rix, R.Janet, P.Caminal, *ITBM* (to be published) (1991).
17. M.E Cain, H.D.Ambos, J.Markham, R.M.Arthur, *JACC* **14** (1989) 1741.

LATE-POTENTIALS STUDY IN POST-INFARCT CARDIAC REHABILITATION

R.MANIEWSKI, E.KANSKA, P.LEWANDOWSKI, M.STOPCZYK
Institute of Biocybernetics and Biomedical Engineering
ul.Trojdena 4, 02-109 Warszawa / Poland

and

H.MOJKOWSKA, S.RUDNICKI
Hospital for Cardiac Rehabilitation
ul.Gasiorowskiego 8, 05-510 Konstancin / Poland

ABSTRACT

Noninvasive detection of the late potentials in the high-resolution ECG records was proposed for selection the patients for various cardiac rehabilitation trainings. A total of 102 patients after myocardial infarction were examined. Analysis in the time domain and frequency domain indicates that post-infarct rehabilitation does not cause significant changes in the late potentials level observed in the ECG records.

1. Introduction

The value of ventricular late potentials (LP) in the detection of patients with a high risk of malignant ventricular arrhythmias is well documented.[1,2] Thus, the post-infarct cardiac rehabilitation of patients with detected LP calls for specially cautious treatment, as well as for very frequent control examinations during the rehabilitation period. The aim of the present studies was to evaluate the influence of cardiac rehabilitation on the level of LP in patients after myocardial infarction, and to single out the patients with a potential risk of ventricular arrhythmia at the beginning of rehabilitation.

2. Methods

Examinations of patients were carried out at the Hospital for Cardiac Rehabilitation in Konstancin near Warsaw. The measurement set-up and data processing system used in the present studies are shown in Fig.1. The

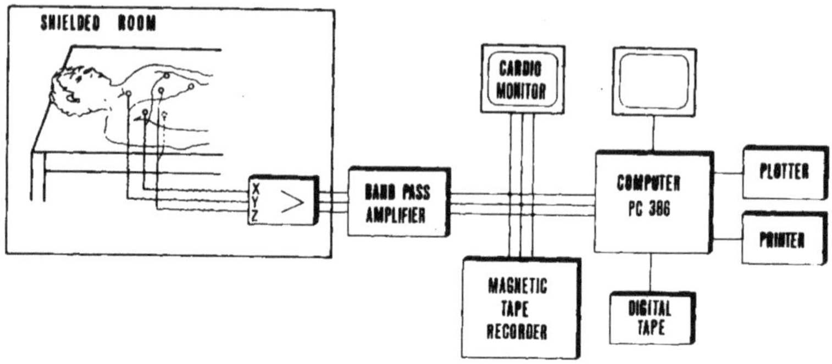

Fig. 1 The measurement set-up and data processing system.

high-resolution ECG recordings are taken in an electrically shielded room, using low-noise amplifiers with inherent noise level below 0.6 μV RMS. Silver-silver chloride electrodes are used; the patient's skin is carefully prepared to maximally increase the signal-to-noise ratio. Signals are measured in a bipolar X, Y, Z lead system with bandwidth from 0.05Hz to 500Hz, recognized as a standard procedure in LP measurements.[3] The measurement data are digitized with a 12 bit A/D converter and transferred to a IBM PC/386 computer, and/or stored in analog form on magnetic tape for off-line processing. Data processing comprises advanced averaging techniques with a cross-correlation procedure, artefact and excessive noise elimination, digital filtering and spectral analysis. Usually about 100 cardiac beats are averaged.

In the present studies, which respect to the time domain analysis we used a bidirectional four-pole Butterworth filter with a high-pass corner frequency of 40Hz. The late potentials were determined by the modified Simson criteria[3] from a filtered QRS vector $\sqrt{X^2+Y^2+Z^2}$, i.e. LP exists when: the filtered QRS vector is longer than 114 ms, the vector magnitude remains below 40μV for more than 38ms, and the vector magnitude in the last 40ms of the signal is below 25μV.

In the frequency domain the measurement data were expressed by the Fast Fourier Transform (FFT). The Kaiser-Bessell window was applied as windowing function to avoid edge discontinuities.[4] The data were padded with zeros to fill the 128-point array for FFT calculation. The spectra were calculated for an 80ms window in the terminal QRS and ST segments of individual X,Y and Z leads, and also for the QRS vector. The window onset was chosen as the time when the QRS vector decreases below 40 μV. The LP-s were recognized as the high-frequency content in the FFT spectrum.

3. Results and Discussion

A total of 102 patients after myocardial infarction were fully examined, i.e. their high-resolution ECG were measured at least twice during the rehabilitation period. At first, the patients were measured immediately after hospitalization (usually ca. 3-4 weeks after infarction), and for the second time - just before completion of 4-week rehabilitation. The basic rehabilitation procedure consists of physical exercise, (e.g. ergometer training), diet and pharmacological treatment.

Late ventricular potentials were found in about 20% of patients. Patients who did not show LP before rehabilitation did not display them after rehabilitation, as well. No disappearance of LP during rehabilitation was observed; however, in a few patients, (as shown in Fig.2 for one case), tendency for LP disappearance was noticed at the 2-nd examination.

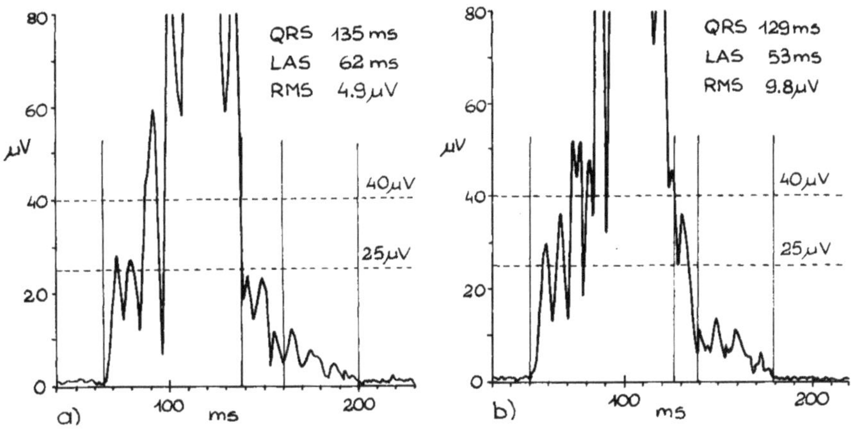

Fig.2. Results of the ECG time analysis, obtained for a post-infarct patient (AS19) at the beginning of rehabilitation (a) and upon completion of the rehabilitation period (b).

Also frequency domain analysis may supply helpful information about the LP behaviour. Fig.3 examplifies the FFT spectra obtained for the same patient as presented in Fig.2 for time domain. There is no evident difference in the high-frequency content in the FFT spectra between the measurements performed at the beginning and at the end of rehabilitation. Slight decrease of the high-frequency content in the spectrum obtained from results of the 2-nd examination as visible only for the QRS vector (Fig.3,b).

Evaluation of the terminal QRS amplitude level by the Simson method in cases without detected evident LP-s is, however, controversial. For improvement of this evaluation, some modified criteria based on spectrotemporal analysis[5] with different filter and on a various data window have to be used.

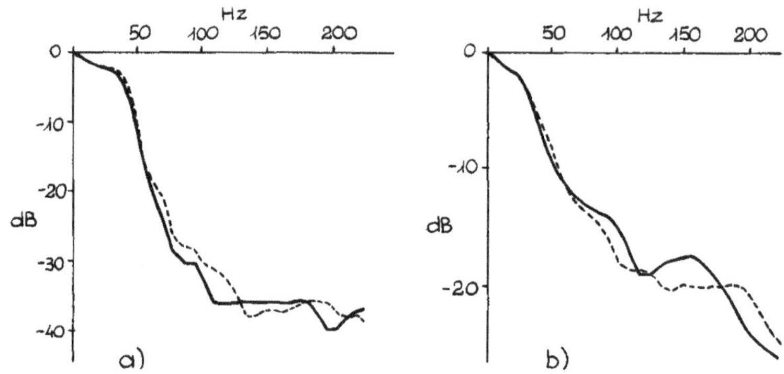

Fig.3. The frequency spectra obtained by the fast Fourier transform (FFT) for post-infarct patient (AS19) at the beginning of rehabilitation (solid line) and at the end of rehabilitation (dashed line). The spectra are presented for individual ECG lead Y (a) and for the QRS vector (b).

4. Conclusion

The present results indicate that post-infarct cardiac rehabilitation training does not cause the occurrence of late potentials in the ECG records; thus, it does not enhance the risk of ventricular arrhythmias. Evaluation of the significance of the observed changes in the amplitude level of late potentials during the rehabilitation period calls for further studies on a greater number of patients, using modified criteria for the time domain and frequency domain.

5. References

1. M.B. Simson, *Circulation,* **64**, 1981, pp 235-242.
2. M.E. Cain, D. Ambados, F.X. Witkowski, B.E. Sobel, *Circulation,* **69**, 1984, pp 711-720.
3. *11ml7*G. Breithardt, M.E. Cain, N. El-Sherif, N.C. Flowers, V. Hombach, M. Janse, M.B. Simson, G. Steinbeck, *Circulation,* **84**, 1991, pp 1481-1488.
4. M. Kohutnicki, T. Palko, R. Maniewski, *in this Volume.*
5. P. Lander, D.E. Albert, E.J. Berbari, *J. Electrocardiology,* **23**, 1990, pp. 95-108.

SPECTRAL ANALYSIS OF LATE POTENTIALS USING PARAMETRIC ESTIMATION

MACIEJ KOHUTNICKI, TADEUSZ PAŁKO
Institute of Precision and Biomedical Engineering, Warsaw University of Technology, Chodkiewicza 8 Warsaw, 02-525 / Poland

and

ROMAN MANIEWSKI
Institute of Biocybernetic and Biomedical Engineering, Trojdena 4 Warsaw, 02-109 / Poland

ABSTRACT

An estimation of power spectral density based on parametric models such as autoregression and minimum variance were proposed for non-invasive detection of late potentials from high-resolution ECG recordings. New approach was compared with fast Fourier transform method by using specially prepared test signals and ECG data. Good detectability of late potentials by means of the autoregression method, especially for short data segments placed at the beginning of the S-T interval, was observed.

1. Introduction

Detection of late potentials (LP) is an important tool for estimation of increased risk of sudden cardiac death. Various methods of analyses in the time domain and in the frequency domain have been applied for that purpose. A classical time domain technique has been proposed by Simson[1] and is still widely used in practice. A frequency domain approach based on fast Fourier transform (FFT), introduced by Cain, is considered to be more efficient.[2,3] An estimation of the Power Spectral Density (PSD) using this procedure has, however, two main limitation:[4]

- -limited frequency resolution which is the reciprocal of time interval over which the sampled data are available
- -'leakage' in the spectral domain caused by implication of windowing of the data.

In order to reduce the shortcoming of classical FFT method one can apply various alternative spectral estimation procedures.[4] In the present studies we applied spectral estimation based on Autoregressive (AR) and Minimum Variance

(MV) models, and compared both these procedures with the conventional FFT method.

2. Methods

The spectral density obtained by the FFT method was calculated directly as a squared modulus of Fourier transform.

$$PSD(f) = |X(f)|^2 \qquad (1)$$

To avoid leakage in the spectrum, the Kaiser-Bessell window was applied as a windowing function of the data sequence. The zero padding technique was used for obtaining 128 length data sequence, for which the Fourier transform was calculated.

The PSD obtained using the AR model was calculated as power spectrum of a linear filter driven by white noise.

$$PSD(f) = \frac{s^2\,\Delta t}{\left| 1 + \sum_{k=1}^{p} a_k \exp(-j2\pi k f \Delta t) \right|^2} \qquad (2)$$

Δt - sampling period f - frequency

n - length of data sequence

In Eq.2 the parameters a_k of the AR model have to be estimated. In this model the output sequence x_k is a linear regression on itself and can be expressed as in Eq 3.

$$x_n = -\sum_{k=1}^{p} a_k x_{n-k} + e \qquad (3)$$

e - driving signal (white noise)

s^2 - total squared error of the model

The parameters a_k and total squared error s^2 of the AR model were estimated using the Yule-Walker algorithm, which provides a better resolution then FFT method[4]. The order p of the AR model was calculated using the Final Prediction Error criterion proposed by Akaike[4].

The PSD obtained by means of the MV model was calculated using the formula relating PSD found by the MV model to PSD given by the AR model:

$$\frac{1}{PSD_{MV}(f)} = \sum_{k=0}^{p} \frac{1}{PSD_{AR}(k,f)} \qquad (4)$$

Using the specially prepared test signals all these methods were verified from the standpoint of detections of the late potentials (LP) which were simulated by a few sine wave of frequency 100 Hz and amplitude 10μV. Two test signals were involved:

-first signal, consisted of simulated LP added to triangle

which was supposed to be a model of QRS complex,
-second signal, consisted of simulated LP added to averaged ECG signal of healthy subject.

The PSD of few data segments of length 20, 40 and 60 ms placed at the end of QRS complex (including and not including the RS slope) were estimated.

Finally, all these methods of PSD estimation were verified with a real high-resolution ECG signal measured from a patient during post-infarct cardiac rehabilitation.[5] The averaged terminal XYZ signal and the QRS vector obtained by Simson procedure were analysed. The PSD was estimated for data segment occurring immediately after the point where the magnitude of the QRS vector decreased to less then 25μV. The data segments with the length of 40 and 80 ms were usually analysed.

3. Results

The results of PSD estimation performed at simulated testing signals has shown good detectability of LP by means of AR method especially for short data segment. This method failed when data segment was placed at a steep slope.

The examples of the PSDs estimations obtained by analysis of real high-resolution ECG are shown at Fig.1 and Fig. 2.

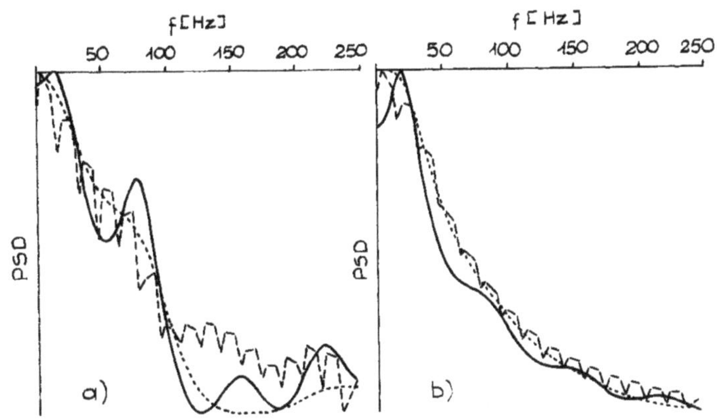

Fig.1 The relative PSDs of the averaged ECG lead Y obtained from two patients: patient with previously detected LP (Fig. 1a) and patient without LP (Fig. 1b). The analised data segment in both cases is 40 ms.

Fig.1 shows the PSDs obtained by all methods for a patients with previously detected LP (using the Simson criteria) and for another patient without LP. The presence of a frequency about 100 Hz in the signal from patient with LP is very well detectable by the AR method and is also evident in the curve of the MV method. The frequency spectrum obtained by FFT procedure is "discontinues" because of very short data segments used and thus it is very difficult to detect the LP frequency by this method.

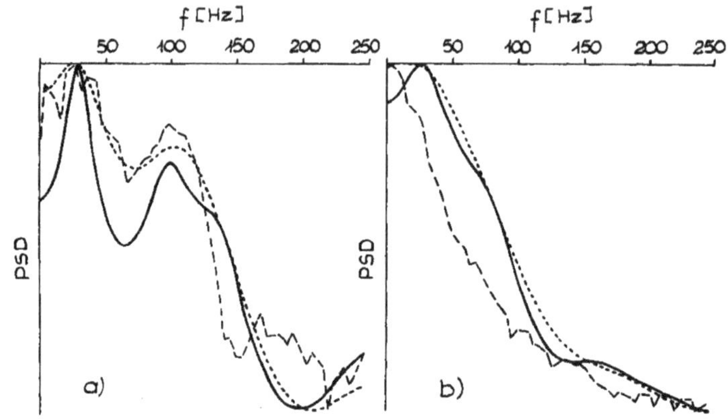

Fig.2 The relative PSDs of the QRS vector obtained according to Simson procedure from the same two patients as in Fig.1. The duration of the data segment was 40 ms.

Fig.2 shows PSDs found for the same patients as in Fig.1 but the spectra were estimated for the QRS vector. Also in this case the frequencies of LP were well detectable by the AR method; both remaining methods gave reasonable results as well. It was also found that the AR method was less suitable when the data segment overlapped the RS slope.

4. Conclusion

According to the present results, spectral estimation of high-resolution ECG can be a useful tool for LP detection. In particular the method based on autoregression model is in some cases very suitable, because it allows for analysing very short data segments. For more extensive conclusions, further studies of greater number of subjects are required.

5. References

1. M.B. Simson, *Circulation* **64** 1981 pp 235-242.
2. M.E. Cain, D. Ambados, F.X. Witkowski, B.E. Sobel, *Circulation* **69** 1984 pp 711-720.
3. R. Haberl, G. Jilge, R. Pulter, G. Steinbeck, *Journal of American College of Cardiology* **12** No 1 1988 pp 150-158.
4. S.M. Kay, S.L. Marple,JR, *Proc. IEEE* **69** No. 11 1981 pp 1380-1419.
5. R. Maniewski, P. Lewandowski, A. Mojkowska, S Rudnicki, M. Stopczyk, *In this Proseedings.*

LATE POTENTIALS DIAGNOSED BY FFT FREQUENCY ANALYSIS IN CHAGAS PATIENTS WITH AND WITHOUT BUNDLE BRANCH BLOCK - COMPARISON OF DIFFERENT AREA RATIOS

Wojciech Zareba*, **Josep Guindo, Cristian Madoery, Xavier Vinolas, Antonio Bayes de Luna**

Dept. of Cardiology, University of Barcelona,
Hosp. Sant Pau, Sant Antoni M. Claret 167,
08-025 Barcelona, Spain.

*Dept. of Cardiology, Medical Academy of Lodz
Sterlinga 1/3, 91-425 Lodz, Poland.

Abstract

The diagnosis of late potentials in signal-averaged ECG by the frequency domain method in relation to ventricular arrhythmias detected on Holter monitoring were studied in 84 patients with Chagas disease. The comparison of frequency analysis results between patients with and without bundle branch block were performed. Frequency analysis revealed the presence of late potentials in 34 patients (40%). In the patients with late potentials and with bundle branch block, higher contents of high-frequency components were observed between 50-150 Hz than in patients with late potentials but without bundle branch block. Ventricular arrhythmias were observed in 82% with late potentials versus 29% without late potentials, and complex arrhythmias in 56% vs 19%, respectively. Thus, frequency analysis of signal-averaged ECG may be useful to predict which patients with Chagas disease are prone to ventricular arrhythmias.

Epidemiological data from WHO estimates, that about 5 million people in South America have Chagas disease with cardiac involvement, with a high incidence of sudden cardiac death in these patients [1,2]. The diagnosis of late potentials in signal-averaged ECG (SA-ECG) can be a marker to predict patients prone to life-threatening ventricular arrhythmias [3]. Time-domain method of signal-averaged ECG (SA-ECG) analysis does not let us assess late potentials in ECG with bundle branch block, common findings in patients with Chagas disease [2,3]. Frequency domain method has been proposed as being independent on conduction disturbances [4].

The aims of our study were: 1) the analysis of late potentials in SA-ECG by the frequency domain method to predict ventricular arrhythmia development in patients with Chagas disease; 2) the comparison of different area ratios in patients with and without bundle branch blocks.

Material and Methods

We studied 84 patients (age: 48 + 16 years) with Chagas disease confirmed by seropositive tests. The patients were divided into: Gr.A consisting of 61 patients (72%) without conduction disturbances, gr.B consisting of 23 patients (28%) with bundle branch blocks. 16 healthy subjects were assessed as controls (gr.C). SA-ECG were performed with ART 1200 Epx device with bipolar X, Y, Z leads. 231±32 (mean ± SD) QRS beats were averaged with noise level < 0.5 uV.

Fast Fourier transform (FFT) frequency analysis of the 120 ms segment beginning 20 ms before the end of QRS complex were made with multiplication by four-term Blackman-Harris window. Three different area ratios (AR) were analyzed for the assessment of various high-frequency components of the ECG signals: area ratio (AR) 1 = 20-50/0-20 Hz, AR 2 = 60-120/0-30 Hz, and AR 3 = 50-150/0-30 Hz. According to the comparison of results of FFT frequency analysis in patients with sustained ventricular tachycardia and in healthy subjects previously made in our laboratory, the following values of mean area ratio were considered as abnormal: AR 1 > 275; AR 2 > 80; and AR 3 > 140. Late potentials were defined according to the presence of an increased content of high-frequency components with an abnormal value in any of studied area ratios.

The comparison between the results of frequency analysis of SA-ECG (presence or absence of late potentials) and ambulatory ECG monitoring findings were made.

Statistical analysis: data are expressed as mean values ± SD. Results were analyzed using unpaired Student's t-test and Chi^2 test where appropriate.

Results

FFT frequency analysis revealed the presence of late potentials in 34 of 84 patients (40%). Late potentials appeared in 24 of 61 patients without bundle branch block, and in 10 of 23 patients with bundle branch block. Area ratio 1 was abnormal in 22 patients, area ratio 2 in 28 patients, and area ratio 3 in 28 patients. However, all three abnormal area ratios were observed in 17 of 84 patients (19%). The comparison of values of studied area ratio for each group of patients is shown in Table 1.

Table 1. Comparison of values of different area ratios (AR) in studied Chagas patients and normals

	AR1	AR2	AR3
Gr.A FFT(-)	202±80	39±18	68±33
Gr.A FFT(+)	338±94*	112±30*	194±48*
Gr.B FFT(-)	159±30	38±20	64±30
Gr.B FFT(+)	363±182*	178±62*	291±112*
Gr.C FFT(-)	166±30	27±8	44±12

AR1=20-50/0-50Hz; AR2=60-120/0-30Hz; AR3=50-150/0-30Hz
FFT(-) - patients and normals without late potentials
FFT(+) - patients with late potentials
FFT(+) vs FFT(-): * $p<0.001$

Normal values of studied area ratios did not differ between all study groups, independently from the presence or absence of bundle branch block. Abnormal area ratio 60-120/0-30 Hz values were significantly higher in patients with bundle branch block than in patients without conduction disturbances (178±62 vs 112±30 respectively, $p<0.01$). Abnormal area ratio 50-150/0-30 Hz for patients with bundle branch blocks also had higher mean value 291±112 vs 194±48 respectively ($p<0.05$). Values of area ratio 20-50/0-20 Hz for these groups did not differ significantly (363±182 vs 338±94 respectively, NS). These findings suggests the patients with late potentials and bundle branch block have higher contents of high-frequency components than patients with late potentials but without bundle branch block.

Ventricular arrhythmias were recorded on Holter monitoring in 36 of 75 patients (48%) with Chagas disease. Simple ventricular arrhythmias (Lown 1-2) were observed in 12 patients (16%). Complex ventricular arrhythmias (Lown 3-4) were detected in 24 patients (32%). Among this last group ventricular runs were recorded in 9 cases (12%). The patients with late potentials revealed significantly higher incidence of ventricular arrhythmias than the patients without late potentials: 82% vs 29% respectively ($p < 0.001$), complex ventricular arrhythmias: 56% vs 19% respectively ($p < 0.01$), and runs 22% vs 6% respectively ($p < 0.05$).

Clinical Implications

Our study demonstrates that 40% of patients with Chagas disease had an increased content of high-frequency components in SA-ECG.

Patients with late potentials and bundle branch block revealed more high-frequency components between 50-150Hz than patients with late potentials but without conduction disorders. However, patients without late potentials had similar contents of high-frequency components independent of the presence or absence of bundle branch block. Lindsay et al. [5] also compared mean values of abnormal area ratio 20-50/10-50Hz in patients with and without bundle branch block. They studied patients with ischemic heart disease or idiopathic cardiomyopathy and sustained ventricular tachycardia. Similar to our findings, there were no significant differences between patients with and without bundle branch blocks in high frequency contents between 20-50Hz, but they did not study other ranges of frequency.

The patients with late potentials detected by frequency-domain method had significantly more frequent ventricular arrhythmias in comparison to the patients without late potentials.

References

1. World Health Organization: *Sixth programme report. Chagas' disease. Special programme for research and training in tropical disease.* (Document TDR, PR-6,83.6-CHA,1983).

2. J.J.Puigbo, H.Acquatella, H.Giordano, C.Suarez, I.Combellas, I.Mendoza, in *Restrictive Cardiomyopathy and Arrhythmias*, ed. E.G.Olsen, M.Sekiguchi (University of Tokyo Press, Tokyo, 1990) p. 347.

3 G.Breithardt, M.E.Cain, N.El-Sherif, N.C.Flowers, V.Hombach, M.Janse, M.B.Simson, G.Steinbeck, *Circulation* **83** (1991) 1481.

4. M.E.Cain, H.D.Ambos, X.Witkowski, B.E.Sobel, *Circulation* **69** (1984) 711.

5. B.D.Lindsay, J.Markham, K.B.Schechtman, H.D.Ambos, M.E.Cain, *Circulation* **77** (1988) 122.

FFT FREQUENCY DOMAIN VERSUS TIME DOMAIN ANALYSIS OF SIGNAL-AVERAGED ECG IN POSTINFARCTION PATIENTS

Wojciech Zareba[*], Josep Guindo, Cristian Madoery, Xavier Vinolas, Antonio Bayes de Luna

Dept. of Cardiology, University of Barcelona,
Hosp. Sant Pau, Sant Antoni M. Claret 167,
08-025 Barcelona, Spain.

[*]Dept. of Cardiology, Medical Academy of Lodz
Sterlinga 1/3, 91-425 Lodz, Poland.

Abstract

Analysis of late potentials in signal-averaged ECG were performed in 126 patients after recent myocardial infarction. Late potentials were recorded by the time domain method in 28 of 110 patients without conduction disturbances and in 46 of 126 patients by the frequency domain method. Increased contents of high-frequency components appeared between different ranges of frequency: 20-200Hz in 34 cases; 20-50Hz in 7 patients; 50-150Hz in 3 patients; 50-200Hz in 2 cases. Clinical analysis revealed significantly higher number of premature ventricular beats recorded in 24-hour ambulatory ECG monitoring in patients with than without late potentials defined by frequency domain method.
Thus, ECG of postinfarction patients require assessment of various ranges of frequency. The presence of late potentials in frequency domain method is associated with a high frequency of ventricular premature beats on Holter monitoring.

Late potentials recorded by the time domain method in signal-averaged ECG in patients after myocardial infarction were confirmed as a predictor of sudden cardiac death [1]. Frequency domain method of signal averaged ECG analysis may be an alternative approach for the detection of patients prone to life-threatening ventricular arrhythmias [2]. The aim of our study was the analysis of late potentials in signal-averaged ECG (SA-ECG) by frequency domain method in 126 patients after recent myocardial infarction.
Special attention was paid to the assessment of different high-frequency components of electrocardiographic signals of postmyocardial patients.

Material and Methods

Study group consisted of 126 patients (97 men, 19 women) age 34 to 79 years (mean 60±10 years), with recent myocardial infarction diagnosed according to conventional criteria. Non-Q wave myocardial infarctions were diagnosed in 33 patients (27%). 16 patients (13%) with bundle branch block were not excluded.

The clinical variables included: localization of myocardial infarction; history of recurrent angina; malignant arrhythmias in acute phase; thrombolytic treatment; ventricular arrhythmias on 24-hour ambulatory monitoring; and ejection fraction (angiographic or radionuclide ventriculography).

Signal-averaged ECG were performed 10-30 days after recent myocardial infarction using ART 1200 Epx device with bipolar X, Y, Z leads. 256±60 (mean ± SD) QRS beats were averaged with noise level below 0.5 uV.

Late potentials were analyzed by the time domain method with 40Hz high-pass filtering and were defined according to at least two of three of the following criteria: root-mean square voltage of the terminal 40 ms of the QRS complex (RMS) < 20 uV; filtered QRS duration (QRS-D) > 114 ms; duration of low amplitude signals below 40 uV in the terminal part of the QRS complex (LAS) > 38ms [1]. Time domain analysis were performed in 110 patients without bundle branch blocks.

In all cases fast Fourier transform (FFT) frequency analysis of the 120 ms segment beginning 20 ms before the end of QRS complex were made with multiplication by 4-term Blackman-Harris window. A 512-point fast Fourier transform was performed. Various high-frequency components were assessed with calculation of the following area ratios (abnormal values defined in our laboratory in brackets): 20-50/0-20 Hz (>275); 60-120/0-30 Hz (>80); 50-150/0-30 Hz (>140); 30-200/0-200 Hz (>220). Late potentials in our FFT frequency domain analysis were defined according to the presence of increased content of high-frequency components with abnormal value of any area ratio recorded in the study patient.

Statistical analysis were performed using unpaired t-Student and Chi^2 where appropriate.

Results

In 110 patients without bundle branch block SA-ECG were assessed by both time domain and frequency domain methods. Late potentials were present in 28 patients (26%) by time domain analysis and in 43 patients (39%) by FFT frequency domain analysis. In 16 patients with bundle branch block, late potentials analyzed only by frequency domain method were recorded in 3 of

them. Finally, late potentials by frequency analysis were recorded in 46 out of 126 studied patients (36%). In 34 of them high-frequency components were observed in all studied ranges of frequency, between 20-200 Hz.
In 7 patients high-frequency components appeared only between 20-50 Hz, in 2 cases between 50-200 Hz, and in 3 cases between 50-150 Hz. Among 46 patients with late potentials detected by frequency domain method, 15 of them presented also late potentials by time domain analysis; 31 patients with late potentials found by frequency domain analysis did not reveal late potentials by the time domain method. Also, in 13 patients with late potentials defined by time domain method frequency-domain analysis did not show an increased content of high-frequency components.

The comparison of clinical data between patients with and without late potentials determined by frequency domain method is shown in Table 1.

Table 1. Results of frequency domain analysis of SA-ECG in relation to the clinical variables in 126 patients after recent myocardial infarction.

Clinical Data		FFT(+) (n=46)	FFT(-) (n=80)	p value
Age (yrs)		62±9	59±11	NS
MI:	non-Q wave	14(30%)	19(24%)	NS
	anterior	14(30%)	10(13%)	<0.02
	inferior	7(15%)	21(26%)	NS
	lateral	3(7%)	3(4%)	NS
	combined	8(18%)	27(33%)	NS
Thrombolysis		16(35%)	37(46%)	NS
Recurrent angina		15(33%)	21(26%)	NS
Acute VT or VF		2(4%)	3(4%)	NS
Holter:				
	couplets/salvos	19(44%)	26(36%)	NS
	mean no. of VPBs/hr	53	14	<0.01
EF(%)		41±14	41±19	NS

FFT(+) - patients with late potentials by FFT;
FFT(-) - patients without late potentials by FFT;
MI - myocardial infarction; VT - ventricular tachycardia; VF - ventricular fibrillation; VPBs - ventricular premature beats; EF - ejection fraction

Clinical Implications

Late potentials were recorded by time domain analysis in 26% of our patients without conduction disturbances. In prior reports, the incidence of late potentials in patients after recent myocardial infarction ranged from 24% to 52% [3,4]. Frequency domain approach for diagnosis of late potentials in postinfarction patients was studied until now by only a few authors, with the assessment of only a single range of frequencies [5,6,7]. Lindsay et al. [6] observed abnormal value of mean area ratio 20-50/10-50 Hz in 21% of 38 postinfarction patients without documented VT but in 91% of 67 patients with sustained VT. In contrast, we analyzed various ranges of frequency of studied SA-ECG diagnosing late potentials in the presence of increased content of high-frequency component in any of studied ranges. This approach let us reveal late potentials in 43% of our 126 patients after myocardial infarction. The number of ventricular premature beats recorded in ambulatory monitoring in patients with late potentials (FFT+) was significantly higher than in the group of patients without late potentials.

Our results indicate, that diagnosis of late potentials by frequency domain analysis of SA-ECG is associated with a high frequency of ventricular premature beats on 24-hour Holter ECG.

The implication of this finding requires further investigations. ECG of postinfarction patient may contain different content of high-frequency components and requires assessment of various ranges of frequency.

References

1. G.Breithardt, M.E.Cain, N.El-Sherif, N.C.Flowers, V.Hombach, M.Janse, M.B.Simson, G.Steinbeck, *Circulation* **83** (1991) 1481.
2. M.E.Cain, H.D.Ambos, F.X.Witkowski, B.E.Sobel, *Circulation* **69** (1984) 711.
3. J.A.Gomes, S.L.Winters, in *Acute Myocardial Infarction*, ed. B.J.Gersh and S.H.Rahimtoola (Elsevier, New York, 1991) p. 423.
4. M.McGuire, D.Kuchar, J.Ganis, N.Samel, Ch.Thorburn, *Am J Cardiol* **61** (1988) 1187.
5. M.E.Cain, H.D.Ambos, J.Markham, A.E.Fisher, B.E.Sobel, *Am J Cardiol* **55** (1985) 1500.
6. B.D.Lindsay, D.H.Ambos, K.B.Shehtman, M.E.Cain, *Am J Cardiol* **62** (1988) 556.
7. T.A.Buckingham, C.M.Thesen, D.Hertweck, D.L.Janosik, H.L.Kennedy, *Am J Cardiol* **63** (1989) 820.

SPECTRAL TURBULENCE ANALYSIS OF THE SIGNAL-AVERAGED ELECTROCARDIOGRAM IN PATIENTS WITH LEFT BUNDLE BRANCH BLOCK.

H. DECOSTER M.D.,
Dept. of Cardiology, University Hospital Antwerp,
Wilrijkstraat 10, B-2650 Edegem,
Belgium.

J. SNOECK M.D., H. GESCHWIND M.D.*, C. VRINTS M.D., M. VERHERSTRAETEN ENG., L. FRANCQUE, M. BERKHOF ENG.
Dept. of Cardiology, University Hospital Antwerp, Wilrijkstraat 10, B-2650 Edegem, Belgium.
*C.H.U. Henri Mondor, University of Paris XII, Créteil, France.

Abstract:

We used a knew technique, the Spectral Turbulence Analysis to detect areas of reentry in human myocardium. We compared this spectral based method with the traditional Time-Domain analysis of Late Potentials. After inducing LBBB by right ventricular pacing, patients became false positive for the presence of Late Potentials but remained negative for Late Potentals with the new technique. This preliminary study shows a higher negative predictive value for the Spectral Turbulence Analysis.

Keywords:

High resolution electrocardiography, Signal-averaged electrocardiogram, Frequency analysis, Bundle branch block, Electrocardiogram, Micropotentials, Late potentials

Introduction:

Signal-averaged electrocardiography (SAECG) is a technique, utilized to detect micropotentials, which are present at the end of the QRS segment but are not identified by the standard 12-lead electrocardiogram [1]. These signals are called late potentials and represent electrical activity in slow conducting areas of abnormal myocard present in patients with sustained ventricular tachycardia. Until now, the presence of a bundle branch block was an exclusionary criterion. Because of the abnormalities associated with bundle branch block, masking or simulation of late potentials may occur.

Different authors have proposed criteria for time-domain SAECG in order to detect those patients with bundle branch block which are at risk for malignant ventricular arrhythmias. Unfortunately, criteria are different from author to author and not always convincing [2,3,4,5].

Cardiologists still disagree regarding the optimal filter characteristics and the numerical criteria of abnormality. Each manufacturer uses a different algorithm [6].

Initial application of frequency analysis techniques of the terminal portion of the QRS complex and early ST segments have been criticized as unreproducible [7, 8, 9, 10, 11, 12].

The frequency-domain analysis technique, applied in this study is different from others, because the whole QRS complex is analyzed. Abnormality criteria are not based on arbitrary values [13].

Methods:

Study subjects: The study was performed on 35 VVI paced patients. From this group, patients with a total pacemaker dependency even at low heart rate, atrial fibrillation or the presence of retrograde conduction on the surface ECG were excluded.

Pacing induced left bundle branch block: Pacing from the right ventricular apex was performed and the L.B.B.B. pattern produced was used for signal averaging in time- and frequency-domain. Therefore the pacemaker was reprogrammed temporary to a heart rate slightly higher than the intrinsic one.

Acquisition of signal-averaged electrocardiograms: Using silver/silver chloride skin electrodes, orthogonal X,Y and Z bipolar leads were recorded on a 3-channel cassette Holter recorder (Del Mar Avionics model 459). The recorder has a flat frequency response of 0,1 to 100 Hz ± 3 dB. The tapes were scanned on a Del Mar Avionics model 750A scanner equipped with the Micropotential Analyzer option for time- and frequency domain analysis. The Simson technique was used for signal averaging.

Time domain analysis was performed using a bidirectional Butterworth filtering at 25-250 Hz. Late Potentials (LP) were considered present if at least 2 of the following 3 parameters were present: HFQRS $\geq$ 120 ms, RMS40$\leq$ 25 μV and LAS40$\geq$ 38 ms (14).

Spectral Turbulence Analysis (STA) was performed with an initial software version, which generates adjacently drawn frequency plots of relatively short, consecutive and overlapping segments of electrocardiographic signals spanning the entire QRS and ST segment from 3 bipolar signal-averaged surface leads [13]. These 3-dimensional frequency plots are called "spectrocardiograms", because they represent the relative contributions of differing frequencies to the electrocardiographic wave form throughout the cardiac cycle.

Study design: In each patient, a recording is made during sinus rhythm with small QRS morphology. Than, the pacemaker is reprogrammed in such a way, it overrides the natural sinus rhythm continuously. At that moment a second recording is obtained. Signal averaged ECG (SAECG) in time-domain and by Spectral Turbulence Analysis is performed in small QRS as well as in paced induced left bundle branch block.

Statistics: Continuous variables are presented as the mean ± one standard deviation.

Results:

Of the initial 35 patients, only 16 were suitable for further investigation.

A first group of 10 patients with a small QRS morphology in sinus rhythm are studied. The mean filtered total QRS duration, RMS40 and LAS40 in small and large QRS complex analysis were 109,7 ± 15,4 ms, 36,2 ± 24,3 μV; 31,5 ± 15,8 ms and 162,9 ± 13,6 ms, 23,6 ± 18,3 μV, 63,3 ± 32,4 ms. When those patients have a small QRS morphology, only two of them have LP. This is confirmed by the Spectro Turbulence Analysis which selected only the same two patients at risk for malignant ventricular arrhythmias. However, when LBBB is induced eight out of ten patients become positive for LP when the standard criteria are used. Applying the criteria for patients with LBBB described by Fontaine et al. seven patients remain positive for Late Potentials. Both sets of criteria induce false positives in patients with RV pacing induced LBBB. Spectral Turbulence Analysis was able to select only four patients out of ten including the initial two patients who were positive for LP after signal averaging of a number of small QRS complexes.

The second group is composed of 6 patients with an intrinsic LBBB. The mean filtered total QRS duration, RMS40 and LAS40 in intrinsic LBBB and paced QRS complex analysis were 162,9 ± 13,6 ms, 23,6 ± 18,3 μV, 63,3 ± 32,4 ms and 241,1 ± 19,5 ms, 14,7 ± 5,6 μV, 86,9 ± 41,4 ms. Applying the standard criteria to the group of patients with intrinsic LBBB, 5 of 6 patients are positive for LP. Using the criteria of Fontaine, only 3 of 6 patients remain positive for LP. The same results are obtained with the Spectro Turbulence Analysis technique. When this group of patients with intrinsic LBBB is paced, all the patients become positive for Late Potentials using the standard criteria, 4 out of 6 patients are positive with the criteria of Fontaine and only 3 out of those 6 patients are at risk for malignant ventricular arrhythmias according to the spectrocardiogram. Fifty per cent of the patients with intrinsic LBBB have changing results using the Fontaine criteria before and after pacing. The results of Spectral Turbulence Analysis before and after pacing are identical.

Discussion and conclusion:

Standard criteria cannot be applied to patients with pacing induced LBBB, because of the development of false positives[14].

Although we used the criteria for detecting late potentials in LBBB of J.M. Fontaine et al, the combination of RMS40≤17 μV and LAS40≥ 55 msec, the results of the Spectral Turbulence Analysis of LBBB correlated better with the time domain analysis of the small QRS complexes. Visual inspection of the Spectral Turbulence graphics added a new dimension to the detection of subjects at risk for developing malignant ventricular arrhythmias. It increases specificity without decreasing sensitivity.

But there are some limitations to this preliminary study: although accepted, pacing induced LBBB may not be the ideal model of intrinsic LBBB[15]. We can demonstrate this by the difference in response to the Fontaine's criteria in patients with intrinsic LBBB and in the same patients after pacing. So, LBBB may not represent only abnormal conduction of the left bundle branch conduction tissue but reflects also the presence of regional myocardial fibrosis. A-V sequential pacing would have excluded

100 % retrograde conduction. Now, only visual inspection of the standard surface ECG was used to exclude these patients. This study was performed with the initial software available and only visual (qualitative) inspection was possible whether LP were present or not. In the final software version, arrhythmogenic abnormality is indicated by a score which reflects the frequent and abrupt changes in the frequency pattern of the QRS wave front velocity as it propagates throughout the ventricle around areas of reentry, resulting in a high degree of spectral turbulence. This should increase sensitivity and specificity.

We correlated this new technique to the well known time domain analysis. In fact it would be better to correlate a new technique to the results of programmed electrical stimulation or even better to the long term natural outcome of this patients. But this was not the issue of the study.

Acknowledgements:

We thank Mrs. Kathy Van Aken for her assistance in the preparation of the manuscript.

References:

1. Simson MB., *Circulation* **64** (1981) 235-246
2. Buckingham TA, Thessen CC, Stevens LL, Redd RM, Kennedy HL. *Am J Cardiol* (1988) 1265-1271
3. Flowers ND. , *J Am Coll Cardiol* **9** (1987) 684-697.
4. S. Kacet, J. Dagano, D. Lacroix, H. Decoster, C. Camier, J. Lekieffre, *PACE*, Ma **10** (1987) nr. 3, abstract 52.
5. Fontaine JM, Ramanath R, Henkin R, Suneja R, Ursell SN, El-Sherif N., *Am Heart J* **121:2** (1991) 494-508.
6. Henkin R, Caref EB, Kelen G, El-sherif N., *J Electrocardiol* **22** (suppl) (1990): 19-24.
7. Haberl R, Jilge G, Pulter R, Steinbeck G., *J Am Coll Cardiol* **12** (1988) 150-158.
8. Buckingham TA, Thessen CM, Hertweck D, Janosik DL, Kennedy HL., *Am J Cardiol* **63** (1989): 820-825.
9. Pierce DL, Easley AR Jr, Windle JR, Engel TR., *J Am Coll Cardiol* **14** (1989) 1731-1740.
10. Kelen G, Henkin R, Fontaine JM, El Sherif N., *Am J Cardiol* **60** (1987) 1282-1289.
11. Haberl R, Jilge G, Pulter R, Steinbeck G. *Eur Heart J* **10** (1989): 316-322.
12. Lindsay B, Ambos H et al. *Am J Cardiol* **62** (1988) 556-561.
13. Kelen G, Henkin R, Starr A-M, Caref E, Bloomfield D, El-Sherif N. *Am J Cardiol* **67** (1991) 965- 975
14. H. Decoster, J. Snoeck, M. Verherstraeten, L. Francque, M. Berkhof, B. Amsel, P. Walter. *Journal of Ambulatory Monitoring* (1990) p 50
15. Vassallo JA, Cassidy DM, Miller JM, Buxton AE, Marchinski FE, Josephson ME. *J Am Coll Cardiol* 7 (1986) 1228-1233.

AUTHORS' INDEX

Cserjes Z.
Daniyarova A.N.
Davidova T.A.
Davydova N.T.
Decoster H.
Devine B.
Dionisio I.
Dorofeeva Z.Z.
Drška Z.
von Dryander S.
Eifrig Th.
von der Emde J.
Endo M.
Esperer H.D.
Fazi A.
Filipová S.
Florian A.
Franca C.C.
Francque L.
Gadzhaeva F.U.
Geschwind H.
Gil V.
Gotti G.
Gremigni C.
Guindo J.
Hain P.
Harumi K.
Hayashi H.
Helfen A.
Heuten H.
Hirai M.
Hirnle T.
Hulin I.
Ichihara Y.
Idini R.
Ignatova E.D.
Inomata F.

www.ingramcontent.com/pod-product-compliance
Lightning Source LLC
LaVergne TN
LVHW071223011026
849280LV00007B/38

9789810209476